RECENT ADVANCES
IN CLINICAL IMMUNOLOGY

R. A. THOMPSON

MBE MBBS BSc MRCP MRCPath
Consultant Immunologist,
Director, Regional Immunology Laboratory,
East Birmingham Hospital;
Senior Clinical Lecturer,
Department of Experimental Pathology,
University of Birmingham

RECENT ADVANCES IN CLINICAL IMMUNOLOGY

EDITED BY

R. A. THOMPSON

NUMBER ONE

CHURCHILL LIVINGSTONE

Edinburgh London and New York

1977

CHURCHILL LIVINGSTONE
Medical Division of Longman Group Limited

Distributed in the United States of America by
Longman Inc., 19 West 44th Street, New York,
N.Y. 10036, and by associated companies,
branches and representatives throughout
the world

First published 1977

ISBN 0 443 01388 8

British Library Cataloguing in Publication Data

Recent advances in clinical immunology
  No. 1
  1. Immunology
  I. Thompson, Ronald Augustine
  616.07'9   QR180.2   77–30129

Printed in Great Britain by
Adlard & Son Ltd, Bartholomew Press, Dorking

PREFACE

Clinical advances are the results of the synthesis of inspirations derived from many sources. Animal experimentation, clinical trials, technological achievements, empirical observations and serendipity all play a part in changing the pattern of medical management.

The main impact of immunology in medicine up to the present time has been in providing a better understanding of mechanisms of disease, with a realisation that immunological factors play a greater or lesser role in many illnesses, and that a consideration of these factors must be added to the evaluation of any pathogenetic process. A better understanding of the role of the immune system in defence against microorganisms has led to new approaches in the control of those parasitic and infectious diseases which still scourge large areas of the world. Immunology has also established a whole new field of techniques by which patients and their responses may be monitored for the purposes of diagnosis and clinical management.

Based on a better understanding of the pathology of disease and more appropriate investigations, rational prophylaxis and therapy of those conditions in which immunological factors play a role should be the natural outcome of progress in this subject. The fact that such measures, often grafted from necessity on to existing more empirical forms of treatment, have yet made only a limited impact on patient management underlines the progress still to be made in fully understanding the complex mechanisms by which the immunological system contributes to the maintenance of the milieu interior.

This book covers some of the areas of immunopathology and applied technology which have taken great strides forward in recent years, and examines some of the problems associated with the institution of therapy based on immunological concepts. No attempt has been made to be comprehensive. Many aspects of clinical immunology have not been included, not because of their lesser consequence, but because of limitations of space, and in some cases recent coverage elsewhere in the immunological literature.

I would like to acknowledge the cooperation and forbearance of the distinguished contributors to this volume, and absolve them from any blame as to its lack of balance. I also wish to acknowledge the help given me in preparation by Miss Alice Bailey of the Immunology Department, East Birmingham Hospital.

Birmingham 1977 R. A. THOMPSON

CONTRIBUTORS

WILLIAM H. ADLER MD
Director of Cellular Immunobiology, Gerontology Research Center, National Institute on Ageing, Baltimore City Hospitals, Baltimore, Maryland, U.S.A.

A. D. BARNES BSc ChM FRCS
Consultant Surgeon, Queen Elizabeth Hospital, Birmingham 15

BENGT BJORKSTEN MD
Assistant Professor of Pediatrics, University Hospital of Umea, Umea, Sweden

REBECCA H. BUCKLEY MD
Professor of Pediatrics and Associate Professor of Immunology, Duke University School of Medicine, Durham, North Carolina, U.S.A.

DANIEL G. COLLEY PhD
Associate Professor of Microbiology, Veterans Administration Hospital and Vanderbilt University, Nashville, Tennessee, U.S.A.

STEVEN D. DOUGLAS MD
Professor of Medicine and Microbiology, University of Minnesota Medical School, Minneapolis, Minnesota, U.S.A.

W. PAGE FAULK BSc MD MRCPath
Professor of Immunology and Pediatrics, Medical University of South Carolina, Charleston, South Carolina, U.S.A.

EDWARD C. FRANKLIN MD
Professor of Medicine, New York University Medical Center, New York, U.S.A.

CHARLES B. FREEMAN DM(Oxon) MA(Oxon) MRCP
[1]MRC Research Fellow, University Department of Medical Genetics, St Mary's Hospital, Hathersage Road, Manchester

M. F. GREAVES PhD MRCPath
Membrane Immunology Department, Imperial Cancer Research Fund, London

A. R. HAYWARD MRCP
Lecturer, Department of Immunology, Institute of Child Health, London

[1]Present: Visiting Associate, Pediatric Oncology Branch, National Cancer Institute, National Institutes of Health, Bethesda, Maryland, U.S.A.

KENNETH H. JONES PhD
Senior Staff Fellow, Gerontology Research Center, National Institute on Ageing, Baltimore City Hospitals, Baltimore, Maryland, U.S.A.

PAUL H. LAMBERT MD
Associate Professor, Department of Medicine, University of Geneve; Head, WHO Immunology Research and Training Centre, Lausanne/Geneve, Switzerland

J. MORRISON SMITH MD FRCP(Edin)
Consultant Physician, Birmingham Chest Clinic and East Birmingham Hospital, Birmingham

HIDEO NARIUCHI PhD
Visiting Fellow, Gerontology Research Center, National Institute on Ageing, Baltimore City Hospitals, Baltimore, Maryland, U.S.A.

PAUL G. QUIE MD
Professor of Pediatrics and Microbiology, American Legion Memorial Heart Research Professor, University of Minnesota School of Medicine, Minneapolis, Minnesota, U.S.A.

C. JULIAN ROSENTHAL MD
Assistant Professor of Medicine, State University of New York, Brooklyn, New York, U.S.A.

R. A. THOMPSON MBE MBBS BSc MRCP MRCPath
Consultant Immunologist and Director, Regional Immunology Laboratory, East Birmingham Hospital; Senior Clinical Lecturer, Department of Experimental Pathology, University of Birmingham

RUDOLPH H. ZUBLER MD
Research Fellow, WHO Immunology Research and Training Centre, Hopital Cantonal, Geneve 4, Switzerland

CONTENTS

1
INTRODUCTION:
TRENDS IN CLINICAL IMMUNOLOGY

R. A. Thompson

The general use of the term clinical immunology in referring to the applications of immunology in medicine has come about in the relatively recent past, and in that sense almost all of clinical immunological practice represents a recent advance. However, the application of immunology in medicine is not new—it has its roots in the beginning of the modern era of scientific medicine heralded by the discoveries of the latter half of the nineteenth century. The prime interest was of course in the mechanism of specific immunity or protection from infectious diseases, and the means by which this could be conferred on otherwise susceptible populations. The application of immunological methods in the diagnosis of infectious disease was also introduced at the beginning of this century, but if any group of medical practitioners was likely to be called clinical immunologists in the era before the 1950s, it was those concerned with enhancing immunity to infection by active immunisation or treating infective disease by the administration of serum from immunised animals.

However, the technological explosion of the post-World War II era led to a greatly increased understanding of the basic mechanisms of the immune response, derived from three sets of factors, and this has considerably broadened the clinical applications of immunology.

Firstly there were new technical achievements. These involved the separation and analysis of proteins, and the separation and analysis of cells, and their preservation in tissue and organ culture. Electrophoresis, ultracentrifugation, chromatography, gel filtration and other techniques have enabled a greater understanding of plasma protein structure and function. The refinements of immunochemical analysis introduced by Oudin, Ouchterlony, Grabar and others in the 1950s allowed the identification and characterisation of these proteins in a manner not previously possible. The determination of the amino acid sequence of proteins has allowed the complete biochemical dissection of many complex molecules including antibodies. Also sensitive techniques for detecting antigen–antibody reactions, such as immunofluorescence and radioimmunoassay, have extended the applications of immunology into many aspects of clinical investigation. Similarly, improvements in methods of tissue culture have enhanced the study of the cells of the immune response; and improved techniques of animal experimentation and animal husbandry, have allowed a deeper understanding of cell biology and the essential role of certain cells, especially lymphoid cells, and organs in the development and maintenance of the immune response and its wider role in physiology and pathology.

Secondly there have been many key observations, both clinical and experimental, which have provided the impetus for a whole series of further investigations. Clinical observations have provided a spur for scientific studies using animal models, or justification of theories based on previously obtained experimental data, or sometimes indeed the raw material from which fundamental scientific data has been obtained. Conversely, the ideas of scientific immunologists, derived from animal experiments, have heightened the understanding of clinical problems and pointed to rational methods of treatment.

The observations of Landsteiner and Chase, on the transfer of delayed hypersensitivity laid the foundations of modern cellular immunology and the concept of the duality of the immune response. The experiments of Miller and his collaborators on neonatally thymec-tomised mice indicated an essential function for the thymus gland, freeing it from the mysticism associated with 'status thymo-lymphaticus'. This together with Glick's work in chickens led to the establishment of the existence of two separate populations of lym-phocytes, B- and T-cells, which were responsible for the humoral and cellular arms of the immune response respectively. These experimental observations were reinforced by the clinical observations of different types of immunodeficiency in patients with recurrent infections. The study of myeloma proteins led to the unravelling of immunoglobulin structure; and the discovery of autoimmune diseases, and the practice of organ trans-plantation each greatly stimulated research into the basic mechanisms of immunity.

Then thirdly there were a number of other original concepts which provided the basis for a completely new approach to problems in fundamental and clinical immunology. Among these must be considered Burnet's clonal selection theory, the Watson–Crick genetic code which had a profound effect on all biological thought, Gell and Coombs' classification of mechanisms of hypersensitivity, and the concept of immune surveillance. More recent ideas on genetic and other control mechanisms of the immune response have still to make their major impact in the clinical field.

Some specific areas of clinical immunology are considered in greater detail.

Immune Deficiency

Following the description (Bruton, 1952; Gitlin and Janeway, 1956) of familial sex-linked antibody deficiency producing an increased tendency to infections, there has been the recognition of a number of primary immunodeficiency syndromes (Fudenberg et al, 1971; Soothill, 1974). These are diagnosed after an assessment of various immunological parameters in patients presenting with recurrent infections, but without some local ana-tomical or constitutional cause. This assessment is based on the physiology of the immune response, and includes an enumeration of the T- and B-lymphocytes (see Ch. 7) and their functional characteristics, evaluation of polymorph leucocyte function (see Ch. 8) and the complement system, in addition to the quantitation of the immunoglobulin levels, antibody responses and other tests which help to differentiate disorders of the various arms of the immune response. Rare symptom complexes have been described (Cooper et al, 1968; Rosen, 1974; Hong, 1974), frequently occurring in families, in which the tendency to infections is one aspect of the conditions; the commonest form of primary immunodeficiency is one in which there are defects of both T- and B-cell functions. It is recognised that this is a heterogeneous group of unclassified conditions and for convenience such cases are referred to as Common Variable Immunodeficiency (CVID). Fundamental enzyme defects have been recognised in some conditions; for example in about one-third of the cases of severe combined immunodeficiency there is a deficiency of the cytoplasmic enzyme adenosine deaminase (ADA) (Giblett et al, 1972; Meuwissen et al, 1975) while in many cases of ataxia telangiectasia, there is a defect in the enzyme responsible for repairing chromosome breaks in the nucleus (Patterson et al, 1976).

Loss of antibody in the gut or through the kidney, or depression of the immune response by reticuloendothelial neoplasia or severe virus infections leads to secondary immune deficiency, which is more common than the primary defects. Malnutrition is another state associated with increased infections, and Drs Douglas and Faulk (Ch. 2) review the recent work on the complex immunological aspects of this problem.

Replacement of immunological capacity is the rationale behind all forms of treatment of primary immunodeficiency states. Passive transfer of normal immunoglobulin has been the most widely used and most successful of the replacement therapies (MRC Report, 1971). More recently the transfer of adoptive immunity by bone marrow grafts (Good and Bach, 1974), has been successful in some patients with severe defects of immunity. Boosting of immune capacity has also been attempted by such expedients as transfer factor (Hitzig et al, 1974; Lawrence, 1974) or thymic hormone (Goldstein et al, 1976) administration, or by the use of the drug levamisole (Renoux and Renoux, 1974; Editorial, 1975) and many of these aspects are discussed by Dr Buckley in her article (Ch. 10).

Autoimmunity

The observation that antibodies against self antigens were present in certain chronic diseases (Gajdusek, 1957; Roitt et al, 1956) was the stimulus which led to the concept of 'self-damage' by an aberrant immune system. Red cell autoantibodies had been detected by the indirect antiglobulin or Coombs test (Weiner, Gordon and Gallop, 1953; Evans and Weiser, 1957), and the observations were extended to a number of other diseases. Gastric antibodies were found in some patients with pernicious anaemia (Schwartz, 1958; Taylor, 1959), adrenal antibodies in primary Addison's disease (Anderson et al, 1957), antibodies to skeletal muscle and myoepithelial cells in myaesthenia gravis (Strauss et al, 1960), and many others, the most recent being antibodies to the islets of Langerhans in some forms of diabetes (Bottazzo, Florin-Christensen and Doniach, 1974; Irvine, Gray and McCallum, 1976).

Accompanying this has been evidence of the ability to induce experimental autoimmune disease in animals by injection of organ extracts (Witebsky and Rose, 1956; Waksman, 1959). Also direct examination of pathological lesions by immunofluorescence has shown the involvement of autoreactive antibodies, e.g. in Goodpasture's syndrome (McPhaul and Dixon, 1970), or cross-reactive antibodies in rheumatic carditis (Kaplan, 1962).

While the ability to form autoantibodies has been documented extensively, the mechanism of tissue damage is seldom clear, and in many instances it is uncertain whether the antibodies are the causes or the consequences of tissue damage, since it has been shown that autoantibody formation frequently follows tissue damage produced by trauma or other means.

Whatever form the autoimmune process takes, treatment is largely symptomatic. In diseases of the endocrine glands whose function is destroyed, hormone replacement is most important; otherwise, anti-inflammatory and immunosuppressive therapy is used empirically.

Autoantibodies against antigens widely dispersed throughout the body occur characteristically in certain diseases, such as rheumatoid arthritis, systemic lupus erythematosus (SLE), coeliac disease, primary biliary cirrhosis and chronic active hepatitis (Doniach,

1972). These so-called non-organ-specific autoantibodies include antibodies to IgG (rheumatoid factor), to nucleoproteins, ribose nucleic acid (RNA), deoxyribose nucleic acid (DNA) and extractable antigen (ENA) (Sharp et al, 1972), to cell organelles such as mitochondria and microsomes, to contractile protein of the cell membrane and to reticulin fibres of basement membranes and connective tissue. The significance of these antibodies in the pathogenesis of the conditions in which they occur is also unknown, although they serve as useful diagnostic markers. The exception is in the case of antibodies to DNA in SLE, in which it has been shown that complexes of DNA and anti-DNA antibodies are deposited in the kidneys and elsewhere, and are responsible for many of the pathological features of the disease (Koffler et al, 1971). Some of these conditions are thought to represent unusual immunological reactions to infective agents and reports of isolation or sometimes direct visualisation in the electron microscope of infective agents (Dubois, 1974; Block and Christian, 1975) have been made.

The tendency to consider autoimmunity as a cause of a disease of obscure aetiology was particularly popular five or more years ago, but has become less so and is being superseded by 'immune complex' theories. The subject has been reviewed recently (Stiller, Russell and Dossetor, 1975). Autoantibodies occur with greater frequency in the aged, and Dr Adler and his colleagues critically review this and other intriguing immunological aspects of ageing in Chapter 4.

Allergy

The clarification of the ways in which immunological responses to certain external non-replicating antigens (allergens) can produce symptoms and pathological features of disease (Coombs and Gell, 1974) has lifted the veil of mystery which surrounded the practice of clinical allergy. The discovery of IgE (Ishizaka and Ishizaka, 1967; Johansson, Bennich and Wide, 1968) and the demonstration of its role in the immediate hypersensitivity reactions (Stanworth et al, 1967) which produce hay fever and allergic asthma, have added considerably to the understanding of these conditions, although as Dr Morrison-Smith illustrates (see Ch. 12), we are still far from controlling such conditions solely by immunological manipulations. Moreover, ways of investigating possible allergic reactions are far from satisfactory, and it is easier to hypothesise than to prove that such a reaction to a food or medication or other extrinsic agent is a cause of symptoms. Clinicians still look to their immunologist colleagues for help in this area.

An interesting concept developed by Soothill and his colleagues (1973) suggests that allergic reactions reflect an underlying partial defect in immune responsiveness, either in the form of a defect in local secretory IgA-mediated responses (Kaufman and Hobbs, 1970; Taylor et al, 1973), or in making low avidity antibody which is inefficient at eliminating antigen (Petty, Steward and Soothill, 1972).

Immune complex diseases

Since the description of serum sickness (von Pirquet and Schick, 1905) and the clarification of its pathogenesis (Dixon, Vazquez and Weigle, 1958; Cochrane, 1971), it has been appreciated that circulating complexes of antigen and antibody produce widespread symptoms ranging from cutaneous vasculitis to arthritis, polyserositis and renal disease. Such conditions can arise acutely or subacutely when the antigen is present in the circulation (e.g. after serum therapy) and the antibody response commences de novo. Many diseases in which such complexes arise are chronic; failure to eliminate antigen due to low affinity antibody (Steward, Petty and Soothill, 1973) or a defective complement system (Lachmann, 1976) could result in persistence of the complexes. This would depend on a number of factors including the genetic make-up of the individual and the nature of the antigen. Microbial antigens derived from organisms which resist the hosts' defences can act as the nidus for immune complex disorders, and the fact that such complexes have been shown to play a part in the pathogenesis of many clinical and experimental infective illnesses (Oldstone and Dixon, 1969; Zuckerman, 1975) rationalises the search for circulating complexes in many diseases of unknown aetiology. However, the techniques are varied and all have their drawbacks, as discussed by Drs Lambert and Zubler in Chapter 6. The interpretation of the results of such tests may also be difficult although this is clearly an advancing front of clinical immunology.

Abnormalities of Complement

The place of the complement system in the interests of immunologists and clinical immunologists has advanced in recent years from being a collection of abstruse biochemical phenomena to a system of fundamental importance in immunogenetics and in the induction of the immune response, and of considerable relevance in immunopathology (McConnell and Lachman, 1976; Pepys, 1976).

Described initially by Bordet (1896) as a system in the blood responsible for the lysis of antibody coated cells, it has been studied ever since by the technique of cell lysis. It was recognised as a complex system of plasma proteins which were normally in proenzyme form and which were sequentially activated to enzymes by antigen–antibody complexes (Ruddy, Gigli and Austen, 1972; Muller-Eberhard, 1975); during this process activated components attached to the red cell or initiating complex, and the activated terminal components effected the cell lysis. There were nine major components in this system of lysis, called C1, C2, etc., to C9. It has become clear that the major biochemical event on activation of the complement system is the activation of the third component (C3) and its physical attachment or fixation to the initiating antigen–antibody complex (Lachmann, 1974) by the action of a complex enzyme, called the C3 convertase, formed from C4 and C2 ($\overline{C42}$).

There exists a second mechanism for fixing C3 by another C3 convertase, generated by another series of plasma proteins. This was initially partially described as the properdin system by Pillemer and his co-workers (1954), but the system has more recently been clarified and called the alternate (or more correctly 'alternative') complement pathway (Gotze and Muller-Eberhard, 1971; Gewurz, 1972). The components of the alternative pathway and their reaction mechanisms are still being actively investigated (Medicus et al, 1976), but the activation of this pathway occurs particularly when bacterial polysaccharides or endotoxin are introduced into serum. The first mechanism is now referred to as the 'classical' pathway of complement activation.

C3 fixation is accompanied by many biological consequences; it results in the opsonisation of the initiating complex for phagocytosis by the reticuloendothelial system, or allows its interaction with macrophages and B lymphocytes. There are also generated chemotactic, anaphylotoxic and kinin-like peptides, and in some instances there may occur the activation of the later components C5–C9 producing cell lysis if the reaction is at the surface of a cell. This 'attack' phase of the system is of uncertain biological significance, for there are many strains of animals, and several humans, genetically lacking one or other of the terminal components (usually C5 or C6). Their serum is unable to lyse sensitised red cells, but the animals and most of the men are otherwise in good health. The complement system has a number of checks and specific inhibitors which modulate the activation process, and confine it to the site of its initiation.

The complement system is involved in pathological processes by two basic mechanisms. Firstly by antibody-initiated reactions, either autoimmune or allergic in nature, with the resultant death of tissue cells or the generation of an inflammatory response by phlogistic peptides. Secondly and more rarely, individuals exist with genetic deficiencies of single components of the system (Alper and Rosen, 1971; Lachmann, 1976), which may have pathological consequences. There may be (i) a tendency to recurrent infections due to a primary or secondary deficiency of C3, (ii) an increased incidence of immune complex diseases because of poor antigen clearance associated with a defect in the early components of the classical system C1, C4 and C2, and (iii) a tendency to chronic or recurrent Neisserian infections due to lack of one of the later components C5–C9 although as mentioned, such individuals may also be completely healthy. Several families have also been described with a genetic defect of the inhibitor to the activated first component (C1 esterase inhibitor); this produces the characteristic clinical syndrome of hereditary angioneurotic oedema (Donaldson and Evans, 1963).

The treatment of complement-deficiency states is in its infancy because of the rarity of the conditions. Therapeutic modulation of the effects of complement in inflammation would produce symptomatic relief and minimise immunologically mediated damage, but as yet reliable and safe means of achieving this in man have not been found, although there are agents which can be used for a short time in animals. Recent interest in the genetics of complement derives from the fact that the genes controlling the synthesis of some of the components, especially C2 and C4, are on the same chromosome, and closely associated with the genes of the HLA system.

Immunosuppression

Therapy to suppress the immune response in those diseases in which over-activity or inappropriate activity of the immune system is thought to be responsible for symptoms, is at present relatively crude and non-specific. Corticosteroids and cytotoxic drugs (Skinner and Schwartz, 1972; Berenbaum, 1974) with antilymphocyte globulin in some cases (see Barnes, Ch. 9) constitute the main armamentarium. To these have recently been added plasmaphoresis, to remove harmful antibodies, immune complexes and inflammatory mediators (Jones et al, 1976; Lockwood et al, 1977). Procedures such as irradiation, lymphoid organ extirpation or thoracic duct drainage, which are effective in experimental animals, have only a very limited application in the treatment of human diseases. The degree of immunosuppression achieved with conventional therapy is seldom assessed and the drugs are used empirically, usually up to the limits of symptomatic relief or side-effects. Achievement of their therapeutic aim is often accompanied by evidence that the abnormal immune reaction, as determined by antibody levels, has declined. However, this is not invariable and the hope for the future is the development of selective suppression of specific immune responses, where these have been identified and defined as the causes of a disease process. Initial success in this direction is likely to be achieved in the management of the allogeneic immune response following organ transplantation.

Alloimmunity

This refers to the immunological reactions against antigens derived from members of the same species; such reactions may have pathological consequences. While a blood transfusion reaction is perhaps an obvious example of this, it also includes such processes as the rejection of an organ homograft, graft versus host disease, and the immunological phenomena associated with pregnancy including rhesus isoimmunisation. Some of the mechanisms involve the interaction between transplantation antigens on the surface of cells, and it is not clear that the nature and specificity of these reactions are exactly comparable to those between sensitised lymphocytes and specific externally derived protein or carbohydrate antigens with which they can interact (Nossal, 1974). In this context it is also reasonable to consider the immune mechanisms which operate against cancer cells, since these are derived from, and bear considerable similarity to, the cells of the host, although possessing new antigens against which it is often possible to detect cellular and humoral immune responses (Currie, 1974).

Transplantation

Organ grafting has been another clinical practice which has stimulated the study of immunological mechanisms. While the technical problems of organ preservation and of the necessary surgical manipulations have largely been overcome (Calne, 1975) in renal, liver and heart transplantation, the rejection process still limits the success of these procedures. Bone marrow transplantation to correct primary immunodeficiency (see Buckley, p. 232) or aplastic anaemia or agranulocytosis (Mathé et al, 1974) has also been successful, but carries the additional hazard of immune damage to the recipient from immuno-competent cells of the donor (graft versus host reaction) (Grebe and Sreilen, 1976). However, transplantation has stimulated the delineation of the HLA antigen system (Festenstein, 1973) and given a considerable boost to immunogenetics, and will undoubtedly receive a feed-back in due course in the form of more effective ways of modulating transplantation immunity, either by the more effective use of immunosuppressive agents (Calne, 1974) or by techniques of specific immunological enhancement of organ grafting (Carpenter, D'Apice and Abbas, 1976).

Cancer

Since Burnet (1965) proposed his theory of immune surveillance there have been many attempts to define the role of the immune system in defence against cancer. There is a variety of experimental and clinical evidence that immunological mechanisms are involved (Currie, 1974) and attempts have been made both to understand the nature of this involvement and to boost the immunological responses of patients to their own tumours. While evidence of immune mechanisms destroying cancer cells in vitro is plentiful, the best results of immunologically mediated cancer regression have been achieved in animal models. In established cases of cancer in man the evidence for a significant role for the immune system in recovery is largely circumstantial, although knowledge of the importance of this system has considerably modified the approach of surgeons and radiotherapists to the treatment of cancer, particularly with regard to the removal or ablation of lymphoid tissue. Immunotherapeutic manoeuvres to enhance the immune response against cancer tissues, and so bring about its regression, is a goal for all those involved in treating this condition (Gray and Watkins, 1975). Such procedures have so far had sporadic and largely uncontrolled trials in patients with a variety of types of cancer, often in the terminal stages of the disease, and the results are largely inconclusive. Dr Freeman (Ch. 11) reports on recent attempts at the immunotherapy of acute myeloid leukaemia, for which the initial results seemed encouraging. His report underlines many of the pitfalls and problems of this approach.

Recent studies have detected in certain types of cancer (Costanza and Nathanson, 1974) new antigens which represent antigens present in abundance in fetal tissue but virtually absent in the adult. This derepression of the cell genome is thought to be a fundamental part of the neoplastic process. Such onchofetal antigens, as they are collectively called, may be released into the circulation where they can be measured, usually in very small micro- or nanogram amounts. This can provide a diagnostic test for cancer, or at least a parameter for monitoring treatment (Booth et al, 1973; Neville and Laurence, 1974).

Myeloproliferative disorders

Since cells of the reticuloendothelial system are those concerned in the initiation and development of the immune reponse, diseases involving those cells have consequences of much interest to the clinical immunologist, particularly to immunohaematologists. Plasma cell neoplasia, besides producing the clinical disease of multiple myeloma, has provided the immunochemist with a phenomenal supply of 'pure' immunoglobulins, which contributed greatly to the present understanding of antibody structure and function (Cunningham et al, 1971; Cohen, 1971; Natvig and Kunkel, 1973). More recently the nature of amyloid substance, which frequently complicates myelomatosis, and occurs under other circumstances of aberrant immunological action, has been appreciably clarified, and this work is reviewed by Drs Rosenthal and Franklin (Ch. 3). Neoplasms of lymphoid cells have been redefined by virtue of their cell membrane characteristics (p. 172), which may assist in providing a prognosis and possibly a more rational therapeutic approach in the future.

Pregnancy

The developing fetus carries antigens derived from both maternal and paternal genes, and thus pregnancy represents a successful temporary allograft. The means by which the fetus escapes immunological rejection have been much investigated in recent years (Beer and Billingham, 1971). Evidence exists for the presence of an antigenic 'barrier' of fibrinoid material in the trophoblast, which keeps maternal immunocompetent cells largely out of contact with fetal tissue antigens. There is also evidence of a non-specific depression of maternal immune responses during pregnancy. However, immunological factors have not been implicated with certainty as operating in any of the common clinical conditions which beset pregnancy, such as recurrent abortions, pre-eclampsia or placental insufficiency. The exception of course, has been haemolytic disease of the newborn, commonly due to rhesus isoimmunisation (and occasionally attributable to other maternal/paternal blood group differences), in which fetal red cells, carrying paternal antigens, gain access to the maternal circulation, usually during labour. They then may stimulate an immune response in the mother with dire consequences for subsequent fetuses of similar antigenic constitution. The introduction and wide acceptance of prophylactic measures against this condition by giving specific human antirhesus D immunoglobulin to rhesus-negative mothers at risk, has been an excellent example of the contribution of clinical practice to immunological understanding (Clarke et al, 1963; Freda et al, 1975).

Infections

The concepts of the pathogenesis of infectious diseases have undergone changes in recent years as a result of immunological ideas and experiments. It is clear that in many instances the pathological effects of infections are as much due to the immune responses of the host as to the invasive and destructive propensities of the infecting organisms. This can be shown in experimental animals, where ablation of part of the host's immune response produces a milder form of the infectious disease than in the intact animal. There is also much evidence for the role of such factors in human infections. The interplay between antigens of the infective agent and the host's immune mechanisms is particularly complex and instructive in parasitic infections, and Dr Colley (Ch. 5) reviews the extensive research which has taken place in the study of schistosomiasis, and the lessons for the study of other similar infections.

HLA and Diseases

The work of Benacerraf, McDevitt, Biozzi and their respective collaborators have helped to establish the genetic basis of the immune response (McDevitt and Benacerraf, 1969; Grumet, 1975), and to show that the genes responsible for this control (Ir genes) are closely linked to those controlling the expression of the HLA antigens. These are on autosome 6 in man, in a region referred to as the Major Histocompatibility Complex (MHC), and are controlled by alleles at four loci, A, B, C and D. The antigens of the A, B, and C loci are determined by serological methods in a manner analogous to the determination of red cell blood group antigens, while D locus antigens are detected by mixed lymphocyte culture.

The HLA antigens achieved particular clinical significance outside the field of organ transplantation, when it became clear that certain antigens occurred more frequently in individuals with certain diseases (Dausset, 1974). This suggested that because of an associated Ir gene abnormality, such individuals were either over-reacting or under-reacting to an environmental antigen, with the clinical disease as a consequence. This association was most clear in the case of antigen B-27 and anklyosing spondylitis (Brewerton et al, 1973), but other associations have been reported in coeliac disease (Stokes et al, 1972; Falchuk, Rogentine and Strober, 1972), in diabetes (Nerup et al, 1974) in asthma (Blumenthal et al, 1974; Rachelefsky et al, 1976) and in multiple sclerosis (Jersild et al, 1975), and other conditions. The association with disease may even be more striking when the means of determining the nature of related antigens which occur only on B lymphocytes and are called Ia (immune-associated) antigens (Shreffler and David, 1975; Moller 1976) become more available. The reagents for detecting the Ia antigens are more scarce and the techniques more exacting than HLA testing, but they hold much promise. At the very least these associations will provide a means of identifying susceptible individuals in the population, while hopefully they will help to elucidate mechanisms of disease, and provide answers as to prophylaxis and therapy.

Organisation of Clinical Immunology

The organisation of the subject has been effected in most countries in a piecemeal fashion. Those engaged in its practice have widely diverse backgrounds and training.

While this has been inevitable and has undoubtedly stimulated the growth of the subject, it has hampered its emergence as a formal discipline with a recognised place in the clinical arena. The definitions of the aims and objectives and modus operandi of clinical immunologists, and of their necessary training and qualifications, have been the subjects of many discussions and papers (WHO Report, 1972; Joint Committee Report, 1972; AAI Report, 1975; Thompson, 1974; IUIS Report, 1976; Reeves, 1976). In the United States and Canada it is a board-certifiable specialty, linked to allergy, in the European Community it is a separately registrable specialty, while in the UK it has emerged clearly as a branch of pathology or laboratory medicine, although not yet firmly established as a subspecialty in clinical medicine.

All those concerned with the subject agree that the immunologist working in the clinical field requires a sound training in basic immunology as well as in clinical medicine, and that particularly for such practitioners, continued research must go hand in hand with service commitments. However, whether the medical educational establishments, and the financial restrictions on the provision of health care, can allow this ideal to be achieved in all areas is another matter. The situation is likely to continue for some time on an ad hoc pragmatic basis, depending for advance largely on the drive and initiative of immunologists and other interested persons bringing pressure to bear at a local level. It is to be hoped that the development of more refined therapeutic and prophylactic measures in immunology over the next decade will transfer attention from interesting laboratory data to the statistics of patient care or cure.

REFERENCES

Alper, C. A. & Rosen, F. S. (1971) Genetic aspects of the complement system. *Advances in Immunology*, **14**, 251.

American Association of Immunologists (AAI) (1975) Report on hospital-based laboratory and clinical immunology. *Journal of Immunology*, **115**, 609.

Anderson, J. R., Goudie, R. B., Gray, K. G. & Turnbury, G. C. (1957) Autoantibodies in Addison's disease. *Lancet*, **i**, 1123.

Beer, A. E. & Billingham, R. E. (1971) Immunobiology of mammalian reproduction. *Advances in Immunology*, **14**, 2.

Berenbaum, M. C. (1974) The clinical pharmacology of immunosuppressive agents. In *Clinical Aspects of Immunology*, 3rd edition, ed. Gell, P. G. H., Coombs, R. R. A. & Lachmann, P. J. Oxford: Blackwell Scientific.

Block, S. R. & Christian, C. L. (1975) The pathogenesis of systemic lupus erythematosus. *American Journal of Medicine*, **59**, 453.

Blumenthal, M. N., Amos, D. B., Noreen, H., Mendell, N. & Yunis, E. S. (1974) Genetic mapping of Ir locus in man—linkage to second locus of HLA. *Science*, **184**, 1301.

Booth, S. N., King, J. P. G., Leonard, J. C. & Dykes, P. W. (1973) Serum carcino-embryonic antigen (CEA) in clinical disorders. *Gut*, **14**, 79.

Bordet, J. (1896) Sur l'agglutination et la dissolution des globules rouges par le serum d'animaux injecties de sang defibrine. *Annales de l'Institut Pasteur (Paris)*, **12**, 688.

Bottazzo, G. F., Florin-Christensen, A. & Doniach, D. (1974) Islet cell antibodies in diabetes mellitus with autoimmune polyendocrine deficiencies. *Lancet*, **ii**, 1279.

Brewerton, D. A., Caffrey, M., Hart, F. D., James, D. C. O., Nicholls, A. & Sturrock, R. D. (1973) Ankylosing spondylitis and HL-A27. *Lancet*, **ii**, 904.

Bruton, O. C. (1952) Agammaglobulinaemia. *Paediatrics*, **9**, 722.

Burnet, F. M. (1965) Somatic mutation and chronic disease. *British Medical Journal*, **i**, 338.

Calne, R. Y. (1974) Immunosuppression and clinical organ transplantation. *Transplant Proceedings*, **6**, 49.

Calne, R. Y. (1975) Organ grafts. *Current Topics in Immunology*, Series No. 4. London: Edward Arnold.

Carpenter, C. B., D'Apice, A. J. F. & Abbas, A. K. (1976) The role of antibodies in the rejection and enhancement of organ allografts. *Advances in Immunology*, **22**, 1.

Clarke, C. A., Donohoe, W. T. A., McConnell, R. B., Woodrow, J. C., Finn, R., Krevans, J. R., Kilke, W., Lehane, D. & Sheppard, P. M. (1963) Further experimental studies on the prevention of Rh haemolytic disease. *British Medical Journal*, **i**, 979.

Cochrane, C. G. (1971). Mechanisms involved in the deposition of immune complexes in tissues. *Journal of Experimental Medicine*, **134**, 75S.

Cohen, S. (1971) Structure and function of immunoglobulins. In *New Concepts in Allergy and Clinical Immunology*, ed. Serafini, U., Frankland, A. W., Masala, C. & Jamar, J. M. Holland: Excerpta Medica.

Coombs, R. R. A. & Gell, P. G. H. (1974) Classification of allergic reactions responsible for clinical hypersensitivity and disease. In *Clinical Aspects of Immunology*, 3rd edn, ed. Gell, P. G. H., Coombs, R. R. A. & Lachmann, P. J. Oxford and Edinburgh: Blackwell Scientific.

Cooper, M. D., Chase, H. P., Lowman, J. T., Krivat, W. & Good, R. A. (1968) Wiskott–Aldrich syndrome. *American Journal of Medicine*, **44**, 499.

Costanza, M. E. & Nathason, L. (1974) Carcino-fetal antigens. In *Progress in Clinical Immunology*, ed. Schwartz, R. S. New York: Grune & Stratton.

Cunningham, B. A., Gohlieb, P. D., Pflumm, M. N. & Edelman, G. (1971) Immunoglobulin structure: diversity, gene duplication and domains. In *Progress in Immunology*, I, ed. Amos, B. New York: Academic Press.

Currie, G. A. (1974) Cancer and the immune response. In *Current Topics in Immunology*, Series No. 2. London: Edward Arnold.

Dausset, J. (1974) Some contributions of the HLA complex to the genetics of human diseases. *Transplantation Reviews*, **22**, 44.

Dixon, F., Vazquez, J. J. & Weigle, W. O. (1958) Pathogenesis of serum sickness. *Archives of Pathology*, **65**, 18.

Donaldson, V. H. & Evans, R. R. (1963) A biochemical abnormality in hereditary angio-neurotic oedema. Absence of serum inhibitor of C1 esterase. *American Journal of Medicine*, **35**, 37.

Doniach, D. (1972) Autoimmune aspects of liver disease. *British Medical Bulletin*, **28**, 145.

Dubois, E. L. (1974) *Lupus Erythematosus*, 2nd edn. Los Angeles: University of Southern California Press.

Editorial (1975) Levamisole. *Lancet*, **i**, 151.

Evans, R. S. & Weiser, R. S. (1957) The serology of auto-immune haemolytic disease; observations on 41 patients. *Archives of Internal Medicine*, **87**, 48.

Falchuk, Z. M., Rogentine, G. N. & Strober, W. (1972) Predominance of histocompatibility antigen HL-A8 in patients with gluten sensitive enteropathy. *Journal of Clinical Investigation*, **51**, 1602.

Festenstein, H. (1973) Histocompatibility testing for organ transplantation. In *Recent advances in Clinical Pathology*, Series 6, ed. Dyke, S. C. Churchill Livingstone.

Freda, V. J., Gorman, J. G., Pollack, W. & Bowe, E. (1975) Prevention of Rh haemolytic disease— ten years' clinical experience with Rh immune globulin. *New England Journal of Medicine*, **292**, 1014.

Fudenberg, H. H., Good, R. A., Goodman, H. C., Hitzig, W., Kunkel, H. G., Roitt, I. M., Rosen, F. S., Rowe, D. S., Seligmann, M. & Southill, J. F. (1971) Primary immunodeficiency; report of a WHO committee. *Paediatrics*, **47**, 927.

Gajdusek, D. C. (1957) An autoimmune reaction against human tissue antigens in certain chronic diseases. *Nature*, **179**, 666.

Gewurz, H. (1972) Alternate pathways to activation of the complement system. In *Biological Activities of Complement*, ed. Ingram, D. G. Basel: Karger.

Giblett, E. R., Anderson, J. E., Cohen, F., Pollera, B. & Meuwissen, H. J. (1972) Adenosine deaminase deficiency in two patients with severe impaired cellular immunity. *Lancet*, **ii**, 1067.

Gitlin, D. & Janeway, C. A. (1956) Agammaglobulinaemia, congenital acquired and transient forms. *Progress in Haematology*, **1**, 318.

Goldstein, A. L., Cohen, G. H., Rossio, J. L., Thurman, G. B., Brown, C. N. & Ulrich, J. T. (1976) Use of thymosin in the treatment of primary immunodeficiency diseases and cancer. *Medical Clinics of North America*, **60**, 591.

Good, R. A. & Bach, F. H. (1974) Bone marrow and thymus transplants. In *Clinical Immunobiology*, ed. Bach, F. H. & Good, R. A., Vol. 2. New York: Academic Press.

Gotze, O. & Muller-Eberhard, H. J. (1971) The C3 activator system: an alternate pathway of complement activation. *Journal of Experimental Medicine*, **134**, 90S.

Gray, B. N. & Watkins, E. (1975) Immunologic approach to cancer therapy. *Medical Clinics of North America*, **59**, 327.

Grebe, S. C. & Sreilen, J. W. (1976) Graft vs. host reactions: a review. *Advances in Immunology*, **22**, 120.

Grumet, F. C. (1975) Genetic control of immune responses. *American Journal of Clinical Pathology*, **63**, 646.

Hitzig, W. (1974) Therapeutic uses of transfer factor. *Progress in Clinical Immunology*, **2**, 69.

Hong, R. (1974) Immunodeficiency: enigmas and speculations. In *Progress in Clinical Immunology*, ed. Schwartz, R. S., Vol. 2. New York: Grune & Stratton.

International Union of Immunological Societies (IUIS) (1976) Report on clinical immunology. *Lancet*, **i**, 796.

Irvine, W. J., Gray, R. S., McCallum, C. J. (1976) Pancreatic islet—cell antibody as a marker for asymptomatic and latent diabetes and pre-diabetes. *Lancet*, **ii**, 1097.

Ishizaka, K. & Ishizaka, T. (1967) Identification of γE antibodies as a carrier of reaginic activity. *Journal of Immunology*, **99**, 1187.

Jersild, C., Dupont, B., Fog, T., Platz, P. J. & Svejgaard, A. (1975) Histocompatibility determinants in multiple sclerosis. *Transplantation Reviews*, **22**, 148.

Johansson, S. G. O., Benwich, H. & Wide, L. (1968) A new class of immunoglobulin in human serum. *Immunology*, **14**, 265.

Joint Committee Report on Clinical Immunology (1972) Published by the Royal Colleges of Physicians, Royal College of Pathologists and British Society for Immunology.

Jones, J. V., Cumming, R. H., Bucknall, R. C., Asplin, C. M., Fraser, I. D., Bothamley, J., Davis, P. & Hamblin, T. J. (1976) Plasmaphoresis in the management of acute systemic lupus erythematosis. *Lancet*, **i**, 711.

Kaplan, M. H. (1962) An immunological cross-reaction between group A streptococcal cells and human heart tissue. *Lancet*, **i**, 706.

Kaufman, H. S. & Hobbs, J. R. (1970) Immunoglobulin deficiencies in an atopic population. *Lancet*, **ii**, 1061.

Koffler, D., Agnello, V., Thorburn, R. & Kunkel, H. G. (1971) Systemic lupus erythematosus— prototype of immune complex nephritis in man. *Journal of Experimental Medicine*, **134**, 169S.

Lachmann, P. J. (1974) Complement. In *Clinical Aspects of Immunology*, 3rd edn, ed. Gell, P. G. H., Coombs, R. R. A. & Lachmann, P. J. Oxford and Edinburgh: Blackwell Scientific.

Lachmann, P. J. (1976) Clinical effects of complement deficiency. *Advanced Medicine*, Vol. 12, ed. Peters, D. K. London: Pitman Medical.

Lockwood, C. M., Pinching, A. J., Sweny, P., Rees, A. J., Russell, B., Uff, J. & Peters, D. K. (1977) Plasma exchange and immunosuppression in the treatment of fulminating immune complex crescentic nephritis. *Lancet*, **i**, 63.

Mathé, G., Schwarzenberg, L., Kiger, N., Florentin, Í., Halle-Panennko, O. & Garcia-Giralt, E. (1974) Bone marrow transplantation for aplasias and leukaemia. In *Clinical Immunobiology*, ed. Bach, F. H. & Good, R. A., Vol. 2. New York: Academic Press.

McConnell, I. & Lachmann, P. J. (1976) Complement and cell membranes. *Transplantation Reviews*, **32**, 72.

McDevitt, H. O. & Benacerraf, B. (1969) Genetic control of specific immune responses. *Advances in Immunology*, **11**, 31.

McPhaul, J. J. & Dixon, F. J. (1970) Characteristics of human antiglomerular basement membrane antibody in the pathogenesis of human glomerulonephritis. *Journal of Clinical Investigation*, **49**, 308.

M.R.C. Report (1971) *Hypogammaglobulinaemia in the United Kingdom*. London: H.M.S.O.

Medicus, R. G., Schreiber, R. D., Götze, O. & Muller-Eberhard, H. E. (1976) A molecular concept of the properdin pathway. *Proceedings of the National Academy of Sciences*, **73**, 612.

Meuwissen, H. J., Pickering, R. J., Pollera, B. & Porter, I. H. (Editors) (1975) *Symposium on Combined Immunodeficiency Disease and Adenosine Deaminase Deficiency; a Molecular Deficit*. New York: Academic Press.

Möller, G. (Editor) (1976) Biochemistry and biology of Ia antigens. *Transplantation Reviews*, **30**.

Muller-Eberhard, H. J. (1975) Complement. *Annual Review of Biochemistry*, **44**, 697.

Natvig, J. B. & Kunkel, H. G. (1973) Human immunoglobulins: classes, subclasses, genetic variants and idiotypes. *Advances in Immunology*, **16**, 1.

Nerup, J., Platz, P., Anderson, O. D., Christy, M., Lyngsøe, J., Poulsen, J. E., Tyder, C. P., Staub Nielson, L., Thomsen, M. & Svegaard, A. (1974) HLA antigens and diabetes mellitus. *Lancet*, **ii**, 864.

Neville, A. M. & Laurence, D. J. (1974) Report of the workshop on the carcinoembryonic antigen: the present position and proposals for future investigation. *International Journal of Cancer*, **14**, 1.

Nossal, G. J. (1974) Principles of immunological tolerance and immunocyte receptor blockade. *Advances in Cancer Research*, **20**, 93.

Oldstone, M. B. A. & Dixon, F. J. (1969) Pathogenesis of chronic disease associated with persistent lymphocytic choriomeningitis virus, *Journal of Experimental Medicine*, **129**, 483.

Patterson, M. C., Smith, B. P., Lohman, P. H. M., Anderson, A. K. & Fishman, L. (1976) Defective excision repair of X-ray damaged DNA in human (ataxia telangiectasia) fibroblasts. *Nature*, **260**, 444.

Pepys, M. B. (1976) Role of complement in the induction of immunological responses. *Transplantation Reviews*, **32,** 93.

Petty, R. E., Steward, M. W. & Soothill, J. F. (1972) The heterogeneity of antibody affinity in inbred mice and its possible immunopathological significance. *Clinical and Experimental Immunology*, **12,** 231.

Pillemer, L., Blum, L., Lepow, I. H., Ross, O. A., Todd, E. W. & Wardlaw, A. C. (1954) The properdin system and immunity. I. Demonstration and isolation of a new serum protein, properdin and its role in immune phenomena. *Science*, **120,** 279.

Rachelefsky, G., Terasaki, P. I., Park, M. S., Katy, R., Siegel, S. & Saito, S. (1976) Strong association between B lymphocyte group 2 specificity and asthma. *Lancet*, **ii,** 1042.

Reeves, W. G. (1976) Clinical immunology; nature of the specialty and provision of facilities. *Lancet*, **i,** 459.

Renoux, G. & Renoux, M. (1974) Modulation of immune reactivity by phenylimidothiazole salts in mice immunised by sheep red blood cells. *Journal of Immunology*, **113,** 779.

Roitt, I. M., Doniach, D., Campbell, P. N. & Hudson, R. V. (1956) Autoantibodies in Hashimoto's disease (lymphadenoid goitre). *Lancet*, **ii,** 820.

Rosen, F. S. (1974) Primary immunodeficiency. *Pediatric Clinics of North America*, **21,** 533.

Ruddy, S., Gigli, I. & Austen, K. F. (1972) The complement system in man. *New England Journal of Medicine*, **287,** 489, 545, 592, 642.

Scheffler, D. C. & David, C. S. (1975) The H_2 major histocompatibility complex and the I-immune response region. *Advances in Immunology*, **20,** 125.

Schwartz, M. (1958) Intrinsic factor inhibiting substance in serum of orally treated patients with pernicious anaemia. *Lancet*, **i,** 61.

Sharp, G. C., Irvin, W. S., Tan, E. M., Gould, R. G. & Holman, H. R. (1972) Mixed connective tissue disease—an apparently distinct rheumatic disease syndrome associated with a specific antibody to an extractable nuclear antigen (ENA). *American Journal of Medicine*, **52,** 148.

Skinner, M. D. & Schwartz, R. (1972) Immunosuppressive therapy. *New England Journal of Medicine*, **287,** 221-227, 281-286.

Soothill, J. F. (1974) Immunity deficiency states. In *Clinical Aspects of Immunology* 3rd edn, ed. Gell, P. G. H., Coombs, R. R. A. & Lachmann, P. J. Oxford and Edinburgh: Blackwell Scientific.

Soothill, J. F. & Steward, M. W. (1973). The relationship of allergic disease to immunodeficiency. *International Archives of Allergy and Applied Immunology*, **45,** 180.

Stanworth, D. R., Humphrey, J. H., Bennich, H. & Johansson, S. G. O. (1967) Specific inhibition of the Prauzuitz–Kustner reaction by an atypical human myeloma protein. *Lancet*, **ii,** 330.

Steward, M. W., Petty, R. E. & Soothill, J. F. (1973) Low affinity antibody—its possible immunopathological significance. *International Archives of Allergy and Applied Immunology*, **45,** 176.

Stiller, C. R., Russell, A. S. & Dossetor, J. P. (1975) Auto-immunity: present concepts. *Annals of Internal Medicine*, **82,** 405.

Strauss, A. J. B., Seegal, B. C., Hsu, K. C., Burkholder, P. M., Natsuk, W. L. & Osserman, K. E. (1960) Immunofluorescent demonstration of a muscle-binding complement fixing serum globulin fraction in myasthenia gravis. *Proceedings of the Society of Experimental Biology and Medicine*, **105,** 184.

Taylor, B., Norman, A. P., Orgel, H. A., Stokes, C. R., Turner, M. W. & Soothill, J. F. (1973) Transient IgA deficiency and the pathogenesis of infantile atopy. *Lancet*, **ii,** 111.

Taylor, K. B. (1959) Inhibition of intrinsic factor by pernicious anaemia sera. *Lancet*, **ii,** 106.

Thompson, R. A. (1974) Report of Workshop on Clinical Immunology. In *Progress in Immunology*, II, Vol. 4. Amsterdam: North-Holland.

Von Pirquet, C. & Schick, B. (1905) *Die serum Kranheit*; English trans. (1951) *Serum Sickness*. Baltimore: Williams & Wilkins.

Waksman, B. H. (1959) Experimental allergic encephalo-myelitis and the autoallergic diseases. *International Archives of Allergy and Applied Immunology*, Suppl. 14.

Weiner, A. S., Gordon, E. B. & Gallop, C. (1953) Studies on autoantibodies in human sera. *Journal of Immunology*, **71,** 58.

Witebsky, E. & Rose, N. R. (1956) Studies on organ specificity; production of rabbit thyroid antibodies in the rabbit. *Journal of Immunology*, **76,** 408.

World Health Organisation (1972) Clinical immunology. *Technical Report Series*, No. 2.

Zuckerman, A. J. (1975) Viral hepatitis: current studies and future prospects. *Monograph on Allergy* **9,** 196.

2
IMMUNOLOGICAL ASPECTS OF PROTEIN CALORIE MALNUTRITION

Steven D. Douglas   W. Page Faulk

Protein energy or protein calorie deficiencies are a major public health problem. Although this is more obvious in developed countries, malnutrition occurs throughout the world. It is estimated that more than 300 million children are affected, this being one of the most important problems in modern pediatrics. Protein calorie malnutrition (PCM)[1] is the most florid clinical manifestation of these deficiencies, and the most advanced condition of PCM is called kwashiorkor. This was first described by Dr Cicely Williams (1933, 1935) who reported a condition in children in the Gold Coast associated with a maize diet. She described a syndrome consisting of 'oedema, chiefly of the hands and feet, followed by wasting, diarrhoea, irritability, sores (chiefly of the mucous membranes) and desquamation of areas of the skin in a manner and distribution which is constant and unique'. This description has changed very little during the intervening 40 years. Kwashiorkor means 'the disease that the deposed baby gets when the next one is born'.

The classification of PCM has been approached in several ways. Waterlow (1972) has proposed that weights be compared to 50 per cent percentile using a standard developed with Boston children. His criteria for kwashiorkor include that the child be at a minimum weight of not less than 60 per cent of the expected weight for age, in association with oedema and either hepatomegaly or dermatosis. Criteria for marasmus are that the child should be less than 60 per cent of the expected weight for age and have no oedema or other specific signs. The clinical syndrome of kwashiorkor is thus characterised by muco-cutaneous lesions, oedema, hepatomegaly and apathy. Laboratory features include hypoalbuminaemia and increased urinary nitrogen excretion.

The interrelationships between proteins, lipids, carbohydrates, vitamins and minerals in malnutrition are not within the scope of this paper (for review see Waterlow and Alleyne, 1971), it should, however, be emphasised that the major dietary deficiency is protein. Although there have been extensive studies of the dietary requirements for protein in man and experimental animals, the precise needs remain complex and largely undefined (Scrimshaw, 1976). The stress which accompanies infection leads to mobilisation of amino acids from the tissues with an increased need for nitrogen to replace protein loss. Moreover, anorexia, vomiting, and diarrhoea are often concomitants of infection thus perpetuating major dietary restrictions during infection. Infection and kwashiorkor may incur a vicious cycle and it may be particularly difficult to distinguish initiating versus secondary factors.

Children with kwashiorkor are usually one to three years old and generally show skin lesions which include dyspigmentation, desquamation and frequently extensive exfoliation

[1]Also known as PEM, protein energy malnutrition.

which resemble burns. Purpura and ecchymoses are often seen (Fig. 2.1). Marasmic children have severe wasting of muscle and adipose tissue, and they are generally somewhat younger than kwashiorkor patients. In marasmus, prognosis on refeeding is good, whereas the treatment of kwashiorkor is more difficult and the prognosis is often poor. Children with kwashiorkor are at higher risk for infection than are marasmic children (Scrimshaw, Taylor and Gordon, 1968; Work et al, 1973; Faulk, Demaeyer and Davis, 1974).

The general characteristics of infection in children with kwashiorkor include absent or mild fever and slight leucocytosis. Skin lesions are frequently necrotising and apurulent, yet, pyogenic microorganisms are often found. Mucous membranes frequently demon-

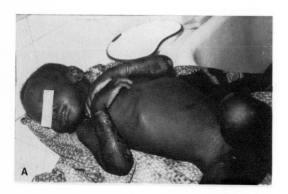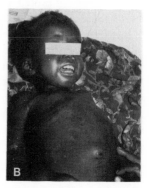

Figure 2.1   Child with severe PCM, kwashiorkor. Note the moon facies, generalised oedema and ecchymotic lesions

strate evidence of fungal infections. Stomatitis, balanitis and vulvitis are frequent. Herpes simplex may occur. Measles in a child with PCM is often associated with giant cell pneumonia and a poor prognosis (Taneja, 1968; Morley, 1969; Douglas and Schopfer, 1976). Protection from measles is thought to be mediated primarily by cellular immune mechanisms (Burnet, 1968) and the rash of measles has been postulated as being a manifestation of cell mediated immunity; its absence may be accompanied by giant cell pneumonia. Malnourished children with measles often have no rash, clinically suggesting impaired CMI.

It has long been known that there is an increased incidence of infectious disease in malnourished populations and these patients sustain greater morbidity and mortality. In severe malnutrition the majority of deaths occur during the first week of clinically apparent kwashiorkor and usually are attributable to infections, electrolyte disturbances, or liver failure (Waterlow and Alleyne, 1971). Substantial biochemical data have indicated that protein deficiency results in profound alterations in many organs, including those of the immune system. Recent studies have included an analysis of the afferent and efferent limbs of the immune response in children with kwashiorkor. These studies have included investigations of the phagocytic system, humoral and cell-mediated immunity, the complement system, and non-specific host defence mechanisms. In this review we shall summarise the present knowledge of immunologic alterations in children with protein calorie malnutrition.

HISTOPATHOLOGIC FEATURES OF THE IMMUNE SYSTEM

Histopathologic examination of tissues from the immunologic system of malnourished children reveal morphologic abnormalities of both central and peripheral lymphoid tissues. These immunopathologic alterations are summarised in Table 2.1. Histologic changes in the thymus vary with the degree of malnutrition (Watts, 1969; Mugerwa, 1971; Schonland, 1972). In intermediate stages of malnutrition there is a loss of corticomedullary differentiation and depletion of lymphocytes (Fig. 2.2), and in advanced PCM the thymus

Table 2.1ᵃ   Immunopathologic features of kwashiorkor

I.   *Histopathology*
    A. Thymus:
        Total weight—reduced
        Lobule architecture—distorted
        Cellularity—diminished
        Hassall's corpuscles—reduced
    B. Lymph nodes, spleen:
        Paracortical and periarteriolar areas—depleted
        Primary follicles and germinal centres—reduced
        Sinus histiocytosis
II.   *Circulating lymphocytes*
    A. Total number—normal or slightly reduced
        Plasmacytoid cells increased (electron microscopy)
    B. Markers:
        'T' (SRBC rosettes)—normal or reduced
        'B' (CRL)—normal?
    C. Mitogen response:
        PHA—decreased
        PWM—normal, elevated
        Antigen streptolysin S—decreased
III. *CMI in vivo*—diminished
IV.   *Immunoglobulin levels*
    IgG, IgA, IgM, IgD, IgE—variable
V.   *Specific antibody production*—decreased/normal/increased, depending on antigen used
    Isoagglutinins—increased
VI.   *Complement component levels*
    Reduced, except C4

ᵃFrom Douglas and Schopfer, 1976

is markedly decreased in size and weight (Faulk et al, 1976), and interlobular spaces are increased and filled with fibrous connective tissue (Fig. 2.2). On the other hand, an increased number of plasma cells have been reported in the bone marrow in PCM (Awdeh et al, 1972). Indeed, in our studies of kwashiorkor children in the Ivory Coast we frequently found increased numbers of plasma cells in the peripheral blood as determined by electron microscopy (Fig. 2.3). This is an unusual finding because plasmacytoid cells have hitherto been reported in the peripheral blood only in conditions such as viral infections, serum sickness, Waldenstrom's macroglobulinaemia, sarcoidosis, following burns, and after ingestion of pokeweed (Schopfer and Douglas, 1976b).

Examination of the spleen from malnourished individuals reveals a depletion of cells in the pericortical areas and in the periarteriolar sheaths of the white pulp (Fig. 2.4). Lymph nodes show a reduction of lymphocytes in primary follicles and germinal centres (Fig. 2.5), and paracortical areas are depleted (Fig. 2.5). The palatine tonsils are also diminished in

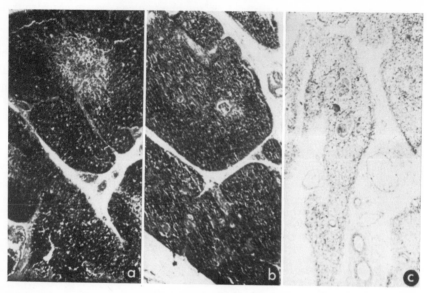

Figure 2.2 Human thymus in health and malnutrition. (a) Normal thymus. Note demarcation between cortex (dark staining) and medulla (light staining). Hassall's corpuscles are found in the medulla, and the thymic cortical cells exhibit intense mitotic activity. (b) Thymus from case of intermediate malnutrition. Note loss of corticomedullary differentiation. (c) Thymus from case of severe PCM. Note absence of lymphoid cells and increased interlobular spaces containing connective tissue elements. Tissues in Figures 2.2, 2.4, 2.5 and 2.6 from children of same age and sex. Haematoxylin-eosin, × 25. (From Faulk et al, 1976)

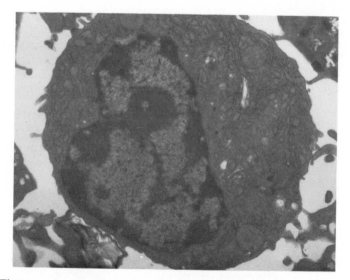

Figure 2.3 Electron micrograph of a plasmacytoid cell in the peripheral blood of a child with kwashiorkor. Note the heterochromatic nucleus. The cytoplasm contains numerous strands of rough-surfaced endoplasmic reticulum which is dilated. × 9000

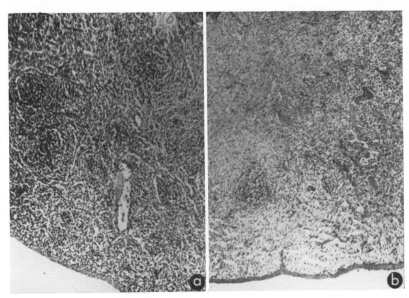

Figure 2.4 Human spleen in health and malnutrition. (a) Normal spleen. Germinal centres are thymus-independent and periarterial lymphatic sheaths of white pulp are thymus-dependent. (b) Spleen from case of severe malnutrition. Note absence of periarterial lymphatic-sheath and sparse germinal centres. Haematoxylin-eosin, × 25. (From Faulk et al, 1976)

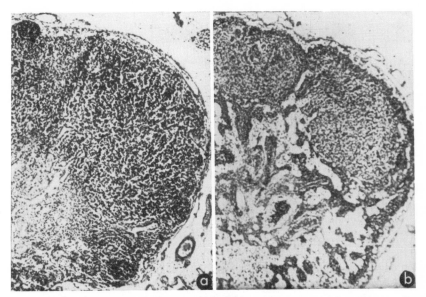

Figure 2.5 Human lymph node in health and malnutrition. (a) Normal lymph node. Germinal centres of cortex and cells of medullary cords are thymus-independent, lymphocytes of the paracortex are thymus-dependent. (b) Lymph node from case of severe malnutrition. Note that the node is virtually empty of lymphocytes and that there is an increase in connective tissue elements. Haematoxylin-eosin, × 25. (From Faulk et al, 1976)

size (Ferguson et al, 1974). Atrophic changes have been reported in Peyer's patches and solitary lymphoid follicles of the large bowel are diminished (Fig. 2.6). Although some studies have reported reduction in circulating lymphocyte counts, lymphocytopenia is not a consistent feature of PCM. The depletion of B-cell areas in lymph nodes and spleen and the observation of circulating plasmacytoid cells suggest a release of B-cells into the circulation in kwashiorkor. The histopathological evidence of thymic involution and loss of thymus-dependent areas in peripheral lymphoid tissues are consistent with reports of

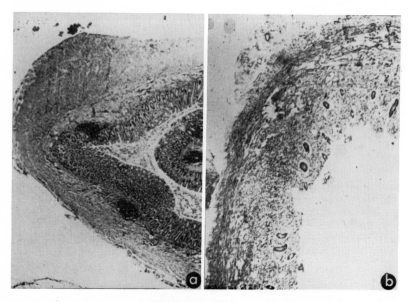

Figure 2.6 Human large bowel in health and malnutrition. (a) Normal bowel. Note solitary lymphoid follicles and intact mucosa. Follicles probably contain a mixed population of lymphocytes. Cells of the lamina propria are responsible for secretory IgA synthesis, and mucosa contributes to non-specific resistance. (b) Bowel from case of severe malnutrition. Note thinning of mucosa and absence of lymphoid follicles. Haematoxylin-eosin, × 25. (From Faulk et al, 1976)

defective cell-mediated immunity in PCM (Geefhuysen et al, 1971; Smythe et al, 1971; Edelman et al, 1973). Although there are major histopathologic changes in malnutrition which are certainly related to impairment in host defence mechanisms, the relative roles of stress, infection, and malnutrition leading to these changes are not known.

IMMUNOGLOBULINS AND ANTIBODIES

Serum immunoglobulin determinations in PCM have been reported from several parts of the world, and the values have been recorded as being low (Aref et al, 1970), normal (Rosen, Geefhuysen and Ipp, 1971) or high (Keet and Thom, 1969). In most studies, the levels of IgG, IgD and IgM have been reported to be normal or elevated, perhaps as a result of repeated and severe infections (Watson and Freesemann, 1970). Serum IgA values tend to be elevated (Mata and Faulk, 1973), again perhaps related to persistent antigenic stimulation via the respiratory and gastrointestinal tract (Sirisinha et al, 1975). Levels of IgE are elevated; however, this finding could be related to parasitism which often is present in patients with PCM (Neumann et al, 1975). In contrast to serum IgA, levels of secretory IgA are reduced in nasopharyngeal washings of patients with PCM, and secretory antibody responses to live attenuated measles and polio vaccines are also diminished (Chandra, 1975a).

Table 2.2 Antibody response in nutritional deficiencies (summary of the reports in the literature)

Antigen	Antibody production Human Normal	Reduced	Animal Normal	Reduced
Bacterial				
Tetanus toxoid	+	+		
Friedlander's bacillus				+
Diphtheria toxoid		+	+	+
Pneumococcus	+			+
E. coli				+
Brucella		+		
Salmonella	+	+	+	+
Cornybacterium kutscheri			+	+
Pasteurella		+		+
Klebsiella				+
Viruses				
Poliomyelitis	+	+		
Yellow fever		+		
Tobacco mosaic		+		
Influenza	+	+	+	+
Western equine encephalomyelitis				+
Miscellaneous				
Heterologous erythrocytes		+	+	+
Keyhole limpet haemocyanin	+			
Rickettsia			+	+
Ascaris				+
Heterologous proteins				+

This table has been modified from Faulk and Chandra (1976); source articles are cited in their publication. Responses indicated by plus in appropriate columns

Studies of specific antibody levels in response to immunisation both in man and in experimental animals have shown variable results (Table 2.2). For example, low responses have been reported to immunisation with yellow fever vaccine and influenza, and salmonella agglutinins have been found to be diminished (for review see Faulk, Mata and Edsall, 1975). The findings reported in Table 2.2 are unfortunately difficult to interpret because many of the reports do not specify the state of the antigen, type of adjuvant, route of administration, or technicalities of the assay system used to measure the antibody response. More precise information relevant to the effects of malnutrition on the immune response could be collected if characterised antigens and standardised reagents were used in future studies. Exact nutritional information is also needed about the patient because deficiencies including thiamine, pyridoxine, cobalamine, pantothenic acid, folate, biotin, ascorbic acid and vitamins A and D may lead to impaired antibody production (for review see Scrimshaw et al, 1968).

THE COMPLEMENT SYSTEM

Immunochemical and functional studies of total haemolytic complement activity in PCM have demonstrated reduced levels (Sirisinha et al, 1973; Chandra, 1975b). Moreover, sera from malnourished individuals have been reported to contain electrophoretically altered complement components (Chandra, 1975b). Analysis of individual complement components in sera of malnourished patients in Thailand demonstrated reduced levels of Cl_q, Cl_s, C3, C5, C8, C9 and C3PA (factor B of the alternative pathway), but C4 values were normal (Sirisinha et al, 1973). This suggests the possibility of in vivo activation of the alternative pathway. Some PCM patients also have elevated levels of immunoconglutinins and positive direct Coomb's tests with anticomplement activity in the sera (Smythe et al, 1971), again suggesting the possibility of in vivo activation of the blood complement system in PCM. The reduction in complement components could occur as a result of consumption as well as being secondary to impairment of protein synthesis in the liver, GI tract, lymphoid system, and macrophages. Also, the possibility of in vivo complement activation by immune complexes and endotoxin would seem to be likely, especially in view of the observation that many children with PCM also sustain an increased burden of infectious diseases.

LYMPHOCYTE FUNCTION

In vivo tests of cell-mediated immunity to purified protein derivative (PPD), dinitro-chlorobenzene (DNCB), dinitrofluorobenzene (DNFB), Candida antigens, keyhole limpet haemocyanin and Trichophyton have shown depressed or absent delayed hypersensitivy reactions in PCM (Harland, 1965; Geefhuysen et al, 1971; Smythe et al, 1971; Chandra, 1972; Edelman, 1977). However, the relative roles of impaired T-cell function, biochemical alterations in the skin, and certain hormones in causing impaired hypersensitivity reactions in PCM are not known. Each of these factors could be important, and it is probably unwise to assign the loss of delayed hypersentivity reactions in the skin to abnormal immune function until their contributions are better understood. For instance, levels of some adrenal hormones are increased in PCM (Abbassy et al, 1967; Alleyne and Young, 1967; Rao, Svikantia and Gopalan, 1968; Beitins et al, 1975), and it has been clinically recognised for many years that skin is abnormal in PCM (Edelman et al, 1973).

Several studies have measured the numbers of T and B lymphocytes in the peripheral circulation of patients with PCM (Chandra, 1974a; Ferguson et al, 1974). Most of these have shown a decrease in the percentage of T lymphocytes as determined by spontaneous rosette formation with sheep erythrocytes (SRBC-R). Studies done in India have reported a greater diminution of circulating T-cells in kwashiorkor than in marasmus and normal numbers of B-cells as determined by complement-receptor rosettes (CRL) in children with kwashiorkor (Bang et al, 1975). Our studies in the Ivory Coast revealed that the absolute number of SRBC-R were reduced in kwashiorkor; however, if both small (i.e. one to two erythrocytes bound) and large (i.e. more than two erythrocytes bound) rosettes were counted, the total number of rosette-forming cells was normal (Schopfer and Douglas, 1976b). Although the significance of decreased large rosettes is unknown, it is interesting to speculate that there may be a plasma membrane abnormality in circulating T-cells.

There have been several studies of the response of lymphocytes from malnourished patients to phytohaemagglutinin (PHA). Some of these reports have indicated that lymphocytes from malnourished individuals do not respond normally to PHA as measured by tritiated thymidine incorporation and blast transformation subsequent to lectin stimulation (Geefhuysen et al, 1971; Smythe et al, 1971; Grace, Armstrong and Smythe, 1972). Indeed, the original studies from South Africa reported a significantly depressed response (Grace et al, 1972; Sellmeyer et al, 1972) and these results have been confirmed by several

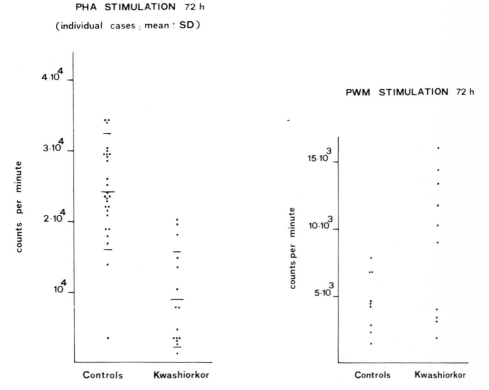

Figure 2.7   Comparison of the response to PHA of lymphocytes from children with kwashiorkor ($n = 15$) to controls ($n = 28$). Cpm/3 × 10⁵ lymphocytes. (From Schopfer and Douglas, 1976a)

Figure 2.8   Comparison of the response to PWM of lymphocytes from children with kwashiorkor ($n = 10$) to controls ($n = 9$). Cpm/3 × 10⁵ lymphocytes. (From Schopfer and Douglas, 1976a)

other laboratories (Sellmeyer et al, 1972; Ferguson et al, 1974; Schopfer and Douglas, 1976b). Other investigators have, however, reported either normal or elevated responses to PHA (Moore, Heyworth and Brown, 1974), and a recent report from the Gambia has suggested that sera from children with PCM may contain factors that inhibit lymphocyte responses to PHA (Heyworth, Moore and Brown, 1975). The pattern which seems to be emerging suggests that PHA responses are normal in marasmus and diminished in kwashiorkor. In our experience with kwashiorkor patients in the Ivory Coast, lymphocyte responses to PHA were decreased (Fig. 2.7), but lymphocyte responses to pokeweed mitogen were either equal to or greater than control responses (Schopfer and Douglas, 1976a) (Fig. 2.8). Detailed studies of the responses of lymphocyte subpopulations to mitogens, antigens and in mixed lymphocyte cultures have not been performed in PCM. Studies of lymphokine production by cells from PCM patients have not been reported and would be of particular interest in view of observations that malnourished persons usually cannot muster adequate inflammatory responses (Edelman et al, 1973).

In summary, available data indicate that T lymphocytes are reduced in number and T-cell function is impaired in severe PCM and similar depressions in T-cell numbers

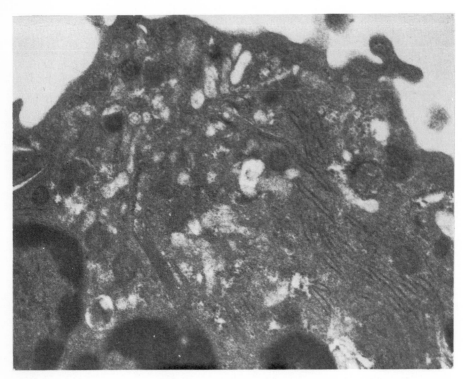

Figure 2.9 Electron micrograph of PMN with strands and stacks of rough endoplasmic reticulum characteristic of Döhle body. × 25 000

and function are not usually seen in marasmus. The number of B-cells and B-cell function appears to be unaltered in human PCM (see later section for comments on Animal Models of Nutrition). Unfortunately, very little data have been gathered in conditions of intermediate malnutrition, and until such information is available it is probably unwise to assume that the above statements are true for all conditions of malnutrition.

PHAGOCYTE FUNCTION

Analysis of the inflammatory response and of the afferent limb of the immune response in malnutrition requires detailed investigations of the events involved in phagocytosis and killing of microorganisms (for review see Bellanti and Dayton, 1975; Douglas and Schopfer, 1976, 1977). This is particularly true in view of observations that malnourished persons sustain high morbidity and mortality from infectious diseases. Although fixed tissue phagocytes (e.g. Kupffer cells, alveolar macrophages) have a major role in host defence, clinical investigations have for technical reasons been largely limited to studies of phagocytic cells in the peripheral circulation. In order for appropriate phagocyte function to occur there must be adequate numbers of phagocytes (neutrophils and mononuclear

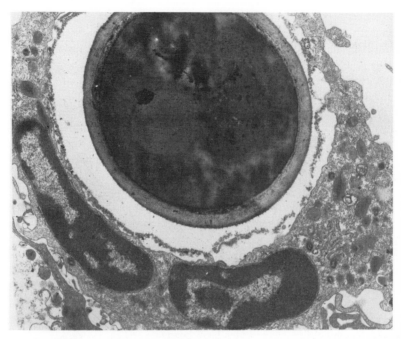

Figure 2.10   PMN from kwashiorkor patient incubated with *Candida albicans* for 60 min. Although some degranulation has occurred, a number of granules remain in the cytoplasm. The yeast cell shows degeneration of the cell wall and the cytoplasm. × 14 000

phagocytes) in tissues as well as in the circulation, and there must also be an adequate capacity of bone marrow to mobilise these cells. Although detailed studies of leucocyte traffic have not been done in children with PCM, the numbers of circulating phagocytes have been reported to be normal or increased (Schopfer and Douglas, 1976c). Electron microscopic studies of neutrophils from malnourished children reveal frequent cytoplasmic vacuolisation and Döhle bodies (Fig. 2.9). Döhle bodies are strands of rough-surfaced endoplasmic reticulum that occur in polymorphonuclear neutrophils (PMNs) from individuals with a variety of infections, and it is thought that these structures are related to the synthesis of lysosomal enzymes by mature neutrophils (McCall et al, 1969; Schopfer and Douglas, 1976b).

Phagocyte function can be divided into three main phases: (1) chemotaxis; (2) engulfment, and (3) postphagocytic events including (a) formation of phagocytic vacuoles or phagosomes, fusion of lysosomes with phagosomes, and release of lysosomal contents (degranulation) into phagosomes with the consequent formation of phagolysosomes, (b) microbial killing, and (c) associated metabolic changes. The morphological events which follow engulfment of microorganisms and other particles include the formation of plasma-membrane derived phagocytic vacuoles and fusion of these vacuoles with lysosomes followed by a release of the lysosomal contents (degranulation). Electron microscopic studies of PMNs from children with kwashiorkor using *Staphylococcus aureus*, *Escherichia coli*, and *Candida albicans* have demonstrated no apparent qualitative abnormality in vacuole formation or degranulation (Fig. 2.10).

The active direct migration of PMNs towards chemotactic stimuli (e.g. bacterial products or certain complement components) is a primary early event in inflammation. Impairment of the in vitro chemotactic response can be correlated with abnormalities in the inflammatory response in certain genetic disorders and malignancies (Bellanti and Dayton, 1975). Children with severe kwashiorkor often have mucocutaneous lesions, cutaneous ulcerations, and superficial necrotising infections. Pyogenic bacteria, mainly *Staph. aureus*, are frequently isolated from these lesions, yet pus formation is rarely seen. In a study of children with malnutrition in Peru, Freyre et al (1973), using a skin-window technique, demonstrated an increased mobilisation of PMNs and a decreased migration of mononuclear cells after 8 h of incubation. Rosen et al (1975) in South Africa reported no difference in the in vitro chemotactic response of PMN from children with kwashiorkor as compared with normals; however, cells from children with infections also had diminished chemotactic responses. Impaired chemotaxis has also been demonstrated for cells from malnourished Australian aboriginal children by Jose et al (1975). Our assessment of PMN chemotaxis using cells from kwashiorkor children in the Ivory Coast demonstrated a diminished number of PMNs migrating toward the chemotactic factor (*E. coli*) at early incubation times (30, 60 and 120 min) when compared to control cells (Schopfer and Douglas, 1976c). This delay in migratory response was however diminished following a 180 min incubation period after which time control and test values were equivalent (Fig. 2.11).

The engulfment of particles, polystyrene latex, *Staph. aureus*, *C. albicans*, and Forssman IgG antibody-coated sheep erythrocytes have been studied for isolated PMNs and blood monocytes of children with PCM (Tejada et al, 1964; Douglas and Schopfer, 1974). These studies indicate that the engulfment of particles by PMNs or monocytes from children with PCM is not adversely affected by malnutrition. Studies of the opsonic activity of plasma obtained from PCM children in both India (Seth and Chandra, 1972) and Australia (Jose et al, 1975) reported slightly increased activity as compared to control sera. Plasma opsonic activity was reported to be reduced for sera from malnourished children in Thailand (Tanphaichitr, Mekanandha and Valyasevi, 1973). In summary, present data suggest that opsonisation and engulfment are not impaired in PCM.

In vitro experiments with isolated PMNs from malnourished children have demonstrated defects in the killing of *Staph. aureus*, *E. coli* (Fig. 2.12), and *C. albicans* (Selvaraj and Bhat, 1972; Douglas and Schopfer, 1974, 1976, 1977). Studies of the hexose monophosphate shunt (HMS) and of glycolysis metabolites in normal and malnourished PMNs revealed no differences between these cells (Schopfer and Douglas, 1976c). Activation of HMS, increased oxygen consumption, and production of superoxide radicals and peroxide are related to microbicidal activity (Klebanoff, 1975). Peroxide generated during the postphagocytic phase is partially used in the intraleucocytic myeloperoxidase-halide-mediated killing system, described by Klebanoff (1975). The activity of this system can be assessed in vitro by measuring the extent of ^{131}I incorporation into trichloroacetic acid (TCA) precipitable proteins after phagocytosis, and studies using this technique have revealed the myeloperoxidase-halide-mediated system to be depressed in PCM (Jose et al, 1975;

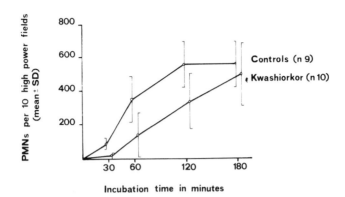

Figure 2.11   Kinetics of neutrophil chemotactic response. The total number of PMNs per 10 high power fields (migrating through the filter) are plotted for each incubation time. (From Schopfer and Douglas, 1976c)

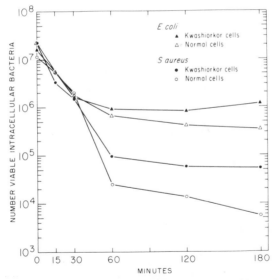

Figure 2.12   Kinetics of neutrophil bactericidal activity with *E. coli* (▲) kwashiorkor cells and (△) normal cells (no antibiotics added) and *S. aureus* (●) kwashiorkor cells and (○) normal cells (penicillin-streptomycin was added at 30 min). (From Douglas and Schopfer, 1974)

Schopfer and Douglas, 1976c) (Fig. 2.13). In our studies the extent of iodination was measured in a kinetic assay and significantly lower iodide incorporation was found in the PMNs from malnourished children at each incubation interval. At present, this is the only biochemical parameter which correlates with the defective in vitro killing of microorganisms by PMNs from children with PCM. It should also be mentioned that, with the exception of Chediak–Higashi syndrome, decreased formation by PMNs of TCA-precipitable iodinated proteins has been found in all clinical conditions that are characterised by decreased in vitro killing of phagocytosed bacteria (Schopfer and Douglas, 1976c). Degradation of thyroxine (T_4) and triiodothyronine (T_3) by phagocytising PMNs is a further assay of neutrophil function (Klebanoff and Green, 1973), and studies using this technique in PCM have shown reduction in thyroid hormone degradation. Decreased

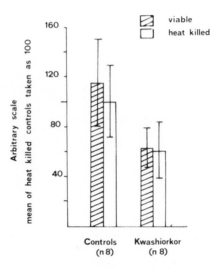

Figure 2.13   Leucocyte iodination by PMN after phagocytosis of viable (H_2O_2 producing) and heat-killed lactobacilli. The mean value for control PMNs incubated with heat-killed lactobacilli was arbitrarily taken as 100

iodination by phagocytising PMNs has been reported in several genetic and acquired granulocytopathies (Klebanoff, 1975).

The elevated levels of baseline hexose monophosphate shunt activity which are reflected by high NBT scores suggest an activation of the phagocytic system in vivo in PCM (Douglas and Schopfer, 1974). This in vitro PMN activation may be a consequence of the presence of infection in children with PCM and indicates normal PMN biochemistry.

Impaired in vitro microbicidal activity of PMNs and reduced iodination during particle ingestion have been reported to be the major consistent characteristic feature of many genetic and acquired disorders of granulocyte function (Table 2.3). Also, the decreased killing function, decreased iodination, and increased basal metabolism of PMNs from children with kwashiorkor are reminiscent of PMN function observed in leukaemic children receiving craniospinal irradiation (Baehner et al, 1973). However, the mechanisms responsible for transient impairment of phagocyte function in PCM, leukaemia, and several other clinical entities are not known.

In summary, correlations between in vitro assessments of phagocyte function such as chemotaxis, microbicidal activity, and biochemical changes with clinical susceptibility to infectious diseases have not been clearly established. Nevertheless, evidence from investigations of patients with genetic granulocytopathies suggests that such in vitro assessments do correlate with the incidence of infectious diseases. These observations support the contention that the increased incidence of infectious diseases in children with malnutrition may at least in part be due to impaired PMN function. In vitro studies of PMN function have revealed impaired chemotaxis, normal phagocytosis, and defective intracellular killing of bacteria and fungi. The prominent characteristics of leucocyte metabolism for cells from children with PCM are an increased resting activity of the hexose monophos-

Table 2.3ᵃ   Functional studies of phagocytes in PCM

	Resting	Phagocytes	References
NBT	Normal	Normal increase	Altay et al (Turkey, 1972)
	Subnormal	Subnormal	Shousa and Kamel (Egypt, 1972)
	Subnormal	N.D.	Kendall and Nolan (Rhodesia, 1972)
	High	N.D.	Avila et al (Venezuela, 1973)
	High	N.D.	Wolfsdorf and Nolan (Rhodesia, 1974)
	Normal/high	N.D.	Rosen et al (S. Africa, 1975)
	High	N.D.	Schopfer and Douglas (Ivory Coast, 1976c)
Hexose Monophosphate shunt (HMS)			
Radiometric	High	Normal	Douglas and Schopfer (Ivory Coast, 1974)
Liquid scintillation	High	Decreased	Selvaraj and Bhat (India, 1972)
	High	Normal	Schopfer and Douglas (Ivory Coast, 1976c)
Iodination	—	Decreased	Schopfer and Douglas (Ivory Coast, 1976c)
Thyroid degradation			
T_3	—	Low to normal	Schopfer and Douglas (Ivory Coast, 1976c)
T_4	—	Normal	Schopfer and Douglas (Ivory Coast, 1976c)

N.D. = not done
ᵃ From Douglas and Schopfer, 1977

phate shunt and a decreased extent of iodination during particle ingestion. These data differ from genetically determined granulocytopathies in that no basic metabolism impairment or lack of key enzyme activity related to killing have been demonstrated. More precise characterisations of these abnormalities of phagocyte function in PCM will hopefully improve our understanding of the decreased resistance to infection in PCM and provide insight into better therapeutic approaches.

RESULTS OF PROTEIN SUPPLEMENTATION

Systematic studies of the effects of supplemental dietary therapy on both cellular and humoral immunological functions in PCM have not been done, but some data are available. Also, studies of the long-term effects of early PCM on the subsequent function of the immune system is not known. However, studies of Egyptian children with early kwashiorkor demonstrated decreased serum IgM concentrations six months after dietary therapy and seemingly complete recovery (Aref et al, 1970). Studies in Ghana (Ferguson et al, 1974) and New Delhi (Bang et al, 1975) indicate that following therapy with high protein and high calorie diets there is recovery of delayed hypersensitivity, and the number of T-cells as assessed by rosette formation return to normal values. A study of malnourished adults showed improvement in delayed hypersensitivity and lymphocyte responses to phytomitogens following nutritional repletion (Law, Dudrick and Abdov, 1973). Serial studies of complement components in sera from malnourished children also showed a restoration of values toward normal (Sirisinha et al, 1973). Finally, a group of 16 malnourished Guatemalan children were treated with transfer factor during recuperation from PCM, but the mortality was the same in both treated and control populations (Walker et al, 1975). Also, no effect of transfer factor was demonstrated on the recovery of both groups from anergy as measured by delayed hypersensitivity reactions. Even though some of the effects of malnutrition on the immune response are correctable by dietary therapy, the long-term effects of PCM on the immune response are unknown, and data on this point are of obvious importance.

The influence of protein intake on serum immunoglobulin (Ig) concentrations has been investigated in children receiving increasing or decreasing amounts of egg protein. The correlation between serum Ig, protein intake and other nutritional parameters was found to be of a very low order, suggesting that Ig levels are not influenced entirely by nutrition (Lechtig et al, 1970). On the other hand, nutritional supplementation of healthy New Guinean schoolchildren with skim-milk powder resulted in the synthesis of significantly more antibody following primary immunisation with flagellin than in a control group of similarly overtly healthy but growth-retarded children (Mathews et al, 1972). Also, supplementation of a natural (inadequate) diet was associated with lower Ig levels (Mathews et al, 1974). Protein and calorie supplementation also has been reported to correct depressed plasma concentrations of complement (Sirisinha et al, 1973).

NON-SPECIFIC FACTORS OF RESISTANCE

There is very little information about non-specific factors in malnutrition, but some attention has focused on the transferrins. These iron-binding proteins reportedly bear a bad prognosis if depressed (Antia, McFarlane and Soothill, 1968; McFarlane et al, 1970). It is not altogether clear why depressed serum transferrin values suggest a poor prognosis, but it is thought to be related to their iron-binding capacity (Bullen, Rogers and Leigh, 1972; Elin and Wolff, 1974; Weinberg, 1975). Certain bacteria require iron to manifest their pathogenecity (Editorial, 1974) and iron is important in the killing of endocytosed bacteria by phagocytes (Chandra, 1973; MacDougall et al, 1975). Indeed, Arbeter et al (1971) have presented data that iron deficiency adversely affects intracellular bacterial killing, and Chandra (1973) has put forward evidence that iron deficiency leads to impaired killing of phagocytosed bacteria. The transferrin–iron relationship may even be important in protecting the human fetus in utero, because transferrin has been reported in trophoblasts as early as the sixth week of development. This persists throughout gestation and is observed in trophoblasts of term placentae (Faulk and Johnson, 1976).

The diets of many malnourished persons also lack adequate vitamins, and several vitamins have been shown to be important in mounting an adequate immune response. This topic has been comprehensively reviewed in a WHO monograph by Scrimshaw et al (1968). Pyridoxine deficiency is associated with defective cell-mediated immunity (Axelrod, 1971) and several effects of vitamin deficiencies on immunoglobulin and antibody synthesis were mentioned in the preceding sections. Regarding non-specific resistance, chickens fed diets deficient in vitamin A demonstrated a replacement of their normal mucociliated epithelium by keratinised squamous cells (Bang and Bang, 1969), and the multiplication of both Newcastle disease and influenza viruses was much higher in these birds (Bang and Foard, 1971). Iron deficiency may alter epithelial structure, which in turn permits the initiation of fungal infections. The consequent antigenic load may contribute to a depression of CMI. Selective vitamin deficiencies are however less common than multiple deficiencies in human malnutrition. These studies are important in terms of understanding the influence of vitamins in augmenting or depressing the immune response. For example, vitamin A can serve an adjuvant-like effect, and its administration in non-toxic doses to well-nourished animals results in an augmentation of humoral immunity as well as a reduction in rejection times of skin grafts (Jorin and Tannock, 1972).

For many years it has been speculated that breast milk contains non-specific factors of resistance, because breast-fed infants seem to thrive better than bottle-fed babies. For instance, significant levels of resistance to enteric infection are observed among breast-fed babies, even if they live in conditions of poor environmental sanitation (Mata and Wyatt, 1971). Mechanisms for this resistance are poorly understood, but one mechanism seems to be related to certain indigenous microflora which form a protective barrier against pathogenic organisms. Breast-fed infants develop a predominant flora comprised of Gram-positive anaerobic bacilli (*Bifidobacterium*) probably as a result of the combined action of bifidus factor(s), lysozyme, secretory IgA, other antibodies and macrophages and lymphocytes present in human milk (Goldman and Smith, 1973). The lysozyme and immunoglobulins are thought to exert a suppressing and/or lytic effect on Gram-negative facultative bacilli (Enterobacteriaceae), and this results in a milieu that is unfavourable for Shigella and other enteropathogenic agents (Mata and Urrutia, 1971). The increased rates of infectious diseases and malnutrition that accompany weaning may be partially due to the loss of natural resistance factors in breast milk.

Fetal Malnutrition

Infants with low birth-weight who are small-for-gestational age represent a fetal form of malnutrition. Several factors are known to contribute to intrauterine growth retardation (Sinclair, 1972). These include (a) maternal variables such as hypertension, metabolic illnesses, toxaemia and infections; (b) fetal factors such as malformations, multiple pregnancy, and infection; and (c) placental factors such as the 'insufficiency' syndromes. In addition, the health–socioeconomic background of the mother is important. This includes factors such as low social class, inadequate prenatal care, ethnic group, high altitude, drug abuse and smoking.

Intrauterine infections significantly affect the morbidity and mortality of low birth-weight infants. The aetiologic agent in these instances may be of low virulence and systemic spread with poor localisation is common. Several aspects of immunocompetence are impaired in such infants (Chandra, 1974b), and thymuses of affected neonates are much smaller than those from appropriately matched controls (Fig. 2.14). Cell-mediated immunity as measured either by delayed hypersensitivity reactions or by lymphocyte responses to in vitro stimulation are often depressed. In addition, quantitative measurements of T-lymphocytes in the blood reveal that they are reduced in number (Ferguson et al, 1974). Hypoimmunoglobulinaemia especially involving IgG is frequent (Papadatos et al, 1970) and the maternofetal transfer of IgG is reduced (Chandra, 1975c). The blood concentration of the third component of complement is low, the opsonic function of plasma is reduced, and the bacterial killing by polymorphonuclear leucocytes is often slightly impaired. It is suspected that these functional defects in the host resistance of infants who have suffered fetal malnutrition can persist for several months in extrauterine life (Chandra, 1977). These babies often sustain repeated infections, and clinically they tend to resemble children with immunodeficiency diseases.

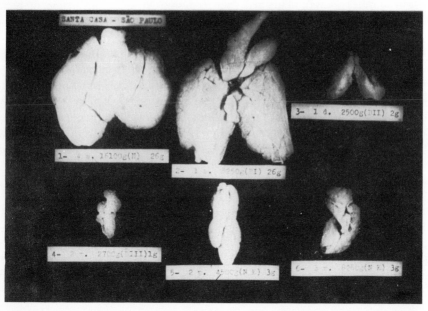

Figure 2.14   Gross morphology of thymuses. From left to right top row: 1, normal thymus—26 g, four year old child; 2, normal thymus—26 g, one year old child; 3, intrauterine malnutrition—2 g thymus. Bottom row: 4, severe malnutrition—two month old child (marasmus); thymus weight 1 g; 5, kwashiorkor—two month old child; thymus weight 3 g; 6, kwashiorkor—eight month old child, thymus weight 3 g.

ANIMAL MODELS OF MALNUTRITION

It is not the intention of this review to deal extensively with data obtained from experimental models, but much of this work is relevant to the immunopathology of PCM in humans. Even in carefully controlled animal experiments, however, it is difficult to rule out the effect of selective deficiencies from PCM in the experimental animals due to anorexia as a result of the selective deficiency. This can be only partially controlled by pair-feeding experiments (Krishnan et al, 1974) and serves to underscore the considerable difficulties of interpreting data acquired from human populations. Immunologic studies in several species have shown that PCM is associated with both cellular and humoral immunologic deficiencies. Aschkenasy (1975) demonstrated that there is a decrease in circulating and tissue lymphocytes and eosinophils in protein-deficient rats. Although there is no decrease in circulating neutrophils, these cells are decreased in inflammatory foci. Bell and Hazell (1975) have demonstrated that mice fed protein-deficient diets have lymphoid cells that show an enhanced capacity to induce graft versus host reactions. They interpret this result as reflecting a decrease in the production of short-lived lymphoid cells having a rapid turnover, such as B-cells. They conclude that long-lived T-cells appear to persist, remaining functionally intact for long periods of time in the face of nutritional insults. Impaired lymphopoiesis has been demonstrated in protein deficiency in several species and this is well illustrated in histological and thymidine uptake studies of Bhuyam and Ramalingaswami (1974a) using guinea-pig mesenteric lymph nodes. These investigators showed a reduction in both mitotic index and thymidine uptake in protein-deficient animals; lymph node germinal centres were reduced in number and size; mitoses were diminished in paracortical areas, but there was no appreciable reduction of plasma cells in the medulla. Bhuyam and Ramalingaswami (1974b) have also demonstrated an impairment of macrophage mobilisation and an inability to form BCG granulomas in protein-deficient rabbits. The granulomas which did form following BCG immunisation were quite small and were characterised by loosely knit epithelioid and giant cells.

Although severe malnutrition usually leads to impairment of host defence mechanisms, moderate forms of nutritional deficiency may enhance certain types of host resistance. Rous (1911) observed that undernourished chickens were resistant to infection with Rous sarcoma virus. Enhanced resistance to vaccinia virus in rabbits, pseudorabies in mice (Cooper, Good and Mariani, 1974), and poliomyelitis in man has also been reported in states of undernutrition. In addition, Fernandes, Yunis and Good, (1976a, b) have shown that protein and calorie restricted diets prolonged the survival time of mice who normally develop life-shortening autoimmune diseases. Jose and Good (1973a, b) reported that animals fed diets containing moderate amounts of protein had a preferential suppression of antibody production, suggesting a compromised ability to produce tumour-specific 'blocking' antibody and augmented cell-mediated immune responses to certain tumour antigens. Much of the experimental work done by this group has been summarised in comprehensive reviews by Good et al (1977) and Fernandes et al (1976a).

Macrophage function and antibody affinity have been shown by Morgan and Soothill (1975a, b) to be closely related to inbred mouse strains, and both of these properties are depressed in moderate protein malnutrition (Passwell, Steward and Soothill, 1974; Coovadia and Soothill, 1976a). Indeed, impaired overall phagocytic function as measured by the clearance of radio-labelled polyvinyl pyrrolidone has been shown by Coovadia and Soothill (1976b) to be depressed in mice receiving phenylalanine and tryptophane restricted diets. These observations are important for several reasons. Firstly, the presence of low affinity antibody in malnutrition could appear in certain antibody assays as a quantitative depression in antibody response, when in fact an alteration in antibody affinity was responsible. Secondly, the effects of protein deprivation on macrophage function and antibody affinity is pertinent to the immune elimination of antigen (Alpers, Steward and Soothill, 1972) and could be very important in determining the vulnerability of some malnourished subjects to immune complex and other immunopathological diseases (Soothill and Steward, 1971). The observation of altered macrophage clearance suggests that the nutritional state may be a significant determinant in antigen processing and in tolerance.

CONCLUDING COMMENTS

The immune system is one of the principal bulwarks of host defence (Good, Finstad and Gatti, 1970). This is not however to be interpreted as being the only aspect of lowered resistance in malnutrition, for the role of hormones (Gardner and Amacher, 1973), trace elements and non-specific factors (Braun and Ungar, 1973) might be equally as important. Studies of malnourished populations are complicated by uncontrollable variables such as concomitant infections, regional diets and customs, weather, altitude and lack of relevant genetic data. Some of these aspects can be controlled in studies of animal models, and this approach continues to add valuable information about basic immunological aspects that are altered by nutritional manipulations. For instance, suppressor T-cell function seems to be importantly affected by dietary restrictions (Fernandes, G., personal communication).

One encouraging observation made in studies of human populations is that some of the immune defects seem to rapidly return to normal following dietary therapy (Mathews et al, 1972, 1974; Chandra, 1974a; Ziegler and Ziegler, 1975) suggesting that the immune lesions may not be irreversible. This has implications for public health programmes that deal with infectious diseases among malnourished populations. For instance, vaccination programmes in certain areas might achieve greater success if they were preceded by a brief period of dietary supplementation. Reports of immunological repair subsequent to dietary therapy must however be tempered with other reports of prolonged suppression of immunoglobulin production in cases of treated PCM and of depressed lymphocyte function in infants who have sustained fetal malnutrition. Indeed, animal studies have shown prolonged effects of malnutrition on the immune response (Jose, Stutman and Good, 1973), and immunological depressions have experimentally been demonstrated in the progeny of malnourished parents (Gebhardt and Newberne, 1974; Chandra, 1975d). Long-term follow-up studies of immunological responses are badly needed in nutritionally supplemented human populations that have sustained various degrees of malnutrition, as well as in children who have been diagnosed as having intrauterine malnutrition.

The clinical and biochemical profiles of malnourished children are extraordinarily complex, and it is unwise to make generalities about their capacities to resist infections. However, several years ago children with immunodeficiency diseases also presented complex clinical and biochemical profiles. Research on these diseases has developed a systematic approach to diagnosis and treatment on the pathophysiology of each deficiency, and this has led to improved prognosis in many immunodeficiency diseases (Cooper, et al, 1974). As research broadens current understanding of the immune response in malnutrition, it seems to be increasingly possible to think of the immune defects in undernutrition as analogous to those in immunodeficiency diseases, and it has been suggested that malnourished children might be considered as having a type of secondary or acquired immunodeficiency disease (Faulk, 1974; Douglas and Schopfer, 1976). This approach may be useful in establishing a better understanding of patterns of host resistance in malnourished children as well as helping to build new concepts in the treatment and prevention of infections in malnourished populations. Thus, immunology has a great deal to offer the science of nutrition, and it would seem that the combined approaches of nutrition, public health, and immunology may have something of value to offer the malnourished child.

The World Health Organisation has coordinated an international collaborative study of the effects of malnutrition on the immune response with particular emphasis on public health aspects of the nutrition–infection cycle (Awdeh et al, 1972; Faulk et al, 1974). Considerable data have accumulated as a result of these studies, and a profile of the immunological capabilities of malnourished children is beginning to emerge.

ACKNOWLEDGEMENT

The authors acknowedge the support of the World Health Organisation and of the Nestle Foundation for Biochemical and Immunological Studies of Phagocytes. We thank Professor Carlos Marigo and Dr Roberto Pinto Paes for Figures 2.2, 2.4, 2.5, 2.6 and 2.14. Studies in the Ivory Coast were done in collaboration with Dr Kurt Schopfer. Dr Douglas' research is supported by USPHS grant AI-12478 from the National Institutes of Health, the National Leukemia Association, and the KROC Foundation. Dr Faulk's research is supported by USPHS grants AM-19201 & HD-09938 from the National Institutes of Health.

REFERENCES

Abbassy, A. S., Mikhail, M., Zeitoun, M. M. & Ragab, M. (1967) The suprarenal cortical function as measured by the plasma 17-hydroxycorticosteroid level in malnourished children. *Journal of Tropical Pediatrics*, **13**, 87–93.

Alleyne, G. A. O. & Young, V. H. (1967) Adrenocortical function in children with severe protein-calorie malnutrition. *Clinical Science*, **33**, 189–200.

Alpers, J. H., Steward, M. W. & Soothill, J. F. (1972) Differences in immune elimination in inbred mice. The role of low affinity antibody. *Clinical and Experimental Immunology*, **12**, 121–132.

Altay, C., Say, B., Dogramaci, N. & Bingol, A. (1972) Nitroblue tetrazolium test in children with malnutrition. *Journal of Pediatrics*, **81**, 392–393.

Antia, A. V., McFarlane, H. & Soothill, J. F. (1968) Serum siderophilin in kwashiorkor. *Archives of Diseases of Childhood*, **43**, 459–462.

Arbeter, A., Echeverri, L., Franco, D., Munson, D., Velez, H. & Vitale, M. (1971) Nutrition and infection. *Federation Proceedings*, **30**, 1421–1430.

Aref, G. H., Badr El Din, M. K., Hassan, A. I. & Araby, I. I. (1970) Immunoglobulins in kwashiorkor. *Journal of Tropical Medical Hygiene*, **73**, 186–191.

Aschkenasy, A. (1975) Dietary proteins and amino acids in leucopoiesis: recent hematological and immunological data. *World Review of Nutrition and Dietetics*, **21**, 151–197.

Avila, J. L., Valesquez-Avila, G., Correa, C., Castillo, C. & Convit, J. (1973) Leukocytic enzyme differences between clinical forms of malnutrition. *Clinica chimica acta*, **19**, 5–10.

Awdeh, Z., Bengoa, J., Demaeyer, E., Dixon, H., Edsall, G., Faulk, W. P., Goodman, H. C., Hopwood, B. E. C., Jose, D., Keller, W., Kumate, J., Mata, L., McGregor, I., Miescher, P., Rowe, D., Taylor, C. & Torrigiani, G. (1972) A survey of nutritional–immunological interactions. *Bulletin of the World Health Organisation*, **46**, 537–546.

Axelrod, A. E. (1971) Immune processes in vitamin deficiency states. *American Journal of Clinical Nutrition*, **24**, 265–276.

Baehner, R. L., Neiburger, R. G., Johnson, D. E. & Murrmann, S. M. (1973) Transient bactericidal defect of peripheral blood phagocytes from children with acute lymphoblastic leukemia receiving craniospinal irradiation. *New England Journal of Medicine*, **289**, 1209–1213.

Bang, B. G. & Bang, F. B. (1969) Replacement of virus-destroyed epithelium by keratinized squamous cells in vitamin A-deprived chickens. *Proceedings of the Society for Experimental Biology and Medicine*, **132**, 50–54.

Bang, F. B. & Foard, M. A. (1971) The effect of acute vitamin A deficiency on the susceptibility of chicks to Newcastle disease and influenza viruses. *Johns Hopkins Medical Journal*, **129**, 100–108.

Bang, B. G., Mahalanabis, D., Mukherjee, K. L. & Bang, F. B. (1975) T and B lymphocyte rosetting in undernourished children. *Proceedings of the Society for Experimental Biology and Medicine*, **149**, 199–202.

Beitins, I. Z., Kowarski, A., Migeon, C. J. & Graham, G. G. (1975) Adrenal function in normal infants and in marasmus and kwashiorkor. *Journal of Pediatrics*, **86**, 302–308.

Bell, R. G. & Hazell, L. A. (1975) Influence of dietary protein restriction on immune competence. *Journal of Experimental Medicine*, **141**, 127–137.

Bellanti, J. A. & Dayton, D. H. (1975) *The Phagocytic Cell in Host Resistance.* New York: Raven Press.

Bhuyan, U. N. & Ramalingaswami, V. (1974a) Lymphopoiesis in protein deficiency. *American Journal of Pathology*, **75**, 315–326.

Bhuyan, U. N. & Ramalingaswami, V. (1974b) Systemic macrophage mobilization and granulomatous response to BCG in the protein deficient rabbit. *American Journal of Pathology*, **76**, 313–320.

Braun, W. & Ungar, J. (1973) *Non-specific Factors Influencing Host Resistance.* Basel: Kargel.

Bullen, J. J., Rogers, H. & Leigh, L. (1972) Iron-binding proteins in milk and resistance to *Escherichia coli* infection in infants. *British Medical Journal*, **i**, 69–72.

Burnet, F. M. (1968) Measles as an index of immunological function. *Lancet*, **ii**, 610–613.

Chandra, R. K. (1972) Immunocompetence in undernutrition. *Journal of Pediatrics*, **81**, 1194–1200.

Chandra, R. K. (1973) Reduced bactericidal capacity of polymorphs in iron deficiency. *Archives of Diseases of Childhood*, **48**, 864–866.

Chandra, R. K. (1974a) Rosette-forming T lymphocytes and cell-mediated immunity in malnutrition. *British Medical Journal*, **iii**, 608–609.

Chandra, R. K. (1974b) Immunocompetence in low-birth-weight infants after intrauterine malnutrition. *Lancet*, **ii**, 1393–1394.

Chandra, R. K. (1975a) Reduced secretory antibody response to live attenuated measles and poliovirus vaccines in malnourished children. *British Medical Journal*, **ii**, 583–585.

Chandra, R. K. (1975b) Serum complement and immunoconglutinin in malnutrition. *Archives of Diseases of Childhood*, **50**, 225–229.

Chandra, R. K. (1975c) In *Maternofetal Transmission of Immunoglobulins*, ed. Hemmings, W. A., pp. 77–90. Cambridge University Press.

Chandra, R. K. (1975d) Antibody formation in first and second generation offspring of nutritionally deprived rats. *Science*, **189**, 289–290.

Chandra, R. K. (1977) In *Malnutrition and the Immune Response*, ed. Suskind, R. M., from Kroc Foundation Series Vol. 7, pp. 111–116, 155–168. New York: Raven Press.

Cooper, M. D., Faulk, W. Page, Fudenberg, H. H., Good, R. A., Hitzig, W., Kunkel, H. G., Rosen, F. S., Seligmann, M., Soothill, J. & Wedgewood, R. J. (1974) Primary immunodeficiency diseases in man. *Clinical Immunology and Immunopathology*, **2**, 416–445.

Cooper, W. C., Good, R. A. & Mariani, T. (1974) Effects of protein insufficiency on immune responsiveness. *American Journal of Clinical Nutrition*, **27**, 647–664.

Coovadia, H. M. & Soothill, J. F. (1976a) The effect of protein restricted diets on the clearance of ^{125}I-labelled polyvinyl pyrrolidone in mice. *Clinical and Experimental Immunology*, **23**, 373–377.

Coovadia, H. M. & Soothill, J. F. (1976b) The effect of amino acid restricted diets on the clearance of ^{125}I-labelled polyvinyl pyrrolidone in mice. *Clinical and Experimental Immunology*, **23**, 562–567.

Douglas, S. D. & Schopfer, K. (1974) Phagocyte function in protein-calorie malnutrition. *Clinical and Experimental Immunology*, **17**, 121–128.

Douglas, S. D. & Schopfer, K. (1976) Host defense mechanisms in protein-energy malnutrition. *Clinical Immunology and Immunopathology*, **5**, 1–5.

Douglas, S. D. & Schopfer, K. (1977) In *Malnutrition and the Immune Response*, ed. Suskind, R. M., pp. 231–244. New York: Raven Press.

Edelman, R., Suskind, R. M., Olson, R. E. & Sirisinha, S. (1973) Mechanisms of defective delayed cutaneous hypersensitivity in children with protein-calorie malnutrition. *Lancet*, **i**, 506–509.

Edelman, R. (1977) In *Malnutrition and the Immune Response*, ed. Suskind, R. M., pp. 47–76. New York: Raven Press.

Editorial (1974) Iron and resistance to infection. *Lancet*, **i**, 325–326.

Elin, R. J. & Wolff, S. M. (1974) The role of iron in nonspecific resistance to infection induced by endotoxin. *Journal of Immunology*, **112**, 737–742.

Faulk, W. P., Demaeyer, E. M. & Davis, A. J. S. (1974) Some effects of malnutrition on the immune response in man. *American Journal of Clinical Nutrition*, **27**, 638–646.

Faulk, W. Page, Mata, L. J. & Edsall, G. (1975) The effects of malnutrition on the immune response in humans: a review. *Tropical Diseases Bulletin*, **72**, 89–103.

Faulk, W. Page (1974) Nutrition and immunity. *Nature*, **250**, 283–284.

Faulk, W. Page & Johnson, P. M. (1976) Immunological studies of human placentae: proteins of mature chorionic villi. *Clinical and Experimental Immunology* **27**, 365–375.

Faulk, W. Page, Pinto Paes, R., Marigo, C. & Verrier-Jones, J. (1976) The immunological system in health and malnutrition. *Proceedings of the Nutrition Society*, **35**, 253–261.

Faulk, W. Page & Chandra, R. K. (1976) Nutrition and resistance to infection. *CRC Handbook of Food and Nutrition*. Cleveland: CRC Press (in press).

Ferguson, A. C., Lawlor, G. J., Neumann, C. G., Oi, W. & Stiehm, E. R. (1974) Decreased rosette-forming lymphocytes in malnutrition and intrauterine growth retardation. *Journal of Pediatrics*, **85**, 717–723.

Fernandes, G., Yunis, E. J. & Good, R. A. (1976a) Influence of protein restriction on immune functions in NZB mice. *Journal of Immunology*, **116**, 782–790.

Fernandes, G., Yunis, E. J. & Good, R. A. (1976b) Influence of diet on survival of mice. *Proceedings of the National Academy of Sciences, U.S.A.*, **73**, 1279–1283.

Freyre, E. A., Chabes, A., Poemape, O. & Chabes, A. (1973) Abnormal Rebuck skin window response in kwashiorkor. *Journal of Pediatrics*, **82**, 523–526.

Gardner, L. I. & Amacher, P. (1973) *Endocrine Aspects of Malnutrition*. Santa Ynez, California: Kroc Foundation.

Gebhardt, B. M. & Newberne, P. M. (1974) Nutrition and immunological responsiveness. T cell function in the offspring of lypotrope and protein deficient rats. *Immunology*, **26**, 489–495.

Geefhuysen, J., Rosen, E. U., Katz, J., Ipp, T. & Metz, J. (1971) Impaired cellular immunity in kwashiorkor with improvement after therapy. *British Medical Journal*, **iv**, 527–529.

Goldman, A. S. & Smith, C. W. (1973) Host resistance factors in human milk. *Journal of Pediatrics*, **82**, 1082–1090.

Good, R. A., Finstad, J. & Gatti, R. A. (1970) In *Infectious Agents and Host Resistance*, ed. Mudd, S. pp. 76–114. Philadelphia: Saunders.

Good, R. A., Jose, D., Cooper, W. C., Fernandes, G., Kramer, T. & Yunis, E. (1977) The influence of nutrition on antibody production and cellular immune responses in man, rats, mice and guinea-pigs. In *Proceedings of the Kroc Foundation Conference on Malnutrition and Immunity*, ed. Suskind, R. M., pp. 169–184. New York: Raven Press.

Grace, H. J., Armstrong, D. & Smythe, P. M. (1972) Reduced lymphocyte transformation in protein calorie malnutrition. *South African Medical Journal*, **46**, 402–403.

Harland, P. S. (1965) Tuberculin reactions in malnourished children. *Lancet*, **ii**, 719–721.

Heyworth, B., Moore, D. L. & Brown, J. (1975) Depression of lymphocyte response to phytohemagglutinin in the presence of plasma from children with acute protein energy malnutrition. *Clinical and Experimental Immunology*, **22**, 72–77.

Jorin, M. & Tannock, I. F. (1972) Influence of vitamin A on immunological response. *Immunology*, **23**, 283–287.

Jose, D. & Good, R. A. (1973a) Quantitative effects of nutritional protein and calorie deficiency upon immune responses to tumors in mice. *Cancer Research*, **33**, 807–809.

Jose, D. G. & Good, R. A. (1973b) Quantitative effects of nutritional essential amino acid deficiency upon immune responses to tumors in mice. *Journal of Experimental Medicine*, **137**, 1–9.

Jose, D. G., Stutman, O. & Good, R. A. (1973) Long term effects on immune function of early nutritional deprivation. *Nature (London)*, **241**, 57.

Jose, D. G., Shelton, M., Tauro, G. P., Belbin, R. & Hosking, C. S. (1975) Deficiency of immunological and phagocytic function in aboriginal children with protein-calorie malnutrition. *Medical Journal of Australia*, **62**, 699–705.

Keet, M. P. & Thom, H. (1969) Serum immunoglobulins in kwashiorkor. *Archives of Diseases of Childhood*, **44**, 600–603.

Kendall, A. C. & Nolan, R. (1972) Polymorphonuclear leucocytic activity in malnourished children. *Central African Journal of Medicine*, **18**, 73–76.

Klebanoff, S. J. & Green, W. L. (1973) Degradation of thyroid hormones by phagocytosing human leucocytes. *Journal of Clinical Investigation*, **52**, 60–72.

Klebanoff, S. J. (1975) Antimicrobial mechanisms in neutrophilic polymorphonuclear leucocytes. *Seminars in Hematology*, **12**, 117–142.

Krishnan, S., Bhuyan, U. N., Talwar, G. P. & Ramalingaswami, V. (1974) Effect of vitamin A and protein-calorie undernutrition on immune responses. *Immunology*, **27**, 383–392.

Law, D. K., Dudrick, S. J. & Abdov, N. I. (1973) Immunocompetence of patients with protein-calorie malnutrition. *Annals of Internal Medicine*, **79**, 545.

Lechtig, A., Arroyave, G., Viteri, F. & Mata, L. J. (1970) Serum immunoglobulins in protein-calorie malnutrition in pre-school children. *Archives Latinam Nutrition*, **20**, 321–332.

MacDougall, L. G., Anderson, R., McNab, G. M. & Katz, J. (1975) The immune response in iron-deficient children: impaired cellular defense mechanisms with altered humoral components. *Journal of Pediatrics*, **86**, 833–847.

Mata, L. J. & Urrutia, J. J. (1971) Intestinal colonization of breast-fed children in a rural area of low socioeconomic level. *Annals of the New York Academy of Sciences*, **175**, 93–109.

Mata, L. J. & Wyatt, R. G. (1971) Host resistance to infection. *American Journal of Clinical Nutrition*, **24**, 976–986.

Mata, L. & Faulk, W. P. (1973) The immune response of malnourished subjects with special reference to measles. *Archives Latinam Nutrition*, **23**, 345–362.

Mathews, J. D., Whittingham, S., Mackay, I. R. et al (1972) Protein supplementation and enhanced antibody-producing capacity in New Guinean children. *Lancet*, **ii**, 675–677.

Mathews, J. D., Mackay, I. R., Tucker, L. & Malcolm, L. A. (1974) Interrelationships between dietary protein, immunoglobulin levels, humoral immune responses and growth in New Guinean school children. *American Journal of Clinical Nutrition*, **27**, 908–915.

McCall, C. E., Katayama, I., Cotran, R. S. & Finland, M. (1969) Lysosomal and ultrastructural changes in human 'toxic' neutrophils during bacterial infection. *Journal of Experimental Medicine*, **129**, 267–293.

McFarlane, H., Reddy, S., Adock, K. J., Adeshina, H., Cooke, A. R. & Akene, J. (1970) Immunity, transferrin, and survival in kwashiorkor. *British Medical Journal*, **iv**, 268–271.

Moore, D. L., Heyworth, B. & Brown, J. (1974) PHA-induced lymphocytic transformation in leucocyte cultures from malarious malnourished and control Gambian children. *Clinical and Experimental Immunology*, **17**, 651.

Morgan, A. G. & Soothill, J. F. (1975a) Measurement of the clearance function of macrophages with ^{125}I-labelled polyvinyl pyrrolidone. *Clinical and Experimental Immunology*, **20**, 489.

Morgan, A. G. & Soothill, J. F. (1975b) The relationship between macrophage clearance of PVP and affinity of anti-protein antibody response in inbred mouse strains. *Nature (London)*, **254**, 711–712.

Morley, D. (1969) Severe measles in the tropics. *British Medical Journal*, **i**, 297–300.

Mugerwa, J. W. (1971) The lymphoreticular system in kwashiorkor. *Journal of Pathology*, **105**, 105–109.

Neumann, C. G., Lawlor, G. J., Stiehm, E. R., Swedseid, M. E., Newton, C., Herbert, J., Ammann, A. J. & Jacob, M. (1975) Immunologic responses in malnourished children. *American Journal of Clinical Nutrition*, **28**, 89–99.

Passwell, J. H., Steward, M. W. & Soothill, J. F. (1974) The effects of protein malnutrition on macrophage function and the amount and affinity of antibody response. *Clinical and Experimental Immunology*, **17**, 491–495.

Papadatos, L., Papaevangelou, G. L., Alexiou, D. & Mendris, J. (1970) Serum immunoglobulin G levels in small-for-dates newborn babies. *Archives of Diseases of Childhood*, **45**, 570.

Rao, K. S. J., Svikantia, S. G. & Gopalan, C. (1968) Plasma cortisol levels in protein-calorie malnutrition. *Archives of Diseases of Childhood*, **43**, 365–368.

Rosen, E. U., Geefhuysen, J. & Ipp, I. (1971) Immunoglobulin levels in protein calorie malnutrition. *South African Medical Journal*, **45**, 980.

Rosen, E. U., Geefhuysen, J., Anderson, R., Joffe, M. & Rabson, A. R. (1975) Leucocyte function in children with kwashiorkor. *Archives of Diseases of Childhood*, **50**, 220–224.

Rous, P. (1911) A sarcoma of fowl transmissible by an agent separable from the tumor cells. *Journal of Experimental Medicine*, **13**, 397.

Schonland, M. (1972) Depression of immunity in protein-calorie malnutrition: a post-mortem study. *Journal of Tropical Pediatrics*, **18**, 217–224.

Schopfer, K. & Douglas, S. D. (1976a) In vitro studies of lymphocytes from children with kwashiorkor. *Clinical Immunology and Immunopathology*, **5**, 21–30.

Schopfer, K. & Douglas, S. D. (1976b) Fine structural studies of peripheral blood leucocytes from children with kwashiorkor: morphological and functional properties. *British Journal of Haematology*, **32**, 569–573.

Schopfer, K. & Douglas, S. D. (1976c) Neutrophil function in children with kwashiorkor. *Journal of Laboratory and Clinical Medicine* **88**, 450–461.

Scrimshaw, N. S. (1976) Shattuck Lecture—Strengths and weaknesses of the committee approach. An analysis of past and present recommended dietary allowances for protein in health and disease. *New England Journal of Medicine*, **294**, 136–142, 198–203.

Scrimshaw, N. S., Taylor, C. E. & Gordon, J. E. (1968) Interactions of nutrition and infection. *World Health Organisation*, Monograph Series 57.

Sellmeyer, E., Bhettay, E., Truswell, H. S., Meyers, O. L. & Hansen, J. D. L. (1972) Lymphocyte transformation in malnourished children. *Archives of Diseases of Childhood*, **47**, 429–435.

Selvaraj, R. J. & Bhat, K. S. (1972) Metabolic and bactericidal activities of leukocytes in protein-calorie malnutrition. *American Journal of Clinical Nutrition*, **25**, 166–174.

Seth, V. & Chandra, R. K. (1972) Opsonic activity, phagocytosis, and bactericidal capacity of polymorphs in undernutrition. *Archives of Diseases of Childhood*, **47**, 282–284.

Shousha, S. & Kamel, K. (1972) Nitroblue tetrazolium test in children with kwashiorkor with a comment on the use of latex particles in the test. *Journal of Clinical Pathology*, **25**, 494–497.

Sinclair, J. C. (1972) In *Pediatrics*, ed. Barnett, H. L. & Einhorn, A. H., pp. 88–116. New York: Appleton-Century-Crofts.

Sirisinha, S., Edelman, R., Suskind, R., Charupatana, C. & Olsen, R. E. (1973) Complement and C3-proactivator levels in children with protein-calorie malnutrition and effect of dietary therapy. *Lancet*, **i**, 1016–1020.

Sirisinha, S., Suskind, R., Edelman, R., Asvapaka, C. & Olsen, R. E. (1975) Secretory and serum IgA in children with protein-calorie malnutrition. *Pediatrics*, **55**, 166–169.

Smythe, P. M., Brereton-Stiles, G. G., Grace, H. J., Mafoyane, A., Schonland, M., Coovadia, H. M., Loening, W. E. K., Parent, M. A. & Vos, G. H. (1971) Thymolymphatic deficiency and depression of cell-mediated immunity in protein-calorie malnutrition. *Lancet*, **ii**, 939–943.

Soothill, J. F. & Steward, M. W. (1971) The immunopathological significance of the heterogeneity of antibody affinity. *Clinical and Experimental Immunology*, **9**, 193–199.

Taneja, P. N. (1968) Measles and malnutrition. *Nutrition Reviews*, **26**, 232–234.

Tanphaichitr, P., Mekanandha, V. & Valyasevi, A. (1973) Impaired plasma opsonic activity in malnourished children. *Journal of the Medical Association of Thailand*, **56,** 118–124.

Tejada, C., Argueta, V., Sanchez, M. & Albertazzi, C. (1964) Phagocytic and alkaline phosphatase activity of leukocytes in kwashiorkor. *Journal of Pediatrics*, **64,** 753–761.

Walker, A. M., Garcia, R., Pate, P., Mata, L. J. & David, J. R. (1975) Transfer factor in the immune deficiency of protein calorie malnutrition. A controlled study with 32 cases. *Cellular Immunology*, **15,** 372–381.

Waterlow, J. C. & Alleyne, G. A. O. (1971) Protein malnutrition in children: advances in knowledge in the last ten years. *Advances in Protein Chemistry*, **25,** 117–241.

Waterlow, J. C. (1972) Classification and definition of protein-calorie malnutrition. *British Medical Journal*, **iii,** 566–569.

Watson, C. E. & Freesemann, C. (1970) Immunoglobulins in protein-calorie malnutrition. *Archives of Diseases of Childhood*, **45,** 282–284.

Watts, T. (1969) Thymus weights in malnourished children. *Journal of Tropical Pediatrics*, **15,** 155–158.

Weinberg, E. D. (1975) Nutritional immunity. Hosts attempt to withhold iron from microbial invaders. *Journal of American Medical Association*, **231,** 39–41.

Williams, C. D. (1933) A nutritional disease of childhood associated with a maize diet. *Archives of Diseases of Childhood*, **8,** 423–433.

Williams, C. D. (1935) Kwashiorkor. A nutritional disease of children associated with a maize diet. *Lancet*, **229,** 1151–1152.

Wolfsdorf, J. & Nolan, R. (1974) Leukocyte function in protein deficiency states. *South African Medical Journal*, **48,** 528–530.

Work, T. H., Ifekwunigwe, A., Jelliffe, D. B., Jelliffe, P. & Neumann, C. G. (1973) Tropical problems in nutrition. *Annals of Internal Medicine*, **79,** 701–711.

Ziegler, H. D. & Ziegler, P. B. (1975) Depression of tuberculin reaction in mild and moderate protein-calorie malnourished children following BCG vaccination. *Johns Hopkins Medical Journal*, **137,** 59–64.

3
AMYLOIDOSIS AND AMYLOID PROTEINS

C. Julian Rosenthal   Edward C. Franklin

Amyloid, an amorphous hyaline extracellular substance, was first noted in the seventeenth century by Bonet, who described white stones in an enormous spleen of a patient with a liver abscess (Schwartz, 1970). It was first recognised and described as a distinct material by Von Rokitansky (1846) in a 'lardaceous liver' and by Virchow (1854) in a 'sago spleen'. The substance which infiltrated these tissues was misnamed amyloid by Virchow because it resembled, after staining with iodine and sulphuric acid, the corpora amylacea of the brain, thought to contain a material similar to cellulose. Although Friedreich and Kekule in 1859 demonstrated that the systemic deposits of amyloid were proteinaceous in nature, the name of amyloid remained for this amorphous material. During the following decades, it was recognised primarily by its histochemical properties, but now it can be more precisely defined by its electron microscopic appearance, staining properties and biochemical characteristics.

On the basis of clinical observation, amyloid deposits were soon found to be widely distributed in many organs, more commonly: kidneys, liver, spleen, tongue and GI tract, etc. At times, amyloid deposits are found unassociated with any underlying pathological conditions. This form was defined as primary amyloidosis in some cases (Wilks, 1856), or as hereditary amyloidosis in few kindreds with either localised or systemic deposition of amyloid. However, more commonly, amyloidosis is seen in association with a large number of apparently unrelated disorders and is therefore classified as the 'secondary type'. The most common among these are: chronic infections such as osteomyelitis, syphilis (Masterson, 1965), bronchiectasis, tuberculosis (Auerbach and Stemmerman, 1944; Wald, 1955), pyelonephritis (Newman and Jacobson, 1953), chronically infected burns (Hoffman et al, 1963), malaria, leprosy (Shuttleworth and Ross, 1956), decubitus ulcers (Newman and Jacobson, 1953) and others.

Amyloidosis also frequently accompanies collagen diseases such as rheumatoid arthritis (Teilum and Lindahl, 1954), periarteritis nodosa, lupus erythematosus (Cohen, 1967), dermatomyositis (Gelderman, Levine and Arndt, 1962), scleroderma (Gardner, 1966), and chronic inflammatory diseases of the bowel such as ulcerative colitis (Moschowitz, 1936), regional enteritis (Cohen and Fishman, 1949), Whipple's disease (Sander, 1964) and a number of neoplastic and lymphoproliferative disorders, such as Hodgkin's disease (Wallace et al, 1950), and renal cell carcinoma (Penman and Thomson, 1972). Amyloidosis only rarely accompanies cases of non-Hodgkin's lymphoma, carcinoma of the rectum, oesophagus, submaxillary glands, cervix, uteri and lung (Kimball, 1961). Amyloid of a different type is found with high frequency in cases of multiple myeloma (10–14 per cent

This work is supported by USPHS Research Grants Nos. AM 01431, AM 02594, AM 05064, AG 00458 and the Helen and Michael Schaffer Fund.

of all cases) and other lymphoid and plasma cell neoplasms. This association has provided significant information regarding the pathogenesis of certain types of amyloidosis (Osserman, Takatsuki and Talal, 1964; Symmers, 1956). Localised amyloid deposits are sometimes seen in certain tumours (apudomas) resulting from the malignant proliferation of endocrine cells in the intestinal tract or in glands or tissues which are derived from the primitive digestive tube (Pearse, 1969), as well as in odontogenic tumours (Vickers, Dahlin and Gorlin, 1965).

Amyloid deposits, often clinically inapparent develop during the ageing process in many tissues. Starting with the original work and hypothesis of Divry (1927), several investigators have documented the presence of amyloid in senile plaques in the brains of individuals without evidence of chronic disorders and in the islets of Langerhans and seminal vesicles in the elderly (Schwartz, 1970). In addition, cardiac amyloidosis has been found in approximately 50 per cent of random autopsies of individuals older than 90 years (Pomerance, 1965). Similar deposits, which may play a role in causing senile degenerative lesions have been noted in several inbred strains of mice when allowed their natural life span (Thung, 1957). Amyloid infiltrations were found in the heart, capillaries, lymphatic spaces, as well as in salivary glands, myometrium fat tissues, spleen and testis. Similar observations were made by Dontenwill, Ranz and Mohr (1960) in hamsters.

Amyloid deposits were noticed to occur spontaneously in the vessels and interstitial connective tissues of various parenchymal or glandular organs of many mammalian species (especially in kidneys, liver and spleen). They were frequently reported in ducks (Jakob, 1960) with a frequency greater than 50 per cent in certain types as well as in horses, cattle and dogs and less frequently in cats, sheep and swine and many other animals. They appear to be rare in other species like goats and rats (for a complete list, see Jakob, 1971). In some species, the amyloid deposits were found only at specific sites (Matthias and Jakob, 1969; Hjarre, 1942; Hjarre and Nordlung, 1942).

As in human pathology, many of the cases of amyloidosis in mammals follow or accompany chronic infections (Jakob, 1971). However, the type that resembles spontaneous senile amyloidosis in man revealed a special predilection for certain inbred species (especially mice) and a characteristic distribution at certain specific sites, e.g. leptomeningeal vessels in canides, islets of Langerhans in felides. Primary amyloidosis was also found to occur, in rare occasions, in certain mammals (Jakob, 1970).

The recognition that amyloid deposition is not just an odd, aberrant pathologic phenomenon, but may reflect relatively common processes in human and mammalian pathology, soon attracted a significant number of investigators to the study of this disorder. Significant progress in elucidating the pathogenesis of amyloidosis, the nature of the amyloid deposits and their origin was slow until 1959 when electron microscopic studies demonstrated that amyloid, previously regarded as a structureless material, consisted of characteristic fibrils (Cohen and Calkins, 1959; Spiro, 1959). This observation was soon followed by the development of several methods of extraction and purification of the amyloid substance, which in turn led to the chemical characterisation of amyloid. The subsequent finding of several chemically distinguishable types of amyloid fibrils provided firm support for the previously suspected existence of several types of amyloidosis, hitherto defined only on the basis of their clinical features.

In spite of many striking advances, numerous questions remain. Most importantly, the obviously complex pathogenetic mechanisms have not yet been resolved. Furthermore, the relationship of the different protein components, their cellular origin, their precise biological function and factors regulating their synthesis remain to be elucidated. Since these uncertainties still preclude a definitive classification for this group of diseases based on a combination of the biochemical, clinical and pathogenetic features of the diseases, we will continue to discuss these disorders on the basis of their clinical and pathological features. Hopefully, it will soon be possible to extend the recently recognised correlation between the clinical and the biochemical features to all types of amyloidosis and to propose a more comprehensive and rational classification of this group of disorders.

This review, due to space limitations, will not attempt an exhaustive coverage of the field of amyloidosis, for which detailed documentation already exists (Cohen, 1967;

Table 3.1   Abbreviations

AA	= amyloid A protein
SAA	= serum amyloid A protein
L chain	= light chain
APUD	= amyloid related to endocrine organs
C1t	= C1t Subcomponent of the first component of complement
CRP	= C-reactive protein
EAC	= red cell coated with antibody and complement
C3	= third component of complement
RER	= rough endoplasmic reticulum
RES	= reticuloendothelial system

Nomenclature suggested at a meeting on amyloidosis, Helsinki, August 1974 (Wigelius and Pasternak, eds.) (in press).

Mandema et al, 1968; Franklin and Zucker-Franklin, 1972a) nor will it describe the various clinical and anatomopathological aspects of amyloidosis recently reviewed in great detail by Brandt, Cathcart and Cohen (1968), Barth et al (1969a) and Kyle and Bayrd (1975). Instead, we will attempt to first define the concept of amyloid in its various presentations, then to discuss in selective fashion current knowledge and in many instances recent and somewhat controversial aspects concerning the morphologic, histochemical, biochemical and immunological characteristics of amyloid, and ultimately try to summarise those facts from the field of human and experimental amyloidosis which may provide insight into factors likely to play a role in the genesis of amyloid and its precursors. Table 3.1 lists the abbreviations used throughout this chapter.

DEFINITION AND CLASSIFICATION OF AMYLOID

During more than a century of investigations into the nature of amyloid, various criteria have been used to define this substance. Initially Virchow (1854) defined amyloid by its macroscopic lardaceous appearance, its amorphous microscopic structure and its histochemical property of staining with iodine and sulphuric acid. Later staining with a variety of other dyes was used. Among them: alcian blue, crystal violet and toluidine blue, dimethylaminobenzaldehyde, trypan blue (Pearse, 1968), and the fluorescence inducers thioflavin S and T (Saeed and Fine, 1967). However, the best known and most widely used has been Congo red which stains amyloid red and gives green birefringence under polarising light (Bennhold, 1922), a characteristic that has been widely used in defining the amyloid substance. It is not surprising that this multitude of empirically derived histochemical tests has generated confusion in the interpretation of the data of various investigators. Thus Schwartz (1965) using thioflavine S fluorescence identified amyloid deposits in various tissues of aged persons with a much higher incidence than that anticipated by previous staining with Congo red. On the other side, Wolman (1971) using toluidine blue in a standardised procedure, did not recognise as amyloid, the fibrillar material found at autopsies in some 'senile' hearts.

In the last two decades, the characteristic fibrillar structure revealed by electron microscopy has been recognised as being common to all types of amyloid substances and is generally considered as characteristic of all forms of amyloidosis (Cohen, 1967). It has also been recognised that the green birefringence under polarising light of the Congo red stained fibrils was related to the antiparallel β-pleated sheet conformation of polypeptide chains making up the amyloid fibrils, as recognised by x-ray crystallographic and infrared spectroscopic analyses (Eanes and Glenner, 1968). Some of the other tinctorial characteristics such as the metachromasia observed with certain dyes and the staining with trypan blue probably represent reactions with associated acid mucopolysaccharides rather than the amyloid substance. Hence, while Congo red staining with green birefringence is, with few exceptions, specific and characteristic of amyloidosis and useful in making the diagnosis clinically, we agree with Glenner et al (1974), that amyloid has to be defined by at least three obligatory criteria:

1. Fibrillar structure detected by electron microscopy with characteristic non-branching linear fibrils of 8–15 nm width.
2. Staining with Congo red associated with green birefringence detected by a polarising microscope or antiparallel β-pleated sheet conformation detected by x-ray crystallography.
3. Destruction of the major protein component by treatment with pronase which leads to the disappearance of the fibrillar structure and the β-pleated sheet conformation. Based on currently available information (see below), it seems likely that a variety of proteins may fulfil these criteria and that amyloid will ultimately prove to be a generic term encompassing a heterogeneous group of substances.

Following all these criteria, fibrillar deposits found in the cerebral corpora amylacea, the concretions of the prostatic corpora amylacea, as well as those described intracellularly in the hearts of patients with several glycogen storage diseases, primarily composed of polysaccharide chains, will not be considered amyloid deposits, despite their Congo red birefringence (Glenner et al, 1974). Also, the deposits giving Congo red birefringence found in the neurofibrillary tangles of Alzheimer's disease should not be considered amyloid. In contrast, the intrafollicular deposits in the parathyroid follicles of some hyperparathyroid patients, the cerebral senile plaques (Terry, Gonatas and Weiss, 1964), the deposits found in the tumours of the APUD series, i.e. medullary carcinoma of the thyroid, insulinoma and pheochromocytoma, and the proteinaceous casts found occasionally in the proximal tubules of patients with myeloma without systemic amyloidosis (Derosena, Koss and Pirani, 1975), fulfil the above criteria (Pearse, Ewan and Polak, 1975; Glenner et al, 1974).

For many years attempts to classify amyloidosis have been made to facilitate the study of its clinical and pathological manifestations. Amyloidosis has been classified primarily on the basis of its clinical features, tissue distribution and associated diseases. While this is obviously not completely satisfactory, we feel that the available chemical information is not sufficient to propose a new and more rational classification at this time. Hence, in this section, we will suggest a classification still based on the above criteria and, when possible, will try to relate the several clinical types to the chemical nature of the amyloid substance (indicated in the last column of Table 3.2). It seems likely that shortly a rational classification based on the nature of the deposits and pathogenetic mechanisms will become feasible, and that this will, in many instances, correlate closely with the clinical features of the diseases.

To the four major categories introduced by Reimann, Kouchy and Eklund (1935), which have served as the basis of virtually all systems of classification, we can add for completeness three others of lower incidence, bringing the total to seven types of amyloid and amyloidosis (Table 3.2).

Table 3.2 Classification of amyloidosis related to the major protein component of its fibrils

	Pathological type	Protein component
1.	Primary amyloid	L (AA)
2.	Amyloid associated with neoplasms of plasma cells and lymphocytes	L (AA)
3.	Secondary amyloid (to infections, etc.)	AA
4.	Localised tumour-forming amyloid	?
5.	Endocrine tumor-associated amyloid	? peptide hormone[a]
6.	Senile amyloid	?
7.	Heredofamilial forms	?[b]

L = protein homologous with immunoglobulin light chains
AA = specific amyloid protein—may form a minor component in categories 1 and 2
[a] Only thyrocalcitonin has been chemically identified (Sletten et al 1976)
[b] Only one—that associated with FMF has been characterised as AA (Levin et al, 1972)

1. Primary amyloid occurring without antecedent or coexistent disease and involving primarily mesodermal tissues and the cardiovascular system.

2. Amyloid associated with neoplasms involving plasma cells or lymphocytes (e.g. multiple myeloma, macroglobulinaemia and heavy chain disease)—with distribution and characteristics similar to those of the primary amyloid.

3. Secondary amyloid associated with a variety of chronic inflammatory and neoplastic conditions already mentioned and involving primarily spleen, liver, kidneys, intestines and adrenals.

4. Tumour-forming (localised) amyloid, characterised by small masses deposited in the skin, eye, bladder, urethra, respiratory tract and generally unassociated with any underlying disease.

5. Amyloid produced in tumours, including those of the APUD series, usually not associated with systemic amyloidosis. This is in contrast to the amyloid associated with other neoplasms (e.g. seminoma, carcinoma of the rectum, Hodgkin's disease) which has a diffuse distribution and characteristics identical to those of secondary amyloid.

6. Senile amyloid found in meningocerebral vessels, brain substance (Divry, 1927), myocardium (Pomerance, 1965), pancreatic Langerhan's islets and seminal vesicles (Schwartz, 1965) in some elderly individuals without evidence of chronic disorders during life or at autopsy.

7. Amyloid found in heredofamilial disorders of extremely rare incidence. Most frequent among them are: the familial Mediterranean fever (FMF) with amyloidosis (Siegel, 1945), the familial amyloidosis with polyneuropathy (Portuguese type) (Andrade, 1952); the familial amyloidosis with polyneuropathy and abnormalities of the serum lipoproteins (Rukavina, Block and Curtis, 1956). Among the many other types which have been des-

cribed only in a few families around the globe are: familial amyloidosis with severe heart disease (Frederisksen et al, 1962); familial amyloidosis with urticaria, deafness and nephropathy (Muckle and Wells, 1962); familial cutaneous amyloidosis (Sagher and Shanon, 1963) and familial cutaneous amyloidosis and thyroid carcinoma. While the first listed type has autosomal recessive inheritance, the others have an autosomal dominant transmission (Heller, Gafni and Sohar, 1966).

A clinical classification recently proposed by Isobe and Osserman (1974), correlating the clinical pattern with the frequency of monoclonal proteins in serum and urine, does not, in our opinion, add sufficient new perspectives to the problem of the nature and origin of amyloid to warrant its use prior to the introduction of a more rational classification. In this classification, pattern I corresponds to the distribution of the primary amyloid and of the amyloid associated with other plasma cell dyscrasias; pattern II corresponds to the distribution of secondary amyloid while the mixed pattern includes all cases with atypical distribution.

For the sake of completeness, one should cite another classification, that of Missmahl and Hartwig (1953) based on the microscopic distribution of amyloid and the conversion to negative of its Congo red birefringence by phenol or glycerol. This distinguishes the perireticular form, which represents a generalised vascular disease with amyloid deposits starting at the basement membrane of the vessels and includes cases of secondary amyloidosis and FMF, from the pericollagenous type with deposition of amyloid first in the adventitia of various vessels as seen in most of the cases of primary amyloidosis and those associated with multiple myeloma and macroglobulinaemia. This classification is difficult to apply in practice and is not widely used at this time.

NATURE OF AMYLOID

In order to determine the nature of amyloid, attempts were first made to study amyloid morphologically in tissue sections and histochemically, using various dyes known to be characteristic for certain chemical components, as well as fluorescent antisera to a variety of serum proteins. This led to the detection of some serum components in the amyloid deposits. Of special interest, in view of the important role that immunologic factors are thought to play in the pathogenesis of amyloidosis, has been the finding of immunoglobulins and certain complement components in the amyloid deposits (Mellors and Ortega, 1956; Lachmann et al, 1962; Milgrom, Kasukawa and Calkins, 1966; Muckle, 1968; Vazquez and Dixon, 1956; Williams and Law, 1960, and others). This approach was soon supplemented by the electron microscopic studies of Cohen and Calkins (1959) and Spiro (1959). A more direct approach has been to try to extract, purify and solubilise the amyloid material from various tissues, and to subject the major constituents to morphological biochemical and immunological analyses. Both approaches have resulted in the identification of two structural components in all types of amyloid deposits. The major structure which makes up more than 90 per cent of the amyloid substance is the amyloid fibril (Shirahama and Cohen, 1967; Pras et al, 1968; Glenner et al, 1971a). These fibrils can be formed of several different protein constituents, but are indistinguishable ultrastructurally in different types of amyloid. A second minor component with the shape of a 'rod' or a 'doughnut' named the P component, has been identified only in partially purified fibril preparations, but was not found in the sections of tissues infiltrated with amyloid

(Bladen, Nylen and Glenner, 1966; Cathcart, Shirahama and Cohen, 1967b). The P component appears to represent a normal serum α_1-globulin, perhaps closely related to C-reactive protein (CRP), and Clt, a subfraction of the first component of complement (Painter, 1976; Osmond, 1976). Since none of the other serum components that have been identified in amyloid tissue sections can be detected after further purification, their specific deposition and their role in the formation of amyloid remains doubtful.

Isolation of Fibrils and P Component

Two methods are commonly employed in the purification of the amyloid fibrils. The method of Cohen and Calkins (1964) subjects the amyloid-laden tissue to homogenisation and maceration in physiologic saline. The homogenate is then centrifuged at 12 000 g for 30 min and the top layer, rich in amyloid fibrils, is subsequently subjected to repeated sucrose gradient centrifugation (Cohen, 1966) to obtain a relatively pure fibril preparation. The method of Pras et al (1968) is based on the observation that amyloid fibrils are insoluble in physiologic saline, but readily extractable as a colloidal suspension which behaves almost like a solution in distilled water. Consequently, the tissue is repeatedly homogenised in 0.15 M sodium chloride and centrifuged at about 9000 g for 30 min. The contaminating proteins including the P component are found in the supernatant from which the P component can then be isolated in several steps including: dialysis against water, lyophilisation, gel chromatography through a Sephadex G-200 superfine column in 0.1 M Tris buffer, pH 8.0, and stepwise elution through DEAE cellulose (Skinner et al, 1974b). The pellets resulting from the centrifugation of the homogenised tissue laden with amyloid fibrils are rehomogenised and recentrifuged until the O.D. of the supernatant at 280 nm is 0. The pellet is then repeatedly homogenised in distilled water and the resultant homogenate is centrifuged at 80 000 g for 1 h. After four or five such extractions, the opalescent supernatant contains 20 to 95 per cent of the amyloid fibrils present in the starting material depending on the tissue used. Further purification can be achieved by column chromatography on Sepharose or Sephadex in solvents containing guanidine with a reducing agent in order to dissociate non-covalently and disulphide bridged polymers (Glenner et al, 1969).

Morphologic and Structural Characteristics

The major morphologic and structural aspects of the amyloid deposits have been defined by electron microscopy and x-ray diffraction combined with infrared spectroscopy.

ELECTRON MICROSCOPIC STUDIES

When the isolated amyloid fibrils are embedded, sectioned and examined in the electron microscope after positive staining with lead and uranium salts (Cohen and Calkins, 1959; Spiro, 1959; Hjort and Christensen, 1961; Boere, Ruinen and Scholten, 1965; Sorenson and Bari, 1968; Zucker-Franklin, 1970, etc.), they appear identical to those in freshly fixed amyloid-laden tissues obtained on biopsy or at autopsy (Fig. 3.1), having a width of 10 to 15 nm. Their length cannot be determined because they criss-cross into and out of the plane of section. Most of them consist of two parallel, longitudinal subunits equal in width, separated by a space of approximately 2.5 nm. Irregularly shaped dots often with a translucent core, scattered among the fibrils probably represent tangential or cross-sections of the fibrils. Electron microscopy of 'soluble amyloid' fibrils, negatively stained, without prior fixation or embedding, very clearly defines the paired, longitudinal subunits

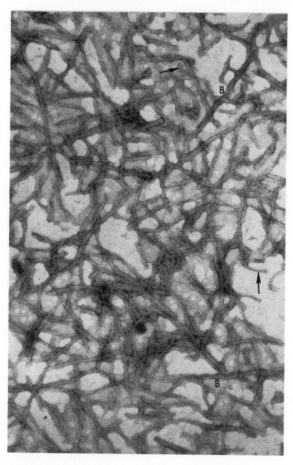

Figure 3.1   Isolated purified amyloid negatively stained with phosphotungstic acid. Arrows point to single filaments. Note that most filaments are paired and end together (half-circles). Some thicker bundles (B) in which filaments are twisting around each other can also be seen. × 62 500. (Franklin, E. C. and Zucker-Franklin, D., 1972a)

or filaments (Fig. 3.1) measuring 5 to 7.5 nm in diameter and separated by a clear space 4 nm wide. The fibrils are several millimicrons in length, often twist around their longitudinal axes (Franklin and Zucker-Franklin, 1972a), and have a beaded or helical sub-structure (Shirahama and Cohen, 1965) which appear to reflect the presence of longitudinal subunits or protofibrils measuring 2.5 to 3.5 nm in width, which in turn may be made up of even smaller subunits (Shirahama and Cohen, 1967). It is of interest that the 'soluble' fibrils, after salt precipitation form thicker bundles that cross and twist more frequently than after precipitation by ultracentrifugation, suggesting that salt promotes aggregation and/or polymerisation of the fibrils (Franklin and Zucker-Franklin, 1972a).

Amyloid fibrils with similar electron microscopic characteristics, including their arrangement in compact bundles and their radial orientation, have also been described in sections of tissues obtained at operation from five types of apudomas: phaeochromocytoma, medullary thyroid carcinoma, insulinoma, gastrin-producing tumours (Pearse et al, 1972) and pituitary adenoma (Schober and Nelson, 1975; Bilbao et al, 1975).

The P component was studied in the electron microscope only after negative staining and was never found in tissue sections (Franklin and Zucker-Franklin, 1972a), perhaps because it is extracted during the embedding procedure. The P component was recognised by EM as a pentagonally structured unit (from where its name was derived) with a diameter of 90 nm for each subunit which may aggregate laterally to form short rods (Bladen et al, 1966; Benditt and Eriksen, 1966).

X-RAY DIFFRACTION AND INFRARED SPECTROSCOPIC STUDIES

A second method, applied to the study of the physical structure of amyloid fibrils, was that of x-ray diffraction, associated frequently with infrared spectroscopy. Studies of human, mouse and duck amyloid by three different groups (Eanes and Glenner, 1968; Bonard, Cohen and Skinner, 1969; Shmueli et al, 1969) have yielded almost identical results, i.e. x-ray diffraction patterns showing a sharp meridional arc at about 0.47 nm and a more diffuse equatorial arc at 0.98 nm, which is characteristic of 'equatorial β' or 'normal β' configuration and distinguishes it from the 'cross β' or 'meridional β' configuration in which the equatorial arcing at 0.98 nm is missing. Within both configurations, various peptide chains can have a parallel or antiparallel direction, which means that their amino and carboxy terminal ends are all in register when parallel or in alternating register when antiparallel. If the association is within the same polypeptide chain, as is the case for amyloid, the β form by necessity must be antiparallel. This assumption has been shown to be correct by infrared spectroscopy (Glenner et al, 1974). The spectroscopic reading showed a shoulder at approximately 1695 cm^{-1} for the antiparallel configuration only, besides the peak at 1630 cm^{-1} which generally reflects the β configuration.

It is of interest that fibrils with the electron microscopic characteristics of amyloid fibrils can be prepared by proteolytic digestion of some Bence Jones proteins (Glenner et al, 1971c; Linke, Zucker-Franklin and Franklin, 1973; Shirahama et al, 1973), as well as by several physical treatments of insulin and glucagon (Waugh 1946; Burke and Rougvie, 1972; Glenner et al, 1973a, 1974), two polypeptide hormones produced by cells frequently associated with apudamyloid. However, the x-ray diffraction pattern of glucagon was that of a 'cross β' type with antiparallel disposition of the peptides, while that of insulin was of 'normal β' type with parallel distribution of the chains. Other synthetic fibrils constituted of poly-α-amino acids, especially poly-1-lysine and poly-1-serine (Davidson, Tooney and Fasman, 1966) have also a β-pleated sheet conformation on x-ray diffraction. All these synthetic fibrils bind Congo red and show green birefringence under polarising light, which suggests that these properties are directly related to their β-pleated sheet conformation and not to the more specific arrangement of their component peptides.

Histochemical Properties

Binding of alkaline Congo red by amyloid was recognised since 1922 (Benhold) and is widely used to detect this substance in various tissues. More recently, it has also been helpful in monitoring the purification of amyloid fibrils (Pras et al, 1968).

In 1965, Wolman and Bubis observed that Congo red augmented the natural birefringence of amyloid under polarising light, causing green birefringence. The Congophilia and green birefringence appeared to be characteristic for all β-pleated sheet fibrils (including insulin, glucagon) (Glenner et al, 1973b) while fibrin and elastin, which do not have β-pleated sheet conformation, do not give birefringence in polarising light although they are Congophilic (Kagan, Hewitt and Franzblau, 1973). Hence, staining with Congo red together with characteristic green birefringence are generally required to definitively identify amyloid in tissue.

The amyloid–Congo red reaction was found to be resistant to various ionic and end-group modifying procedures (e.g. acetylation, dinitrophenylation, nitrosation, and methylation) (Cooper, 1974), but was abolished after brief treatment with concentrated HCl. It appears likely that the dye molecules are regularly oriented with their long axes parallel to that of the fibrils and that the binding of the dye is affected by non-specific close range forces (Cooper, 1974), perhaps hydrophobic interactions, and is dependent on the β-pleated sheet conformation. The fact that Congo red staining does not change the infrared spectrum of amyloid fibrils (Glenner et al, 1974) suggests that the dye does not form an inclusion compound with the amyloid fibrils.

Using a new method, phase modulation microspectrophotometry, Taylor, Allen and Benditt (1974) explained the green birefringence under polarising light of the Congo red stained amyloid fibrils by a combination of optical effects, the strongest of which are the dispersion of birefringence and linear dichroism superimposed on the smaller effects of circular dichroism and optical rotatory dispersion.

Another histochemical characteristic of amyloid, the red birefringence noted with toluidine blue under polarising light can be explained by a mechanism similar to that of Congo red binding and birefringence (Wolman, 1971), and has been called 'para' or 'orthochromasia'.

Toluidine blue, crystal violet and trypan blue, when added to amyloid cause a shift in the absorption peak from about 600 to 550 μm measured by spectrophotometry (Pras and Schubert, 1968). This histochemical property called metachromasia is associated with yellow birefringence under polarising light and can be abolished by prior methylation of the stained material or by saturation of the dye solution with salt. This suggests electrostatic binding of dye cations to tissue polyanions. The relevant polyanions in amyloid, like heparitin sulphate (Bitter and Muir, 1966; Mowry and Scott, 1967) and certain other sulphated glycosaminoglycans (Cooper, 1974), are probably not an integral part of the fibril protein, but rather attached to it and easily extracted from it (Pras et al, 1971).

Another well-known histochemical property of amyloid, that of giving a blue colour as well as green birefringence under polarising light after treatment with iodine, appears to be primarily determined by the conformational aspects of the glycoprotein constituents of the deposits which may constitute an interfilamentous matrix between the fibrils (Wolman, 1971).

The above-mentioned histochemical and crystallographic studies indicate that the macromolecular structure of amyloid fibrils may be similar to that of a helix, as previously suggested by Cooper (1974) and support the model proposed by Emerson, Kikkawa and Gueft (1966) that twin fibrils form a double helix with 100 nm periodicity surrounding a central space of about 2 nm in diameter. An electron microscopic analysis of negatively stained amyloid fibrils (Cohen and Shirahama, 1973) has revealed the helical intertwining of filaments. The twisting of the faces of the pleated sheet suggested by the x-ray diffraction studies widens the spaces between the longitudinal rows of residues on one face of the pleated sheet and permits Congo red, toluidine blue or other planar dye molecules to fit edgewise into the grooves of this face of the sheet, and to bind it by close range forces (Cooper, 1974). Iodine instead, probably binds the mucopolysaccharides in the central hollow. These, according to Wolman (1971), may also exist as snake-like wires which twist through and surround the fibrils.

Physicochemical and Biochemical Properties

Physicochemical characteristics of amyloid fibrils

Among the properties of amyloid, its solubility characteristics are of special interest. Pras et al (1968) found that amyloid fibrils polymerise and precipitate in the presence of salt, proportionally to its concentration. This ultimately led to their isolation.

The isoelectric point of these proteins was found between 4.5 and 5 (Carnes and Forbes, 1956; Goldberg and Deane, 1960) while their electric charge appeared to be negative (Pras et al, 1968). Their exact electrophoretic mobility was not obtainable due to their precipitation in salt. For the same reason it was difficult to determine by ultracentrifugation the sedimentation coefficients of amyloid preparations. When examined shortly after extraction they were homogeneous and had a major component with a 45S sedimentation coefficient. After prolonged standing, 75S polymers appeared and rapidly began to precipitate spontaneously. A few preparations contained 8 to 15S components (Pras et al, 1968).

In order to obtain soluble subunits of amyloid protein, the effect of alkali on extracted amyloid was studied (Newcombe and Cohen, 1964). Ultimately, small 1 to 2S subunits soluble in 0.15 M-NaCl were obtained after their degradation in 0.1 M-NaOH (Pras et al, 1968). These were called degraded amyloid proteins (DAM).

The use of reducing agents together with 6 to 8 M urea or guanidine combined with Sephadex separation offered the best dissociative procedure for the isolation of pure subunits. The use of proteolytic enzymes like papain and pepsin did not succeed in splitting the amyloid fibrils (Sorenson and Binington, 1964; Ruinen et al, 1968) perhaps due to their antiparallel β-pleated sheet conformation. Trypsin was able to split these fibrils only in small pairs of trypsin-resistant filaments. Only pronase can degrade them completely. The fibrils degraded by alkali are more susceptible to proteolysis.

Specific amyloid components

THE IMMUNOGLOBULIN RELATED COMPONENT

Although immunoglobulins and complement were identified in tissue sections by immunofluorescence (Mellors and Ortega, 1956; Lachman et al, 1969; Vazquez and Dixon, 1956) initial attempts to determine the chemical nature of purified amyloid fibrils using specific antibodies, did not recognise human gammaglobulins or their components as integral parts of the fibrils (Paul and Cohen, 1963; Cathcart and Cohen, 1966). However, using chemical dissociative techniques previously mentioned, Glenner and collaborators demonstrated that the major constituent subunits of certain amyloid fibrils, especially those of primary or myeloma associated type, had structural homologies to the variable region of immunoglobulin light chains (Glenner et al, 1970, 1971a, b, c; Skinner and Cohen, 1971). This was indicated by finding pyrrolidone carboxilic acid (PCA), Asp or Glu as the most common amino terminal residues, as well as by the N-terminal amino acid sequence obtained from amyloid protein subunits with unblocked N-termini. These proteins showed a striking homology with the first 30 residues of the variable region of a κ light chain. Studies of many other such proteins confirmed their structural identity with parts of κ light chains of variable size and in some cases with that of the whole light chain (Glenner, Ein and Terry, 1972) or even with light chain polymers (Glenner et al, 1973b). Similar structural homologies were found for other subunits with the λ light chains (Kimura et al, 1972; White et al, 1975). These were more difficult to establish due to the blocked N-terminus of the λ light chain. It should be noted that for reasons that remain obscure, λ-related proteins occur in patients with amyloidosis with an unexpectedly higher frequency than in patients with myeloma. The κ/λ ratio is about $3:2$ among myeloma cases and $3:5$ among patients with amyloidosis (Glenner et al, 1973b).

Finally, in support of the findings indicating that some amyloid fibrils can be exclusively constituted of light chain fragments containing the variable region, was the demonstration by Glenner et al (1971c) and Linke et al (1973) that fibrils with histochemical electron microscopic and x-ray diffraction characteristics of amyloid can be produced by digestion of some Bence Jones proteins with trypsin or pepsin. In light of the difficulty of demonstrating L chain determinants in amyloid, it is notable that in the synthetic amyloid fibrils, the antigenic properties of the native Bence Jones protein were also lost. In a more physiologic manner Tan and Epstein (1972) demonstrated that similar fibrils can be produced from certain light chains by the action of naturally occurring lysosomal enzymes from the kidney, a mechanism that may be important in the formation of amyloid in vivo. Of interest also is the recent report (Pruzanski, Katz and Nyburg, 1974) of the in vitro production of an amyloid-like substance from a heavy chain protein. Except for one case of amyloidosis associated with epidermolysis bullosa and tuberculosis, all the other cases in which the predominant protein was found to be homologous to a light chain, had primary amyloidosis or amyloidosis associated with multiple myeloma or macroglobulinaemia (Glenner et al, 1973b).

AMYLOID A PROTEIN (AA)

In studies carried out mainly on amyloid preparations obtained from patients with secondary amyloidosis and with amyloidosis associated with familial Mediterranean fever (FMF), Benditt et al (1962, 1964, 1966, 1968) accumulated evidence for the existence of another type of low molecular weight subunit extractable from amyloid tissue with acid and urea, which were defined as amyloid A protein. Benditt and Eriksen (1971a) found that the amino acid analysis of three of these subunits with a MW of approximately 7000 daltons, was strikingly different from that of the variable region of immunoglobulins, lacking cysteine and threonine and having very little proline. This was later confirmed (Benditt and Eriksen, 1971b) by the lack of homology to any known immunoglobulin of the amino acid sequence of the first 24 residues of two amyloid A proteins, one of which was from a patient with amyloid associated with tuberculosis. The same unique amyloid A proteins were found in the amyloid extracted from tissues of patients with various other chronic diseases such as juvenile rheumatoid arthritis, ulcerative colitis, bronchiectasis, etc. (Benditt and Eriksen, 1971a). A similar protein was noted but not further defined by Glenner et al (1970) in a preparation from a patient with secondary amyloidosis. In an independent study, Pras and Reshef (1972) extracted a homogeneous protein of approximately 8000 daltons MW, using 0.02 M-HCl. This acid-soluble, water-insoluble component was found in amyloid fibrils from patients with FMF, and other chronic diseases (in which it constituted up to 60 per cent of their weight. It could be reconstituted into a fibrillar shape with vermiform fibrils, 35 to 45 nm thick, which did not resemble the EM ultrastructure of the native amyloid fibrils (Franklin and Zucker-Franklin, 1972a). When the complete amino acid sequence of the A protein was obtained from a patient with FMF (Franklin et al, 1972; Levin et al, 1972), the A protein was shown to be a hitherto un-described polypeptide chain of 76 amino acid residues, without cysteine and without any homology to any immunoglobulin chain (Fig. 3.2). A similar sequence with several differences in the carboxy terminal half was obtained from a patient with rheumatoid arthritis and amyloidosis by another group (Sletten and Husby, 1974), and additional

1
Arg-Ser-Phe-Phe-Ser-Phe-Leu-Gly-Glu-Ala-Phe-Asp-Gly-Ala-Arg-Asp-Met-Trp-Arg

Ala-Tyr-Ser-Asp-Met-Arg-Glu-Ala-Asn-Tyr-Ile-Gly-Ser-Asp-Lys-Tyr-Phe-His-Ala

Trp*
Arg-Gly-Asn-Tyr-Asp-Ala-Ala-Lys-Arg-Gly-Pro-Gly-Gly-Ala-Arg-Ala-Ala-Ala-Glu-Val

76
Ile-Ser-Asn-Ala-Arg-Glu-Asn-Ile-Gln-Arg-Leu-Thr-Gly-Arg-Gly-Ala-Glu-Asp-Ser

Figure 3.2 The complete amino acid sequence of amyloid A protein from a patient with familial Mediterranean fever. *The automatic sequencer yielded tryptophan in position 53 while the cor-responding tryptic peptide contained arginine in this position. This discrepancy could not be re-solved due to lack of material (Levin et al, 1972)

partial amino acid sequence analyses of various amyloid fibrillar proteins isolated from patients with secondary amyloidosis associated with various disorders (Franklin et al, 1972; Levin et al, 1972; Ein et al, 1972b) have presented striking homologies towards the N-terminal end. However, it should be noted that the amino terminus of all of these proteins presented some heterogeneity with arginine or serine as the first residue, a feature which raised the possibility that the AA protein might be the product of proteolytic digestion of a larger molecule.

It is not yet certain whether the fibrils consisting mainly of the amyloid A protein also contain light chains. While some of the peptides noted in their peptide maps bore some similarities to those characteristic of light chains of immunoglobulins (Levin et al, 1972) direct evidence for the presence of small amounts of light chain related material was obtained only for three preparations (Levin et al, 1972; Westermark et al, 1976).

Attempts to extract the amyloid A protein from patients with macroglobulinaemia and multiple myeloma were unsuccessful in our hands (Franklin and Rosenthal, 1974) and those of Glenner et al (1973b) but AA was identified in several preparations by Husby et al (1973c). It appears likely that the fibrillar amyloid proteins from most patients with plasma cell disorders, are exclusively constituted of light chain related peptides, but the possibility that some may contain a small amount of A-related peptides cannot yet be excluded.

The sequence of the amyloid fibril proteins from a monkey with amyloidosis and chronic granulomatous disease (Hermodson et al, 1972), from ducks with amyloidosis (Eriksen, Fowler and Ericsson, 1974; Pras et al, 1977) as well as that of the fibrillar amy-loid proteins from guinea-pigs and mice (Skinner et al 1974a; Eriksen et al, 1976) have also shown numerous similarities to the human AA protein.

HORMONE RELATED AMYLOID

While much has been learned about the nature of these two types of amyloid, less is known about the amyloid associated with tumours of a number of endocrine cells secreting peptide hormones. This material has been referred to as apudamyloid because it contains fluorogenic amines (A), retains the amine precursors (precursor uptake PU); and contains amino acid decarboxylase (D) (Pearse, 1969). APUD amyloid has been most clearly defined in association with medullary carcinoma of the thyroid (Hazard, Hawk and Crile, 1959), and insulin, glucagon and gastrin producing tumours of the pancreas (Porta, Yerry and Scott, 1962), but it seems possible that similar deposits may be seen with carotid body tumours (Capella and Solcia, 1971) phaeochromocytomas (Paloyan et al, 1970), bronchial carcinoids (Sterba, 1968) and pituitary adenomas (Pearse, 1969). Using histochemical techniques, Pearse et al (1972) concluded that apudamyloid fibrils from pancreas are probably constituted of peptides of the C chain of the insulin prohormone which lacks tyrosine and tryptophan. This last amino acid was thought to be absent due to the lack of yellowish autofluorescence of the apudamyloid fibrils under quartz iodine illumination, which is known to result from the oxidation of some of the tryptophan residues to N'-formylkynurenine.

However, in a recent study Westermark (1974) found that tyrosine was present in the apudamyloid fibrils from a β-cell pancreatic insulinoma as indicated by the positive diazotisation-coupling reaction for tyrosine. Glenner et al (1974) proved that the fibrils obtained from insulin at a low pH have identical histochemical and electron microscopic properties as the fibrils containing the variable region of light chains, obtained after the proteolytic degestion of Bence Jones proteins, even if they are not as straight or 'rigid' as the native amyloid fibrils on EM pictures. Westermark (1974) also found that antibodies against insulin reacted with the degraded (alkali-treated) apudamyloid fibrils. All these data led to the conclusion that fibrillar apudamyloid proteins of insulinomas might be made up of part of the insulin molecule which has retained the antigenic properties of insulin but not its biologic activity.

Significant progress has been made recently in defining the amyloid deposits associated with medullary carcinoma of the thyroid. Using immunofluorescence, Tashjian, Wolfe and Voelkel (1974) showed that these deposits stained with fluorescent antisera to thyrocalcitonin; Sletten et al (1976) were able to isolate these fibrils and establish sequence homologies with this hormone. Based on the molecular weight of the subunit which was larger than that of the hormone, they postulated that the amyloid fibrils may be derived from the prohormone.

Further support favouring a possible role for fragments of peptide hormones in the genesis of the various types of apudamyloid is provided by the conversion of insulin (Waugh, 1946; Burke and Rougvie, 1972; Glenner et al, 1973a, 1974) and glucagon into characteristic β-pleated sheet fibrils by treatment with acid and proteolytic enzymes.

CARBOHYDRATE CONSTITUENTS

The question of the presence of carbohydrate as an integral part of amyloid proteins is still controversial. Even though the mucopolysaccharide content of highly purified fibrils was found to be greater than that of the surrounding tissue (Muir and Cohen, 1968), Pras et al (1971) reached the conclusion that these carbohydrates were derived by trapping from adjacent connective tissues and not integral components of the amyloid protein because the metachromatic properties of amyloid did not correlate with the chemical composition of the extracted mucopolysaccharides. Furthermore, neither the purified A protein nor most of the L chain related amyloid proteins contain carbohydrate. Nevertheless, a recent study (Brandt, Skinner and Cohen, 1974), without being able to prove carbohydrate linkage to the amyloid fibrillar proteins, pointed out a close and constant association of heparitin sulphate, chondroitin sulphate, and dermatan sulphate with a fraction of amyloid fibrils bearing homology to immunoglobulin light chains, and raised the possibility that mucopolysaccharides may play a role in determining the structure of the amyloid fibrils without the proteins being glycoproteins.

P COMPONENT

Another protein found in all tissue amyloid preparations including the apudamyloid of pancreatic islet cells (Westermark, 1974) is the P component which has been thought to be a bystander trapped from the serum. Recently, a procedure has been developed (Skinner et al, 1974b) to isolate the P component from the saline washes of amyloid-laden tissues. The purified protein was found to have a MW of 180 000 daltons which fell to 36 000 after mild reduction, thus confirming previous electron microscopic observations which suggested that the molecule is composed of five subunits. Its amino acid analysis revealed histidine at the N-terminal; the sequence of its 23 amino terminal residues was reported. The composition was almost identical for the P components found in the amyloid of various tissues, including pancreatic islet cell apudamyloid (Westermark, Skinner and Cohen, 1975). Recently additional importance has been attributed to the P component by the observation of Painter (1976) that it was similar, and perhaps identical to C1t, a subfraction of the first component of complement, and by the observation of Osmond (1976) of structural homologies to C-reactive protein. The observation that these proteins have molecular weights of 220 000 and are composed of subunits of 22 000 daltons raised the possibility that each of the pentamers may be composed of two subunits and that the P component contains 10 subunits.

A component immunologically identical to the P component was isolated from the human plasma by affinity chromatography (Benson et al, 1976). It was found to have an identical mobility on polyacrylamide gel and immunoelectrophoresis with the P component extracted from tissues, and to migrate in the α_1-globulin fraction. If its identity with the above-mentioned complement fraction is confirmed, the role of complement in amyloid formation should be further investigated.

IMMUNOLOGICAL PROPERTIES

It has long been recognised that specific antibodies to amyloid are difficult to prepare because amyloid fibrils are poorly immunogenic (Ram, DeLellis and Glenner, 1968; Franklin and Pras, 1969), perhaps due to their large size and fibrillar structure and their marked resistance to phagocytosis (Zucker-Franklin, 1970) and proteolysis (Sorenson and Binington, 1964; Pras et al, 1968; Kim et al, 1969). In order to overcome this difficulty, partially or completely degraded amyloid extracts have been used for immunisation. Degradation by exposing new antigenic sites and increasing the solubility of the amyloid fibrillar proteins may make processing by the cells involved in the immune response easier. Initially, Franklin and Pras (1969) used as antigen alkali-degraded amyloid (DAM) which retained part of the amyloid fibrillar structure in the EM but became soluble in saline buffer solutions, even at neutral pH as antigen. Others degraded amyloid with the same agent (Husby and Natvig, 1972) or concentrated urea and guanidine (Glenner et al,

1969). The resultant antibodies were found to react specifically with amyloid and failed to react with serum proteins including γ-globulins and normal tissues and often did not distinguish A protein and immunoglobulin-related amyloids. Hence, it appears that these antibodies recognise some features of the tertiary structure of amyloid fibrillar proteins rather than the amino acid sequence. This conclusion was supported by the observation that the reactivity of DAM with these antisera was abolished after complete reduction and alkylation in 6 M-guanidine, concomitant with the loss of the last traces of fibrillar structure, while similar treatment of Bence Jones proteins did not abolish their reaction with antisera to Bence Jones proteins (Franklin and Zucker-Franklin, 1972b).

The antisera to DAM reacted best with the antigen used for immunisation, but cross-reacted with most other DAMs and generally reacted well with the native amyloid fibrils. For these reasons, they were found useful as reagents to detect amyloid in tissues (Zucker-Franklin and Franklin, 1970).

With the recognition and characterisation of AA protein and immunoglobulin-related component in different amyloid preparations, antisera have been produced that react specifically with the AA protein or with κ- or λ-chain-related amyloid components. Initially working with the protein subunits of amyloid from patients with primary amyloidosis, Isersky et al (1972) demonstrated both an idiotypic reaction with the protein used for immunisation as well as varying degrees of cross-reaction with other amyloid proteins and with Bence Jones proteins belonging to either the κ or λ class and the same variable region subclass. These cross-reactivities offered strong support for the chemical analyses showing that these amyloid proteins are closely related to immunoglobulin light chains (Glenner et al, 1971a, b, c). The antisera to amyloid proteins with aspartic amino terminals reacted with other aspartic amino terminal amyloid proteins and with most κ Bence Jones proteins (Glenner et al, 1972) while the antiserum to an amyloid fibril protein with a blocked amino terminus reacted with other blocked amyloid proteins and with several λ Bence Jones proteins, but not with κ Bence Jones proteins (Isersky et al, 1972). Cohen's group obtained similar results of cross-reactivity in the case of κ-related proteins (Cohen and Cathcart, 1974). These antisera appear to be directed against determinants associated with the primary structure of amyloid protein and are helpful in studying the relationships between different amyloid proteins. The failure to observe cross-reactivity between antisera to light chains and to γ-globulins and the basic amyloid subunit, or the synthetic amyloid fibrils prepared from Bence Jones proteins by proteolysis may be due to the poor immunogenicity of the variable region of light chains, or to the possibility of the antigenic determinants associated with amyloid being hidden within the molecule.

The immunologic properties of the P component have also been well studied. It was found to be very immunogenic in its native state (Glenner and Bladen, 1966; Cathcart et al, 1967b). Specific antibodies against the P component were used to identify and isolate the component from the serum (Benson et al, 1976) and to study its relationship to Clt and CRP.

PATHOGENESIS OF AMYLOID

During the last few years some progress has been made in understanding the processes leading to amyloid formation. Precursors of the amyloid fibrillar proteins have been isolated from the human sera and partially characterised; new information has been obtained concerning the possible sites of origin of the amyloid precursors, as well as regarding enzymes which may induce the formation of amyloid, and a variety of immunologic aberrations accompanying both naturally occurring and experimental amyloidosis have been catalogued. However, numerous links in the chain of events leading to the creation of amyloid are still missing; the cellular events leading to the formation and assembly of the fibrils are unknown, even the identity of the cell of origin of the amyloid precursors still raises significant debate; and very little is known about the function and the metabolic fate of amyloid precursors, and the significance of defects in T-cell and B-cell function in terms of pathogenesis.

In this section we will try to briefly review some of the recent data concerning the amyloid precursors in human sera, analyse the way in which information obtained from the study of experimentally induced amyloidosis could be applied to an understanding of the disease in man, and finally, we will try to advance some hypotheses concerning the possible role of amyloid precursors as well as some of the events leading to amyloid deposition.

Serum Precursors of Amyloid

In a somewhat mechanistic, but not very fundamental sense, the discovery of precursors of amyloid fibrils has thrown some light on the mechanisms of amyloid deposition.

SERUM IMMUNOGLOBULIN LIGHT CHAIN PRECURSOR

The structural homology of the amyloid fibrillar proteins and immunoglobulin light chains in cases of primary amyloidosis and amyloidosis associated with myelomatosis as well as their immunologic cross-reactivity identify light chains as precursors of at least some types of amyloid fibrillary proteins (Glenner et al, 1970, 1973b). In most instances, only fragments consisting of the amino terminal region of light chains were found in the amyloid fibrils (Isersky et al, 1972; Kimura et al, 1972; Glenner et al, 1973b). In a few instances, a whole light polypeptide chain, or a whole light chain and additional amino terminal light chain fragments were found in these fibrillar proteins (Glenner et al, 1973b; White et al, 1975), and in one instance (Terry et al, 1973) the amyloid subunit was found to be identical to the Bence Jones protein isolated from the urine of the patient. Some insights into possible mechanisms of degradation were recently contributed by the observation of Tan and Epstein (1972) and Epstein and Tan (1974) that lysosomal enzymatic digestion of intact light chains frequently causes polymeric precipitates constituted of the whole light chain and either their variable or constant region having the tinctorial and electron microscopic characteristics of amyloid fibrils. These observations add potentially important physiological significance to the previously documented in vitro degradation of L chains by proteolytic enzymes. Large circulating covalent polymeric forms of light chains of high molecular weight were noticed in the sera of several patients with amyloidosis (Parr et al, 1971) and were found, at least on one occasion, to have idiotypic determinants in common with the amyloid fibril proteins of the respective patients.

SERUM AMYLOID A PRECURSOR (SAA)

During the last five years, significant data have been accumulated concerning the existence in human and animal sera of a precursor of the AA protein. Levin, Pras and Franklin (1973) detected, with a monospecific antiserum produced against the alkali-degraded acid soluble fraction of amyloid protein (AA protein), a circulating component in some human sera that migrated in the α-globulin region on immunoelectrophoresis, and was eluted from a Sephadex G100 column at a MW level of approximately 80 000 to 90 000 daltons. This circulating component gave a line of identity with degraded AA by double immunodiffusion. Concomitant studies by Husby, Natvig and their collaborators led to similar findings (Husby et al, 1973a, b; Husby and Natvig, 1974). Both groups found the presence of the serum precursors of the AA protein (SAA) in 50 to 80 per cent of sera from patients with chronic diseases known to be frequently associated with amyloidosis in cases of hypogammaglobulinaemia and in a relatively large number of apparently normal individuals, 80 years of age and older. Later when a sensitive radioimmunoassay

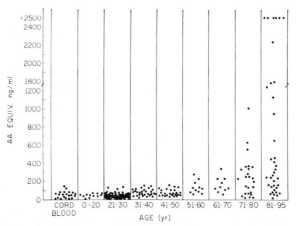

Figure 3.3   Concentration of SAA in the normal population in relation to age (Rosenthal C. J. and Franklin, E. C., 1975)

was developed (Rosenthal and Franklin, 1974b, 1975) using the displacement of radioactively iodinated AA protein, the SAA protein was established as a normal component of human blood, and was quantitated at an average level of 90 ± 50 ng/ml of equivalent AA protein. It seems likely, based on recovery of SAA from sera, that use of the AA protein yielded values that were too low, and that the actual concentration may be at least 10-fold greater.

VARIATIONS OF THE SAA LEVEL

The concentration of SAA was found to increase significantly with age (especially in the sixth to ninth decades) (Fig. 3.3), and in an unexpected number of pathological conditions (Rosenthal and Franklin, 1974a, b, 1975) (Table 3.3). Thus, values higher than 200 ng/ml AA equivalent were found in the sera of most of the patients suffering of chronic inflammatory or infectious disorders with and without apparent amyloidosis, such as tuberculosis, rheumatoid arthritis, as well as in lymphoproliferative disorders in which it correlated with disease activity. Also high values were found in a significant number of patients with neoplastic diseases, in which the elevation was remarkable, especially in cases with diffuse metastases and was unrelated to the site of origin and histologic type of the neoplastic process (Rosenthal and Franklin, 1974b). Elevated levels were also found in patients with leprosy (Kronvall et al, 1975) and with systemic lupus erythematosus

(Benson et al, 1975b). Of interest was the finding (Rosenthal and Franklin, 1975) of a significant elevation of SAA levels in most of the patients with macroglobulinaemia and IgA myeloma, as well as in approximately 50 per cent of those with IgG myeloma and with primary amyloidosis. These data are somewhat intriguing, in view of the inability of most investigators to detect the AA protein in the amyloid tissue deposits of patients with similar disorders. Because of the high frequency with which elevated SAA levels are found in a variety of disease states, the almost invariable increase in the SAA level noted in patients with all types of amyloidosis cannot be used to diagnose the disease as we had

Table 3.3   SAA concentration in various disease states in patients under the age of 70[a]

	No. subjects	SAA ng/ml Mean	s.d.	*P* value
Pulmonary tuberculosis	26	761	894	< 0.01
Rheumatoid + psoriatic arthritis	11	677	788	< 0.05
Acute infections	27	> 5000	ND	< 0.01
Lymphoma	21	749	851	< 0.01
Carcinoma	29	647	798	< 0.05
IgG multiple myeloma	12	303	481	< 0.05
IgA multiple myeloma	6	1465	1152	< 0.01
Macroglobulinaemia	6	1432	1176	< 0.01
Primary amyloidosis	11	235	105	< 0.01
Secondary amyloidosis	8	1150	1029	< 0.01
Atherosclerotic heart disease	25	178	244	—
Diabetes mellitus	5	65	38	—
Other endocrine diseases	5	46	46	—
Chronic liver diseases	6	105	114	—
Chronic obstructive lung diseases	9	155	139	—
Healthy adults (15–70 years)	67	95	58	—

[a] Data combined from Rosenthal and Franklin (1974a, b) and Gorevic, Rosenthal and Franklin (1976)

originally hoped. In contrast, normal SAA levels were found in patients with chronic inactive osteoarthritis, chronic obstructive lung disease without bronchitis, various endocrine diseases, as well as chronic liver disease except for biliary cirrhosis and chronic active hepatitis. Of interest, also, is the finding that in conditions like medullary thyroid carcinoma and diabetes mellitus, in which only localised amyloid deposits were found in the respective endocrine glands, the SAA levels were generally normal (Gorevic, Rosenthal and Franklin, 1976; Rosenthal et al, 1974a). In these cases, as previously mentioned, the composition of amyloid tissue proteins appears to be different from that of all other cases.

Of interest, in relation to the elevation of SAA in plasma cell disorders, is the recent observation (Rosenthal, 1976) that in patients with myeloma complicated by renal failure the SAA was significantly increased in all cases except those with nephrotic syndrome, while it was elevated only in 20 per cent of cases with IgG myeloma uncomplicated by renal failure. So far, it has not been possible to detect SAA protein in the urine (unpublished observation).

The initial screening of the SAA level in various disorders by radioimmunoassay uncovered a significant elevation of SAA in patients with acute inflammatory and infectious diseases such as pneumonia, meningitis, diverticulitis, cholecystitis, subacute bacterial endocarditis, Gram-negative sepsis, septic arthritis, etc. (Rosenthal and Franklin, 1974a 1975; Gorevic et al, 1976). The fact that this elevation was found to resolve rapidly with therapy and improvement of clinical status and that the SAA appeared to behave like an acute phase reactant, may provide significant insights into its role in the formation of amyloid.

Consistent with this finding is the rapid rise in SAA long before the appearance of amyloid in endotoxin-treated mink (Anders et al, 1976). As yet, preliminary studies measuring other acute phase reactants showed that the SAA levels did not correlate strictly with the C-reactive protein or with C3 and serum immunoglobulins. Also, no cross-reactivity of the anti-AA serum with the C-reactive protein or C3 component was found (Rosenthal and Franklin, 1975).

All these data seem to indicate that SAA is significantly increased in all situations in which some foreign antigens (bacterial, viral, tumour-specific antigens, etc.) stimulate the immunologic system, and that it decreases when such antigens are cleared. Since many of these conditions, if they persist, can eventuate in amyloidosis, it seems attractive to consider the possibility that the body can cope with the transient production of SAA but that persistent liberation of this component will lead to amyloid deposits. Consistent with this interpretation is the occasional disappearance of amyloid in rare cases where the primary disorder is cured. The role of overproduction or possible decreased degradation and clearance in these conditions cannot yet be evaluated.

CHEMICAL CHARACTERISATION OF SAA

A complementary approach to study the significance of these proteins in the genesis of amyloid is their isolation, chemical characterisation and ultimately the elucidation of their possible physiologic function. The recent efforts of investigators in three laboratories have led to the practically concomitant isolation and partial characterisation of the SAA protein. Using acidic solutions, which induced the precipitation of part of serum components, it was found (Rosenthal and Franklin, 1974b) that in the presence of 0.01 M-HCl or 5 per cent formic acid, the SAA molecule, which in physiologic conditions had a MW of 85 000, yielded a subunit with a MW of 12 500 daltons and antigenic identity with the AA protein as determined by double immunodiffusion. It was possible to isolate this component in a homogeneous state by a two-step gel filtration procedure. In most of the patients, however, a small fraction of the SAA molecule was eluted in acidic conditions as a probable polymer of 160 000 to 180 000 daltons. Linke et al (1975) obtained a similar 12 500 dalton subunit after treatment with 5 M-guanidine and elution in a Sephadex G-100 column from a patient with secondary amyloidosis, whose intact SAA protein had a molecular weight level of 200 000 daltons in phosphate buffer. Anders et al (1975) have also succeeded in obtaining in high yield a 14 000 dalton SAA subunit using a double step gel filtration chromatography procedure (Bio-Gel P 100 followed by Sephadex G-75 in 10 per cent formic acid).

Biochemical analyses of this subunit (Anders et al, 1975; Rosenthal et al, 1976) have shown identity of the amino terminal 20 residues of SAA and AA. On comparing the peptide maps, all the peptides of AA were present in SAA which contained seven to eight additional ones including two with cysteine residues. Studies are currently in progress to further characterise this carboxy terminal unique region of SAA. Based on its physiologic behaviour together with the biochemical data, there can be little doubt that the SAA subunit must be the precursor of tissue AA protein. It still remains to be established if in the circulating blood, this component is present in a polymerised form, or if the large 90 000 or 180 000 MW proteins identified in physiologic conditions may be made up by the SAA subunit bound to some other large carrier. The possibility of an even larger precursor suggested by the amino terminal heterogeneity has recently received support by the finding of a 25 000 dalton AA protein in the tissues of one subject with amyloidosis (Lian et al, 1975).

A component similar to human SAA was also found in the α-globulin fraction of the sera from mice and guinea-pigs with casein-induced amyloidosis (Benson et al, 1975a) and in endotoxin-treated mink (Anders et al, 1976). This component cross-reacted with antisera to autologous tissue AA protein, but was found to be species specific. The specific functional activity of this circulating SAA protein in humans and animals is far from well defined. Preliminary studies in our laboratory have indicated that human SAA at a concentration of 100 to 500 ng/ml caused a moderate inhibition of lymphocyte response to pokeweed mitogen stimulation and a significant inhibition of EAC rosettes of B lymphocytes, but that it did not have any activity on E rosette formation of T-cells and on the lymphocyte response to PHA (Rosenthal, 1977). Benson et al (1975a) have found that serum from amyloidotic mice markedly suppresses in vitro antibody response to sheep red blood cells in the Mishell–Dutton culture system. This suppression was reversed by absorbing the serum with rabbit antiserum specific for murine amyloid AA protein, but not by normal rabbit serum. From these preliminary data, which have to be confirmed, it appears possible that the SAA protein may act on the B lymphocytes, suppressing their humoral as well as cellular immune activity and that it may be liberated as an autoregulatory substance in states of potent antigenic stimulation.

Site of Origin of Amyloid

The precise origin and place of assembly of the amyloid fibrils have not yet been completely defined despite a considerable number of electron microscopic and histologic studies, perhaps because multiple sites and mechanisms may be involved. In light of recent chemical studies, indicating that the immunoglobulin light chain is an important and sometimes the sole component of amyloid fibrillar protein, the plasma cell is thought to play an important role in the production of amyloid or its precursors. It seems likely that in some cases the fibrils may be formed in these cells, whereas in other instances, a precursor may be secreted and converted by proteolysis at sites distant from their synthesis. As early as 1956, Teilum, based on histochemical studies, implicated plasma cells and reticuloendothelial cells in the genesis of amyloid. Later, Zucker-Franklin and Franklin (1970) recognised on electron microscopy, intracellular amyloid fibrils in well-delineated plasma cells and have since seen them in the rough endoplasmic reticulum, Golgi apparatus, and cytoplasm of these cells. However, similar fibrils have been described since 1962 in the reticuloendothelial cells (Heefner and Sorenson, 1962; Teilum, 1968; Zucker-Franklin and Franklin, 1970) as well as in their liver and nervous system counterparts, the Kupffer and the glial cells respectively. All the cells mentioned up to now are of mesenchymal origin, and may be potentially capable of synthesising the same protein as a result of dedifferentiation. The identity of the intracellular fibrils to amyloid, which is difficult to establish morphologically, is supported by the presence of extracellular deposits of amyloid surrounding the cells. Some reports have mentioned the presence of structurally identical fibrils in epithelial cells, where they are defined as tonofibrils or stress fibrils (Fawcett, 1966). Their function and biochemical composition are unknown and, hence, their possible relationship to amyloid remains unknown.

In experimentally induced renal amyloidosis, Cohen and Calkins (1960) found the earliest amyloid deposits in the endothelial cells. Shibolet et al (1967) concluded that fibroblasts of the interstitial spaces were the initial source of hamster kidney amyloid, while Sorenson and Shimura (1964) first described them in the mesangial area of glomeruli of murine renal amyloidosis.

Data concerning the site of origin of the other main component of the amyloid fibrils, the AA protein, are even less precise. Preliminary data from our laboratories seem to indicate a peripheral blood mononuclear cell, perhaps a subset of T lymphocytes as the primary source of the SAA component as indicated by specific fluorescent staining using rabbit antibody against AA protein in a sandwich technique with fluorescent goat anti-rabbit IgG antibody (Zucker-Franklin, 1976, and unpublished observation). A search of liver, spleen, kidney and other organs has failed to reveal positive cells.

Recent studies by Tan and Epstein (1972) have shown that lysosomal enzymes may have a determinant role in the production of amyloid fibrillar protein since they can digest intact light chains to generate fragments, which subsequently precipitate, usually as polymeric components with all the characteristics of amyloid. These enzymes are found in large amounts in monocytes and reticuloendothelial cells and may be involved in the generation of amyloid fibrils recently detected in the urine (Derosena et al, 1975). Recent electron microscopic studies (Shirahama and Cohen, 1973) of spleen, liver, and kidney amyloid tissues from mice with casein-induced amyloidosis, are consistent with a major role for lysosomes in the genesis of amyloid.

Not much has been learned about the removal of amyloid deposits which has on occasions been noted to occur in man and experimental animals since the original observation by Waldenstrom (1928) who demonstrated regression of amyloid by means of serial splenic biopsies after excision of tuberculous fistulas or amputations of limbs afflicted with osteomyelitis. While lysosomes undoubtedly play a role and are at times seen in proximity to phagocytosed amyloid, native amyloid fibrils have a marked resistance to proteolysis, and are not readily engulfed by peripheral blood phagocytes under the same conditions as bacteria, foreign particles or denatured serum proteins. Only after treatment of amyloid with specific antibodies to amyloid, were they phagocytised by macrophages (Zucker-Franklin, 1970). These factors may explain the long persistence of amyloid and the absence of a marked inflammatory response in proximity to the tissue deposits. Recently, Kedar, Sohar and Gafni (1974a) have demonstrated that normal human serum has an amyloid degrading activity, not affected by heating to $100°C$ for 15 min while the activity appeared markedly decreased in three patients with FMF and amyloidosis. This serum factor may have an important role in determining the engulfment of amyloid fibrils by macrophages.

Experimental Amyloidosis

Unlike the situation in most other diseases, a multitude of experimental measures can induce amyloidosis in a large number of animal species. While this would be expected to accelerate an understanding of the pathogenesis of the disease, the situation has proved so complex that it has not been possible to clearly define the underlying factors responsible for the disease. While almost all of these measures appear to affect the immunologic and reticuloendothelial systems, the studies have provided few profound insights into the pathogenesis. Nevertheless, many phenomena have been described which ultimately can perhaps be fashioned into a meaningful pattern.

INDUCTION OF AMYLOIDOSIS IN EXPERIMENTAL ANIMALS

Since the first induction by Bailey (1916) of amyloidosis in rabbits by repeated administration of living bacilli, numerous procedures have been used for the production of amyloidosis in various animals (guinea-pigs, rabbits, mink and mice). Among these are the administration of killed bacteria (Hass, Huntington and Krumdieck, 1943; Howes et al, 1963) and the repeated injections of various macromolecular substances such as serum proteins (Jaffe, 1926; Dick and Leiter, 1941), ribonucleic acid (Bohle, Hartmann and Pola, 1950), adjuvant (Rothbard and Watson, 1954) and the one most commonly used, casein (Smetana, 1925; Jaffe, 1926). The latter is usually injected subcutaneously in mice as a 5 per cent solution on 20 consecutive days and results in amyloid deposits especially in the spleen, and to a lesser extent and somewhat later, in the liver and kidneys. After 10 injections of casein, the spleens show intense perifollicular proliferation of pyroninophilic (large) lymphoid cells, concomitant with a marked decrease in the number of small lymphocytes (pyroninophilic or preamyloidotic stage). After 20 injections, the pyroninophilia decreases and a large number of PAS-positive mesenchymal cells appear (mesenchymal or amyloidotic stage). Barth et al (1969b) have presented data suggesting that endotoxin may ultimately be the substance inducing amyloid deposition after injecting casein and other macromolecular proteins.

In part because of the nature of the stimuli and the histopathology of the lesions, and in part because of the association of amyloidosis with a variety of disorders of the immune system both in man and the animal kingdom, efforts have been directed primarily at an elucidation of defects in immunologic function and their possible role in the pathogenesis of the disease. These studies have been of two major types; one approach has been to modify the immune function of the experimental animal and to measure its effect on the induction of amyloidosis; the second has been an effort to measure the specific and nonspecific immunologic function in animals developing amyloidosis.

IMMUNOLOGIC MANIPULATIONS IN THE INDUCTION OF AMYLOIDOSIS

Conflicting results have been obtained concerning the role of the thymus and T-cell function in the induction of experimental amyloid. Adult thymectomy alone, or in combination with irradiation before casein injection, were found by Ranlov (1966) to accelerate amyloidosis; while antilymphocyte serum, if administered to adult mice during casein administration, reduced amyloid formation (Ranlov, 1967). Neonatal thymectomy has been shown to have either no effect (Rohde, 1965) or more often, an enhancing effect (Ebbesen, 1971). Deposition of amyloid appeared somewhat inhibited in adult mice after irradiation or thymectomy alone (Nielsen et al, 1973). Grafting of T lymphocytes from syngeneic donors sensitised with casein to mice given casein did not accelerate amyloid formation (Clerici et al, 1969), whereas transfer of sensitised spleen cells (Hardt, 1971b), and unsensitised lymph node cells (Hardt, Ebbesen and Moesner, 1972) had some enhancing effect. Recently, it has been shown in mice connected by parabiosis that intact cellular immunity of a healthy mouse was able to inhibit induction of amyloidosis in another mouse if parabiosis was established no later than the tenth injection of casein (Hardt and Claësson, 1973). Also it was found that amyloidosis could not be transferred from an amyloidotic mouse to a healthy one connected with the first one by parabiosis.

While it is tempting to postulate that B-cells and antibody production are important in amyloid formation, there is little evidence in support of that contention. Thus, in the casein model, there is no parallel between antibody formation and amyloid deposition. Of even greater significance is the observation by Pierpaoli and Clerici (1964) that amyloidosis appeared with equal severity and rapidity in animals tolerant to casein as in control animals. So far, no studies have been carried out to specifically ablate B-cell function, but it should be stressed that amyloidosis is not uncommonly seen in patients with agammaglobulinaemia (Teilum, 1968).

Another group of substances that has been widely investigated and shown to have an effect on amyloid formation are corticosteroids. Though they have a variety of effects, it has been long recognised that they significantly alter both the immune system and the RES and hence they will be discussed here. Here, too, the results are conflicting. Teilum (1952) and Hardt (1971a) concluded that cortisone stimulated the production of experimental amyloidosis, whereas the opposite conclusion was reached by Grayzel et al (1956), and Laufer, Tal and Kolander (1968). Fields, Laufer and Pollack (1973) have recently noticed that when cortisone acetate was given at various time intervals after six weekly injections of complete Freund's adjuvant, the mice presented a decrease of the amyloid deposited in spleen and liver, and a somewhat increased deposition of amyloid at the level of renal glomeruli, possibly due to an increase of cathepsin D and acid phosphatase activity and a decrease of β-glucuronidase activity. Perhaps some of the observed differences may be related to dose, time of administration, and differences in species reaction.

CHANGES IN PARAMETERS OF IMMUNE FUNCTION

The first suggestion of a change in T-cell function during amyloid deposition was the finding by Druet and Janigan (1966) of a marked depletion of lymphocytes in the thymic-dependent areas of the spleen, and the later observation by Hardt and Claësson (1971) of a decrease in the θ-positive cells in spleens of casein-treated C3H mice as amyloid deposition began to be noted. This was followed by the demonstration by Ranlov and Jensen (1966) that the development of amyloidosis was accompanied by delayed homograft rejection, by the report by Hardt and Claësson (1972) of a decrease in the ability of spleen cells to initiate a GVH reaction in F_1 hybrids and by similar observations by Scheinberg and Cathcart (1974). Ranlov and Hardt (1970) provided further evidence for deficiency in cellular immunity in this condition through leucocyte migration inhibition studies and Cathcart, Mullarkey and Cohen (1971), utilising the macrophage migration inhibition tests on cells isolated from the peritoneal cavity, demonstrated an initial response followed by marked inhibition of cell migration in response to casein but not to other antigens, such as diphtheria toxoid, mumps vaccine, and horseradish peroxidase, during the development of amyloidosis. The authors' conclusion that tolerance to a specific immunogen may play an important role in the pathogenesis of casein-induced amyloidosis may not be justified, however, since the three antigens to which the animal remained responsive are all 'strong' antigens, while sodium caseinate is a 'weak' antigen. The significance of the decreased response of splenic lymphocytes to three T-cell mitogens (concavalin A, phytohaemagglutinin and pokeweed mitogen) (Scheinberg and Cathcart, 1974) is difficult to interpret since it was observed in both amyloid sensitive CBA/J mice and amyloid resistant A/J strains, and because of the finding of Baumal, Ackerman and Wilson (1975) that the diminished response was limited to spleen cells and could not be observed when thymic and peripheral blood cells were studied.

Studies of B-cell function in the casein model are even more difficult to interpret since casein has been shown to be a non-specific B-cell mitogen which acts more strongly on spleen cells from amyloid susceptible than resistant mice (Britton, 1975). In the studies of

Cathcart et al the response to lipopolysaccharide, a B-cell mitogen, was almost completely abolished in the amyloid-resistant A/J strain, but unaltered in the CBA/J strain which suggests the possibility that amyloidogenesis may stem from an imbalance between the T-cell and B-cell response to prolonged antigenic stimulation. Perhaps a defect in suppressor T-cells allows B-cell function to escape from normal regulatory controls.

A provocative observation implicating depression of T-cell function in amyloidogenesis is the finding by Scheinberg, Goldstein and Cathcart (1976) that administration of thymosin, a substance that causes the differentiation of T-cell precursors, to mice receiving serial injections of sodium caseinate reduced the frequency and severity of amyloidosis. A possible role for AA and SAA in immunoregulation is suggested by the recent, but as yet unconfirmed report by Benson et al (1975a) that serum obtained from mice developing experimental amyloidosis suppressed the antibody response utilising the Jerne haemolytic plaque technique of spleen cells of mice immunised with SRBC while normal serum did not and that the responsible factor could be removed by an antiserum to AA protein. Since antibody response to sheep red blood cells is thymus dependent, SAA which is present in high concentration in conditions known to predispose to amyloidosis such as prolonged infection, multiple myeloma, ageing, etc., may exert a 'feedback' suppression on either T-cell or perhaps B-cell function. These findings which await confirmation raise the possibility that the various manifestations of T-cell dysfunction, which have been observed during the development of experimental amyloidosis, may in fact, represent a secondary response to the elevation in the SAA protein.

While the observed impairment of various T-cell effector functions during casein-induced experimental amyloidosis may play a role in its pathogenesis (Muckle, 1968; Cathcart et al, 1971; Hardt and Claësson, 1972), perhaps through its influence on B lymphocytes (Dennert and Lennox, 1972), the possibility that many of the T-cell function abnormalities are the result, rather than the cause of amyloid disease cannot be excluded because they were found to also occur in strains of inbred mice that are relatively resistant to amyloid induction after casein administration (Scheinberg and Cathcart, 1974). Recent data of Scheinberg and Cathcart (1976) indicated that B-cell activation may play a more important and decisive role in the genesis of experimental amyloidosis than had hitherto been suspected. These investigators found B-cell abnormalities (i.e. enhanced response to B-cell mitogens) more pronounced in amyloid-susceptible CBA/J than in amyloid-resistant A/J mice. They noted that CBA/J amyloid spleen cell suspensions were enriched with immature B-cells which did not form EAC or EA rosettes (characteristic for B and T lymphocytes respectively), but had readily detectable surface immunoglobulin and good response to B-cell mitogens. These B-cell changes are perhaps the result of depletion of a subset of T-cells.

MISCELLANEOUS EXPERIMENTAL DATA

A number of observations of potential interest which are still difficult to fit into an immunologic concept of amyloid pathogenesis have been made in recent years. Probably, potentially, the most significant one is the effect of colchicine in preventing the induction of amyloid. During the last few years, various attempts were made to block the induction of experimental amyloidosis using various pharmacologic or physiologic agents. Colchicine, for a total dose of 0.1 mg (0.015 mg/day), appears up until now to be the only substance which inhibits the amyloid induction in the experimental mouse model during its final stages, but does not significantly affect amyloid already deposited in tissues (Kedar et al, 1974b; Shirahama and Cohen, 1974). Through its specific binding to the cytoplasmic protein subunit 'tubulin', colchicine is known to disrupt the microtubules and this may inhibit the suspected endocytic activity of RE cells leading to amyloid fibril formation, secretion of the amyloid precursor, or, perhaps by analogy to its effect on microtubules, it may interfere with the polymerisation of amyloid proteins, inhibiting fibril formation.

Recent studies have shown that polycations like DEAE-dextran and polybrene (Ebbesen, 1972) accelerated the formation of casein-induced amyloid, perhaps by facilitating several membrane functions. As expected, cyclic AMP and the phosphodiesterase inhibitor theophyline, were found to produce similar acceleration (Ebbesen, 1974). Based on these data, one can speculate that external membrane stimuli (Teilum, 1956), and endogenous alterations, causing a sustained elevation of the intracellular cyclic AMP level, may lead to amyloid formation by as yet unknown mechanisms.

One other aspect of experimental amyloidosis deserves mention though its precise significance remains unclear. Several groups of workers have identified in spleens and other tissues of amyloidotic animals, a factor, which, if injected into other animals, induces amyloid or accelerates its formation with casein. Keizman et al (1972) reported that this activity was associated with a glycopeptide of 10 000 daltons MW, which accelerated the amyloid production induced by casein in mice.

CONCLUSIONS

From what has been said above, several tentative conclusions can be expressed which are subject to change and modification as new information becomes available, perhaps even before this review appears. Firstly, and perhaps most importantly, it should be emphasised that amyloid is a generic term and that the typical fibrillar appearance can be assumed by a number of different proteins, some of which are now known while others may still defy detection, as for example, many of the familial forms and the amyloid of ageing.

Of the currently recognised types of amyloid, one type, that derived from peptide hormones (apudamyloid), appears to be unrelated to disorders of immune function while the two others, those related to L chains, and those made of the AA protein obviously are associated with such disorders. Nevertheless, the final mechanism of fibril formation appears to be similar in all and to involve the digestion of a precursor protein by proteolytic enzymes, perhaps often in close association with cells of the RES. Even in those instances, where fibrils are seen inside non-phagocytic cells, presumably active in the synthesis of the proteins, it seems likely that some such mechanisms may initiate the process of fibril formation. While excess synthesis of the precursor molecule seems almost indisputable in the light chain associated types of amyloid, it is not possible to exclude alterations in the degradative mechanisms normally involved in removal of the affected molecule although such a possibility seems less attractive especially in the case of endocrine tumours.

In the two types of amyloidosis associated with disorders of immune function, certain common features emerge. Primary among these are their association either with neoplasms of the lymphoid system producing homogeneous immunoglobulins or with a stimulus in excess of the capacity of the immune system, as is the case in the AA associated form of the disease. In both instances, the serum levels of the SAA protein appear elevated. If the recently demonstrated immunoregulatory function for the SAA protein can be confirmed and if the T-cell should prove to be its source, one could postulate that its production is stimulated in conditions of excessive or autonomous B-cell function with the purpose of providing a feedback control. When this production continues for prolonged periods, the protein may be deposited in the tissues in the form of amyloid. While this is commonly observed in association with long-term antigenic stimulation, it is only rarely seen in plasma cell tumours, possibly because the duration of the disease before death ensues is shorter. Perhaps in the few instances where the AA protein is found in deposits of L chain amyloid excessive production of AA has persisted for a time sufficiently long to allow conversion to amyloid fibrils.

The experimentally observed changes in B-cell and T-cell function, if indeed causally related to amyloid formation, are difficult to implicate directly at this time due to the enormous complexity of B-cell and especially T-cell function. Nevertheless, based on the observed depression of T-cell function in experimentally induced and perhaps also human amyloidosis and the disordered B-cell function which is generally seen, one can postulate the existence of an aberration of immune regulatory function of one of several components of the immunologic system, predominantly of the suppressor T-cell fraction.

Two other points deserve emphasis. One deals with the tissue localisation of different types of amyloid. While this may reflect in part the sites of synthesis of the precursor as is the case for many of the apudamyloids and some of the L chain amyloids, involving lymphoid organs, other factors must be involved when amyloid is deposited at sites distant from those of biosynthesis of the precursor. As suggested by Osserman, Takatsuki and Talal (1964), this may reflect the propensity of certain amyloid precursors to react specifically with certain tissues or tissue components.

Lastly, the discovery that colchicine and possibly other drugs can prevent the formation of amyloid and perhaps reverse it once deposited, makes it imperative to study the mechanisms by which this occurs in the hope of finding ways to alleviate this dread disease. Perhaps, in the not too distant future, ways will have been found to prevent or cure this disease. Furthermore, if some of the speculations prove to be correct and the SAA protein can be proven to have a physiologic function as an immunosuppressive factor released by T lymphocytes, the study of the nature of amyloid, which at the beginning seemed unappealing due to the impression that amyloid is an end product of metabolism, may in fact open the door to a whole new field of immunology—that of the molecular biology of immunosuppression, and may also lead to new therapeutic applications.

REFERENCES

Anders, R. F., Natvig, J. B., Michaelsen, T. E. & Husby, G. (1975) Isolation and characterisation of amyloid-related serum protein SAA as a low molecular weight protein. *Scandinavian Journal of Immunology*, **4**, 397–401.

Anders, R. F., Nordstoga, K., Natvig, J. B. & Husby, G. (1976) Amyloid related serum protein SAA in endotoxin induced amyloidosis of the mink. *Journal of Experimental Medicine*, **143**, 678–683.

Andrade, C. (1952) Peculiar form of peripheral neuropathy: familial atypical generalized amyloidosis with special involvement of peripheral nerves. *Brain*, **75**, 408–427.

Auerbach, O. & Stemmerman, M. G. (1944) Renal amyloidosis. *Archives of Internal Medicine*, **74**, 244–253.

Bailey, C. H. (1916) The production of amyloid disease and chronic nephritis in rabbits by repeated intravenous injections of living colon bacilli. *Journal of Experimental Medicine*, **23**, 773–790.

Barth, W. F., Willerson, J. T., Waldman, T. A. & Decker, J. L. (1969a) Primary amyloidosis. Clinical, immunochemical and immunoglobulin metabolism studies in fifteen patients. *American Journal of Medicine*, **47**, 259–268.

Barth, F. W., Willerson, J. T., Asofsky, R., Sheagren, J. N. & Wolf, S. M. (1969b) Experimental murine amyloid, III. Amyloidosis induced with endotoxins. *Arthritis and Rheumatism*, **12**, 615–626.

Baumal, R., Ackerman, A. & Wilson, B. (1975) Immunoglobulin biosynthesis in myeloma associated and casein and endotoxin induced murine amyloidosis. *Journal of Immunology*, **114**, 1785–1791.

Benditt, E. P., Lagunoff, D., Eriksen, E. & Iser, O. A. (1962) Amyloid. Extraction and preliminary characterization of some proteins. *Archives of Pathology*, **74**, 323–330.

Benditt, E. P. & Eriksen, N. (1964) Amyloid, II. Starch gel electrophoresis analysis of some proteins extracted from amyloid. *Archives of Pathology*, **78**, 325–331.

Benditt, E. P. & Eriksen, N. (1966) Amyloid, III. A protein related to the subunit structure of human amyloid fibrils. *Proceedings of the National Academy of Sciences, U.S.A.*, **55**, 308–316.

Benditt, E. P. & Eriksen, N. (1971a) Chemical classes of amyloid substances. *American Journal of Pathology*, **65**, 231–249.

Benditt, E. P. & Eriksen, L. H. (1971b) The major proteins of human and monkey amyloid substance: common properties including unusual N terminal amino acid sequences. *FEBS Letters*, **19**, 169–173.

Benditt, E. P., Eriksen, N. & Berglund, C. (1968) In *Amyloidosis—Proceedings of the Symposium on Amyloidosis*, ed. Mandema, E., Ruinen, L., Scholten, J. H. & Cohen, A. S., pp. 206–216. Amsterdam: Excerpta Medica Foundation.

Benditt, E. P., Eriksen, N. & Berglund, C. (1970) Congo Red dichroism with dispersed amyloid fibrils and extrinsic cotton effect. *Proceedings of the National Academy of Sciences, U.S.A.*, **66**, 1044–1051.

Bennhold, H. (1922) Eine spezifische Amyloidfärbung mit Kongorot. *Münchener medizinische Wochenschrift*, **69**, 1537–1549.

Benson, M. D., Aldo-Benson, M. A., Shirahama, T., Borel, I. & Cohen, A. S. (1975a) Suppression of in vitro antibody response by a serum factor (SAA) in experimentally induced amyloidosis. *Journal of Experimental Medicine*, **142**, 236–242.

Benson, M. D., Skinner, M., Lian, J. & Cohen, A. S. (1975b) 'A' protein of amyloidosis. *Arthritis and Rheumatism*, **18**, 315–322.

Benson, M. D., Skinner, M., Shirahama, T. & Cohen, A. S. (1976) P component of amyloid: isolation from human serum by affinity chromatography. *Arthritis and Rheumatism*, **19**, 749–755.

Bilbao, J. M., Horvath, E., Hudson, A. R. & Kovacs, K. (1975) Pituitary adenoma producing amyloid-like substance. *Archives of Pathology*, **99**, 411–414.

Bitter, T. & Muir, H. (1966) Mucopolysaccharides of whole human spleens in generalized amyloidosis. *Journal of Clinical Investigation*, **45**, 963–975.

Bladen, H. A., Nylen, M. U. & Glenner, G. G. (1966) The ultrastructure of human amyloid as revealed by the negative staining technique. *Journal of Ultrastructure Research*, **14**, 449–455.

Boere, H., Ruinen, L. & Scholten, J. H. (1965) Electron microscopic studies on the fibrillar component of human splenic amyloid. *Journal of Laboratory and Clinical Medicine*, **66**, 943–951.

Bohle, A., Hartmann, F. & Pola, W. (1950) Elektrophoretische Serumeiweissuntersuchungen bei experimentellem mauseamyloid. *Virchows Archiv (Pathologische Anatomie)*, **319**, 231–246.

Bonard, L., Cohen, A. S. & Skinner, M. (1969) Characterization of the amyloid fibril as a cross-β-protein. *Proceeding of the Society for Experimental Biology and Medicine*, **131**, 1373–1375.

Brandt, K., Cathcart, E. S. & Cohen, A. S. (1968) A clinical analysis of the course and prognosis of forty-two patients with amyloidosis. *American Journal of Medicine*, **44**, 955–969.

Brandt, K. D., Skinner, M. & Cohen, A. S. (1974) Characterization of the mucopolysaccharides associated with fractions of guanidine-denatured amyloid fibrils. *Clinica chimica acta*, **55**, 295–305.

Britton, S. (1975) Experimental amyloidosis: the inducer is a polyclonal B cell activator. *Journal of Experimental Medicine*, **142**, 1564–1569.

Burke, M. I. & Rougvie, M. A. (1972) Cross B protein structure. I. Insulin fibrils. *Biochemistry*, **11**, 2435–2439.

Capella, C. & Solcia, E. (1971) Optical and electron microscopical study of cytoplasmic granules in human carotid body, carotid body tumours and jugular tumours. *Virchows Archiv Abt. B*, **7**, 37–53.

Carnes, W. H. & Forbes, B. R. (1956) Metachromasy of amyloid. *Laboratory Investigation*, **5**, 21–43.

Cathcart, E. S. & Cohen, A. S. (1966) The relation between isolated human amyloid fibrils and human gammaglobulins and its subunits. *Journal of Immunology*, **96**, 239–245.

Cathcart, E. S., Wollheim, F. A. & Cohen, A. S. (1967a) Plasma protein constituents of amyloid fibrils. *Journal of Immunology*, **99**, 376–385.

Cathcart, E. S., Shirahama, T. & Cohen, A. S. (1976b) Isolation and identification of a plasma component of amyloid. *Biochimica et biophysica acta*, **147**, 392–393.

Cathcart, E. S., Mullarkey & Cohen, A. S. (1971) Cellular immunity in casein induced amyloidosis. *Immunology*, **20**, 1001–1008.

Cathcart, E. S., Rodgers, O. G. & Cohen, A. S. (1972) Amyloid inducing factor and immunologic unresponsiveness. *Annals of Rheumatic Diseases*, **31**, 303–307.

Clerici, E., Mocarelli, P., de Ferrari, F. & Villa, M. L. (1969) Studies on the passive transfer of amyloidosis by cells. *Journal of Laboratory and Clinical Medicine*, **74**, 145–152.

Cohen, A. S. (1966) Preliminary chemical analysis of partially purified amyloid fibrils. *Laboratory Investigation*, **15**, 66–71.

Cohen, A. S. (1967) Amyloidosis. *New England Journal of Medicine*, **277**, 522–530, 574–582, 628–638.

Cohen, A. S. & Calkins, E. (1959) Electron microscopic observations on a fibrous component in amyloid of diverse origins. *Nature*, **183**, 1202–1203.

Cohen, A. S. & Calkins, E. (1960) Study of fine structure of kidney in caseine induced amyloidosis in rabbits. *Journal of Experimental Medicine*, **112**, 479–490.

Cohen, A. S. & Calkins, E. (1964) Isolation of amyloid fibrils and study of the effect of collagenase and hyaluronidase. *Journal of Cell Biology*, **21**, 481–486.

Cohen, A. S. & Cathcart, E. S. (1974) Amyloidosis and immunoglobulins. *Advances in Internal Medicine*, **19**, 41–55.

Cohen, H. & Fishman, A. P. (1949) Regional enteritis and amyloidosis. *Gastroenterology*, **12**, 502–508.

Cohen, A. S. & Shirahama, T. (1973) Electron microscopic analysis of isolated amyloid fibrils from patients with primary, secondary and myeloma associated disease: a study utilizing shadowing and negative staining technique. *Israel Journal of Medical Sciences*, **9**, 849–857.

Cooper, J. H. (1974) Selective amyloid staining as a function of amyloid composition and structure. *Laboratory Investigation*, **3**, 232–238.

Davidson, B., Tooney, N. & Fasman, G. D. (1966) The optical rotatary dispersion of the β structure of poly-1-lysine and poly-1-serine. *Biochemistry and Biophysics, Research Communications*, **23**, 156–165.

Dennert, G. & Lennox, E. (1972) Cell interaction in humoral and cell-mediated immunity. *Nature New Biology*, **238**, 114–115.

Derosena, R., Koss, M. N. & Pirani (1975) Demonstration of amyloid fibrils in urinary sediments. *New England Journal of Medicine*, **293**, 1131–1133.

Dick, G. F. & Leiter, L. (1941) Some factors in the development and reabsorption of experimental amyloidosis in rabbit. *American Journal of Pathology*, **17**, 741–753.

Divry, P. (1927) Etude histochimique des plaques séniles. *Journal de Neurologie and Psychiatrie*, **27**, 643–657.

Dontenwill, W., Ranz, H. & Mohr, U. (1960) Experimentelle Untersuchungen zur Amyloid entstehung beim Goldhamster. *Beiträge pathologischen Anatomie*, **122**, 390–405.

Druet, R. L. & Janigan, D. T. (1966) Experimental amyloidosis. Rates of induction, lymphocyte depletion and thymic atrophy. *American Journal of Pathology*, **49**, 911–916.

Eanes, E. D. & Glenner, G. G. (1968) X-ray diffraction studies of amyloid filaments. *Journal of Histochemistry and Cytochemistry*, **16**, 673–681.

Ebbesen, P. (1971) Amyloid induction with casein in mice of different ages and investigations for casein antibodies using the single radial diffusion technique. *Virchows Archiv Abt. und Zellpathologie*, **7**, 263–268.

Ebbesen, P. (1972) On the influence of two polycations and a polyanion on casein-induced amyloidosis, with a hypothesis on membrane alterations during amyloidogenesis. *Acta pathologica et microbiologica scandinavica* Section A, Suppl., **233**, 158–161.

Ebbesen, P. (1974) On the influence of exogenous cyclic AMP (3′,5′-adenosine monophosphate) on amyloid formation in casein treated C_3H mice. *Acta pathologica et microbiologica scandinavica*, Section A, **82**, 455–458.

Ein, D., Kumura, S. & Glenner, G. G. (1972a) An amyloid fibril protein of unknown origin; partial amino acid sequence analysis. *Biochemistry and Biophysics, Research Communications*, **46**, 498–502.

Ein, D., Kimura, S., Terry, W. D., Magnotta, J. & Glenner, G. G. (1972b) Amino acid sequences of an amyloid protein of unknown origin. *Journal of Biological Chemistry*, **247**, 5653–5655.

Emerson, E. E., Kikkawa, Y. & Gueft, B. (1966) New features of amyloid found after digestion with trypsin. *Journal of Cellular Biology*, **28**, 570–574.

Eriksen, N., Fowler, S. & Ericsson, L. H. (1974) Origin of amyloid protein A. *Federation Proceedings*, **33**, 1563 (Abstract).

Eriksen, N., Ericsson, L. H., Pearsall, N., Lagunoff, D. & Benditt, E. P. (1976) Mouse amyloid protein AA: homology with non-immunoglobulin protein of human and monkey amyloid substance. *Proceedings of the National Academy of Sciences, U.S.A.*, **73**, 964–967.

Epstein, W. V. & Tan, M. (1974) Formation of 'amyloid' fibrils in vitro by action of human kidney lysosomal enzymes on Bence Jones proteins. *Journal of Laboratory Clinical Medicine*, **84**, 107–110.

Fawcett, D. W. (1966) In *The Cell*, pp. 247–258. Philadelphia: Saunders.

Fields, M., Laufer, A. & Pollack, A. (1973) Lysosomal enzyme studies in experimental amyloidosis of mice treated with cortisone. *Acta pathologica et microbiologica scandinavica*, Section A, Suppl. **236**, 45–66.

Franklin, E. C. & Pras, M. (1969) Immunologic studies of water-soluble human amyloid fibrils. *Journal of Experimental Medicine*, **130**, 797–805.

Franklin, E. C. & Rosenthal, C. J. (1974) Chemical heterogeneity of human amyloid. *Federation Proceedings*, **33**, 758 (Abstract).

Franklin, E. C. & Zucker-Franklin, D. (1972a) Current concepts of amyloid. *Advances in Immunology*, **15**, 249–304.

Franklin, E. C.· & Zucker-Franklin, D. (1972b) Antisera specific for human amyloid reactive with conformational antigens. *Proceedings of the Society of Experimental Biology and Medicine*, **140**, 565–568.

Franklin, E. C., Pras, M., Levin, M. & Frangione, B. (1972) The partial amino acid sequence of the major low molecular weight component of two human amyloid fibrils. *FEBS Letters*, **22**, 121–123.

Frederiksen, T., Gotzsche, H., Harboe, N., Kiaer, W. & Mellemgaard, K. (1962) Familial primary amyloidosis with severe amyloid heart disease. *American Journal of Medicine*, **33**, 328–348.

Friedreich, N. & Kekule, A. (1859) Zur Amyloidfrage. *Virchows Archiv (Pathologische Anatomie)*, **16**, 50–67.

Gardner, D. I. (1966) *Pathology of the Connective Tissue Diseases*, pp. 480–481. Baltimore: Williams and Wilkins.

Gelderman, A. H., Levine, R. A. & Arndt, K. A. (1962) Dermatomyositis complicated by generalised amyloidosis. *New England Journal of Medicine*, **267**, 858–861.

Glenner, G. G. & Bladen, H. A. (1966) Purification and reconstitution of the periodic fibril and unit structure of human amyloid. *Science*, **154**, 271–272.

Glenner, G. G., Cuatrecasas, P., Isersky, C., Bladden, H. A. & Eanes, E. D. (1969) Physical and chemical properties of amyloid fibers, II. Isolation of a unique protein constituting the major component from human splenic amyloid fibril concentrates. *Journal of Histochemistry and Cytochemistry*, **17**, 769–780.

Glenner, G. G., Harbaugh, J., Ohms, J. J., Harada, M. & Cuatrecasas, P. (1970) An amyloid protein: the amino-terminal variable fragment of an immunoglobulin light chain. *Biochemistry and Biophysics, Research Communications*, **41**, 1287–1289.

Glenner, G. G., Page, D., Isersky, C., Harada, M., Cuatrecasas, P., Eanes, E. D., DeLellis, R. A., Bladen, H. A. & Keiser, H. R. (1971a) Murine amyloid fibril protein: isolation, purification and characterisation. *Journal of Histochemistry and Cytochemistry*, **19**, 16–28.

Glenner, G. G., Terry, W., Harada, M., Isersky, C. & Page, D. (1971b) Amyloid fibril proteins: proof of homology with immunoglobulin light chains by sequence analysis. *Science*, **171**, 1150–1151.

Glenner, G. G., Ein, D., Eanes, E. D., Bladen, H. A., Terry, W. & Page, D. (1971c) The creation of 'amyloid' fibrils from Bence Jones proteins in vitro. *Science*, **174**, 712–714.

Glenner, G. G., Ein, D. & Terry, W. D. (1972) Editorial. The immunoglobulin origin of amyloid. *American Journal of Medicine*, **52**, 141–144.

Glenner, G. G., Eanes, E. D., Termine, J. D., Bladen, H. A. & Linke, R. P. (1973a) The structural characteristics of some proteins having the properties of Congo red stained amyloid fibrils. *Journal of Histochemistry and Cytochemistry*, **21**, 406 (Abstract).

Glenner, G. G., Terry, W. D. & Isersky, C. (1973b) Amyloidosis. Its nature and pathogenesis. *Seminars in Hematology*, **10**, 65–86.

Glenner, G. G., Eanes, E. D., Bladen, H. A., Linke, R. P. & Termine, J. D. (1974) β-pleated sheet fibrils; a comparison of native amyloid with synthetic protein fibrils. *Journal of Histochemistry and Cytochemistry*, **22**, 1141–1158.

Goldber, A. F. & Deane, H. W. (1960) A comparative study of some staining properties of crystals in a lymphoplasmacytoid cell, of Russell bodies in plasmocytes and of amyloids—with special emphasis on their isoelectric point. *Blood*, **16**, 1708–1721.

Gorevic, P. D., Rosenthal, C. J. & Franklin, E. C. (1976) Amyloid related serum component (SAA) —studies in acute infectious, medullary thyroid carcinoma and post surgery. Behavior as an acute phase reactant. *Clinical and Experimental Immunology* (in press).

Grayzel, H. G., Grayzel, D. M., Heimer, R. & Saremsky, I. (1956) Amyloidosis—experimental studies, IX. The effect of corticotropin (ACTH) and amyloidosis in albino mice. *Experimental Medicine and Surgery*, **14**, 332–343.

Harada, M., Isersky, C., Cuatrecasas, P., Page, D., Bladen, H. A. & Eanes, E. D. (1969) Physical and chemical properties of amyloid fibers, II. Isolation of a unique protein constituting the major component from human splenic amyloid fibril concentrates. *Journal of Histochemistry and Cytochemistry*, **17**, 769–780.

Hardt, F. (1971a) Acceleration of casein induced amyloidosis in mice by immunosuppressive agents. *Acta pathologica et microbiologica scandinavica*, Section A, **79**, 61–64.

Hardt, F. (1971b) Transfer amyloidosis. *American Journal of Pathology*, **65**, 411–422.

Hardt, F. & Claësson, M. H. (1971) Graft versus host reactions mediated by spleen cells from amyloidotic and non-amyloidotic mice. *Transplantation*, **12**, 36–39.

Hardt, F. & Claësson, M. H. (1972) Quantitative studies on the T cell populations in spleens from amyloidotic and non-amyloidotic mice. *Immunology*, **22**, 677–683.

Hardt, F. & Claësson, M. H. (1973) Experimental amyloidosis. *Acta pathologica et microbiologica scandinavica*, Section A, **81**, 770–774.

Hardt, F., Ebbesen, P. & Moesner, J. (1972) The effect of syngeneic transfer of normal lymphoid cells on the development of casein-induced amyloidosis in mice. *Acta pathologica et microbiologica scandinavica*, Section A, **80**, 471–476.

Hass, G. M., Huntingdon, R. & Krumdieck (1943) The properties of amyloid deposits occurring in several species under diverse conditions. *Archives of Pathology*, **35**, 226–241.

Hazard, J. B., Hawk, W. A. & Crile, G., Jr (1959) Medullary (solid) carcinoma of the thyroid. A clinico-pathological entity. *Journal of Clinical Endocrinology*, **37**, 205–209.

Heefner, W. A. & Sorenson, G. D. (1962) Experimental amyloidosis. Light and electron microscopic observations of spleen and lymphnodes. *Laboratory Investigation*, **11**, 585–593.

Heller, H., Gafni, J. & Sohar, E. (1966) The inherited systemic amyloidoses. In *Metabolic Basis of Inherited Diseases*, 2nd edn, ed. Stanbury, J. B., Wyngaarden, J. B. & Fredrickson, D., p. 995. New York: McGraw-Hill.

Hermodson, M. A., Kuhn, R. W., Walsh, K. A., Neurath, H., Eriksen, C. & Benditt, E. P. (1972) Amino acid sequence of monkey amyloid protein A. *Biochemistry*, **11**, 2934–2938.

Hjarre, A. (1942) Uber Amyloidose bei Tieren mit besonderer Berücksichtigung atypisher Formen. *Berlin–München tierärztliche Wochenschrift*, **16**, 331–334.

Hjarre, A. & Nordlund, J. (1942) On atypisk amyloidos hos djuren. *Skandinavisk Veterinärtidskrift*, **32**, 385–441.

Hjort, G. H. & Christensen, H. E. (1961) Electron microscopic investigations on secondary renal amyloidosis. *Acta rheumatologica scandinavica*, **7**, 65–68.

Hoffman, S., Simon, B. E., Fischel, R. A. & Gribetz, D. (1963) Renal amyloidosis resulting from chronically infected burn. *Pediatrics*, **32**, 888–894.

Howes, E. L., Jr, Pincus, T., McKay, D. G. & Christian, C. L. (1963) A model of amyloidosis. *Arthritis and Rheumatism*, **6**, 278–285.

Husby, G. & Natvig, J. B. (1972) Individual antigenic specificity and cross reactions among amyloid preparations from different individuals. *Clinical Experimental Immunology*, **10**, 635–646.

Husby, G. & Natvig, J. B. (1974) A serum component related to non-immunoglobulin amyloid protein AS, a possible precursor of the fibrils. *Journal of Clinical Investigation*, **3**, 1054–1061.

Husby, G., Natvig, J. B., Michaelsen, T. E., Sletten, K. & Host, H. (1973a) Unique amyloid protein subunit common to different types of amyloid fibril. *Nature (London)*, **244**, 362–365.

Husby, G., Michaelsen, T. E., Sletten, K. & Natvig, J. B. (1973b) Immunochemical characterization of a non-immunoglobulin amyloid fibril subunit and a structurally related serum component. *Scandinavian Journal of Immunology*, **2**, 319–327.

Husby, G., Sletten, K., Michaelsen, T. E. & Natvig, J. B. (1973c) Amyloid fibril protein subunit 'protein AS': distribution in tissue and serum in different types of amyloidosis, including that associated with myelomatosis and Waldenstrom's macroglobulinaemia. *Scandinavian Journal of Immunology*, **2**, 395–406.

Isersky, C., Ein, D., Page, D. L., Harada, M. & Glenner, G. G. (1972) Immunochemical cross reactions of human amyloid proteins with immunoglobulin light polypeptide chains. *Journal of Immunology*, **108**, 486–492.

Isobe, T. & Osserman, E. F. (1974) Patterns of amyloidosis and their association with plasma cell dyscrasia, monoclonal immunoglobulins and Bence Jones proteins. *New England Journal of Medicine*, **290**, 473–477.

Jaffe, R. H. (1926) Amyloidosis produced by injections of proteins. *Archives of Pathology*, **1**, 25–36.

Jakob, W. (1970 Untersuchungen uber die Amyloidose der Katze. *Zeitblatt Veterenerisher Medizin*, A, **17**, 261–272.

Jakob, W. (1971) Spontaneous amyloidosis of mammals. *Veterinarian Pathology*, **8**, 292–306.

Kagan, H. M., Hewitt, N. A. & Franzblau, C. (1973) A microenvironmental probe of elastin properties of a solubilized Congo red elastin complex. *Biochimica et biophysica acta*, **322**, 258–263.

Katenkamp, D. & Stiller, D. (1972) Polarisationosoptisch-histochemische Untersuchungen Zur Kongorot farbung des Amyloid. *Histochemie*, **29**, 37–43.

Katenkamp, D. & Stiller, D. (1973) Comparisons of the texture of amyloid, collagen and Alzheimer cells. *Virchows Archiv (Pathologische Anatomie)*, **359**, 213–221.

Kedar, I., Sohar, E. & Gafni, J. (1974a) Demonstration of amyloid degrading activity in normal human serum. *Proceedings of the Society for Experimental Biology and Medicine*, **145**, 343–345.

Kedar, I., Ravid, M., Sohar, E. & Gafni, J. (1947b) Colchicine inhibition of casein induced amyloidosis in mice. *Israel Journal of Medical Sciences*, **10**, 787–789.

Keizman, I. Rimon, A., Sohar, E. & Gafni, J. (1972) Amyloid accelerating factor: purification of a substance from human amyloidotic spleen that accelerates the formation of casein induced murine amyloid. *Acta pathalogica et microbiologica scandinavica* (A), Suppl., **233**, 172–177.

Kim, I. C., Franzblau, C., Shirahama, T. & Cohen, A. S. (1969) The effect of papain, pronase, Nagarse and trypsin on isolated amyloid fibrils. *Biochimica et biophysica acta*, **181**, 465–467.

Kimball, K. G. (1961) Amyloidosis in association with neoplastic diseases. *Annals of Internal Medicine*, **55**, 958–974.

Kimura, S., Gayer, R., Terry, W. D. & Glenner, G. G. (1972) Chemical evidence for lambda type amyloid proteins. *Journal of Immunology*, **109**, 891–892.

Kronvall, G., Husby, G., Samuel, D., Bjune, G. & Wheate, H. (1975) Amyloid related serum component (protein ASC) in leprosy patients. *Infections and Immunity*, **11**, 969–976.

Kyle, R. A. & Bayrd, E. D. (1975) Amyloidosis: review of 236 cases. *Medicine*, **54**, 211–239.

Lachmann, P. J., Müller-Eberhard, H. J., Kunkel, H. G. & Paronetto, F. (1962) The localization of in vivo bound complement in tissue sections. *Journal of Experimental Medicine*, **115**, 63–71.

Laufer, A., Tal, C. & Kolander, N. (1968) Experimental amyloidosis and the effect of cortisone treatment. *Pathological Microbiology*, **31**, 85–92.

Levin, M., Franklin, E. C., Frangione, B. & Pras, M. (1972) The amino acid sequence of the major non-immunoglobulin component of some amyloid fibrils. *Journal of Clinical Investigation*, **51**, 2773–2776.

Levin, M., Pras, M. & Franklin, E. C. (1973) Immunologic studies of the major non-immunoglobulin protein of amyloid. *Journal of Experimental Medicine*, **138**, 373–380.

Lian, J. B., Benson, M. D., Skinner, M. & Cohen, A. S. (1975) A 25,000 dalton protein constituent of human amyloid fibrils related to protein AA. *Archives of Biochemistry and Biophysics*, **171**, 197–202.

Linke, R. P., Zucker-Franklin, D. & Franklin, E. C. (1973) Morphologic, chemical and immunologic studies of amyloid like fibrils formed from Bence Jones proteins by proteolysis. *Journal of Immunology*, **111**, 10–17.

Linke, R. P., Sipe, J. D., Pollock, P. S., Ignaczak, T. F. & Glenner, G. G. (1975) Isolation of a low molecular weight serum component antigenically related to an amyloid fibril protein of unknown origin. *Proceedings of the National Academy of Sciences, U.S.A.*, **72**, 1473–1476.

Magnus-Levi, A. (1952) Amyloidosis in multiple myeloma: progress noted in 50 years of personal observation. *Journal of Mount Sinai Hospital*, **19**, 8–27.

Mandema, E., Ruinen, L., Scholten, J. H. & Cohen, A. S. (eds) (1968) *Amyloidosis*. Amsterdam: Excerpta Medica Foundation.

Masterson, G. (1965) Cardiovascular syphilis with amyloidosis and periods of alternating heart block. *British Journal of Venereal Diseases*, **41**, 181–185.

Matthias, D. & Jakob, W. (1969) Untersuchungen über die Altersamyloidose des Hundes und ihre Stellung zur sog typishen Amyloidose. *Zeitblatt Veterenerisher Medizin*, A, **16**, 477–494.

Mellors, R. C. & Ortega, L. G. (1956) Analytical pathology, III. New observations on the pathogenesis of glomerulonephritis, lipid nephrosis, periarteritis nodosa and secondary amyloidosis in man. *American Journal of Pathology*, **32**, 455–463.

Milgrom, F., Kasukawa, R. & Calkins, E. (1966) Studies on antigenic composition of amyloid. *Journal of Immunology*, **99**, 245–252.

Missmahl, H. P. & Hartwig, M. (1953) Polarisationsoptische Untersuchungen an der Amyloidsubstanz. *Virchows Archiv, Pathologische, Anatomie und Physiologie*, **324**, 489–508.

Moschowitz, E. (1936) Clinical aspects of amyloidosis. *Annals of Internal Medicine*, **10**, 73–88.

Mowry, R. W. & Scott, J. C. (1967) Observations on the basophilia of amyloids. *Histochemie*, **10**, 8–32.

Muckle, T. J. & Wells, M. (1962) Urticaria, deafness and amyloidosis: new heredo-familial syndrome. *Quarterly Journal of Medicine*, **31**, 235–248.

Muckle, T. J. (1968) Impaired immunity in the etiology of amyloidosis. A speculative review. *Israel Journal of Medical Sciences*, **4**, 1020–1026.

Muir, H. & Cohen, A. S. (1968) In *Amyloidosis*, ed. Mandema, E., Ruinen, L., Scholten, F. H. & Cohen, A. S., pp. 280–288. Amsterdam: Excerpta Medica Foundation.

Newcombe, D. S. & Cohen, A. S. (1964) Solubility characteristics of isolated amyloid fibrils. *Biochimica et biophysica acta*, **104**, 480–486.

Newman, W. & Jacobson, A. S. (1953) Paraplegia and secondary amyloidosis, report of six cases. *American Journal of Medicine*, **15**, 216–222.

Nielsen, G., Leuchars, E., Doenhoff, M. & Ebbesen, P. (1973) Casein induced amyloidosis in T cell deprived mice. *Acta pathologica et microbiologica scandinavica* (B), **81**, 242–244.

Osmond, R. (1976) Communication presented at the 6*th International Workshop in Complement*, Sarasota, Florida.

Osserman, E. F. (1965) Amyloidosis and plasma cell discrasia. In *Immunopathology IVth International Symposium*, Monte Carlo, ed. Grabar, P. & Miescher, P. New York: Grune and Stratton.

Osserman, E. F., Takatsuki, K. & Talal, N. (1964) The pathogenesis of amyloidosis. *Seminars in Hematology*, **1**, 3–85.

Painter, R. H. (1976) Communication presented at the 6*th International Workshop in Complement*, Sarasota, Florida.

Paloyan, E., Scand, A., Straus, F. H., Pickleman, J. R. & Paloyan, D. (1970) Familial pheochromocytoma, medullary thyroid carcinoma and parathyroid adenomas. *Journal of American Medical Association*, **214**, 1443–1447.

Parr, D. M., Pruzanski, W., Scott, J. G. & Mills, D. M. (1971) Primary amyloidosis with plasmacytic dyscrasia and tetramer of Bence Jones type lambda globulin in the serum and urine. *Blood*, **34**, 473–479.

Paul, W. E. & Cohen, A. S. (1963) Electron microscopic studies of amyloid fibrils with ferritin conjugated antibody. *American Journal of Pathology*, **43**, 721–726.

Pearse, A. G. E. (1968) *Histochemistry: Theoretical and Applied*, Vol. I. Boston: Little Brown & Co.

Pearse, A. G. E. (1969) The cytochemistry and ultrastructure of polypeptide hormone producing cells of the APUD series and the embryologic, physiologic and pathologic implications of the concept. *Journal of Histochemistry and Cytochemistry*, **17**, 303–313.

Pearse, A. G. E., Ewen, S. W. B. & Polak, J. M. (1972) The genesis of apudamyloid in endocrine polypeptide tumours: histochemical distinction from immunamyloid. *Virchows Archiv B, Zellpathologie*, **10**, 93–107.

Penman, H. G. & Thomson, K. J. (1972) Amyloidosis and renal adenocarcinoma; a post mortem study. *Journal of Pathology*, **107**, 45–47.

Pierpaoli, W. & Clerici, E. (1964) Immunological aspects of experimental amyloidosis. *Experientia*, **20**, 693–694.

Pomerance, A. (1965) Senile cardiac amyloidosis. *British Heart Journal*, **27**, 711–718.

Porta, A. E., Yerry, R. & Scott, R. F. (1962) Amyloidosis of functioning islet cell adenoma of the pancreas. *American Journal of Pathology*, **41**, 623–627.

Pras, M. & Reshef, T. (1972) The acid-soluble fraction of amyloid—a fibril forming protein. *Biochimica et biophysica acta*, **271**, 193–205.

Pras, M. & Schubert, M. (1968) Metachromatic properties of amyloid in solution. *Journal of Histochemistry and Cytochemistry*, **17**, 258–265.

Pras, M., Schubert, M., Zucker-Franklin, D., Rimon, A. & Franklin, E. C. (1968) The characterization of soluble amyloid prepared in water. *Journal of Clinical Investigation*, **47**, 924–933.

Pras, M., Nevo, Z., Schubert, M., Rotman, J. & Matalon, R. (1971) The significance of mucopolysaccharides in amyloid. *Journal of Histochemistry and Cytochemistry*, **19**, 443–449.

Pras, M., Gorevic, P., Franklin, E. C. & Frangione, B. (1977) The amino acid sequence of the duck amyloid A protein (manuscript in preparation).

Pruzanski, W., Katz, A. & Nyburg, S. C. (1974) In vitro production of an amyloid like substance from gamma 3 heavy chain disease protein. *Immunology Communications*, **3**, 469–474.

Ram, J. S., DeLellis, R. A. & Glenner, G. G. (1968) Amyloid, IV. Is human amyloid immunogenic? *International Archives of Allergy and Applied Immunology*, **34**, 269–282.

Ranlov, P. J. (1966) The role of the thymus in experimental amyloidosis. *Acta pathologica et microbiologica scandinavica*, **67**, 42–54.

Ranlov, P. J. (1967) Effect of heterospecific antisera against lymphnode cells on the development of experimental amyloidosis in mice. *Acta pathologica et microbiologica scandinavica*, **69**, 534–542.

Ranlov, P. & Hardt, F. (1970) In vitro evaluation of cell mediated immunity in mice: experiments with soluble and cellular antigens in a spleen thymus cell leukocyte migration test (LMT). *Clinical and Experimental Immunology*, **8**, 163–171.

Ranlov, P. & Jensen, E. (1966) Homograft reaction in amyloidotic mice. *Acta pathologica et microbiologica scandinavica*, **67**, 161–164.

Reimann, H. A., Kouchy, R. F. & Eklund, C. M. (1935) Primary amyloidosis limited to tissue of mesodermal origin. *American Journal of Pathology*, **11**, 977–988.

Rohde, R. (1965) Über die experimentelle Amyloidose bei thymektomierten Mäusen. *Zeischrift für Immunitäts- und Allergie-forschung*, **129**, 268–277.

Rosenthal, C. J. (1977) Serum amyloid A(SAA) effect on human B lymphocytes. *Clinical Research*, **25**, 366 (Abstract).

Rosenthal, C. J. & Franklin, E. C. (1974a) Age associated changes of an amyloid related serum component. *Transactions of the Association of American Physicians*, **87**, 159–168.

Rosenthal, C. J. & Franklin, E. C. (1974b) Isolation and characterization of an amyloid related component from human serum (ARSC). Increased level in lymphoproliferative and neoplastic disorders. *Blood*, **44**, 907 (Abstract).

Rosenthal, C. J. & Franklin, E. C. (1975) Variation with age and disease of an amyloid A protein-related serum component. *Journal of Clinical Investigation*, **55**, 746–753.

Rosenthal, C. J., Franklin, E. C., Frangione, B. & Greenspan, J. (1976) Isolation and partial characterization of SAA—an amyloid related protein from human serum. *Journal of Immunology* (in press).

Rothbard, S. & Watson, R. F. (1954) Amyloidosis and renal lesions induced in mice by injection with Freund type of adjuvant. *Proceedings of the Society for Experimental Biology and Medicine*, **85**, 133–137.

Ruinen, L., Van Bruggen, E. F. J., Scholten, J. H., Gruber, M. & Mandema, E. (1968) A comparison of the structure observed in the human splenic amyloid fibrils by electron microscopy. In *Amyloidosis*, ed. Mandema, E., Ruinen, L., Scholten, F. H. & Cohen, A. S., pp. 194–199. Amsterdam: Excerpta Medica Foundation.

Rukavina, J. G., Block, W. D. & Curtis, A. C. (1956) Ultracentrifugal analyses of serum lipoproteins in familial primary systemic amyloidosis. *Journal of Laboratory and Clinical Medicine*, **47**, 365–369.

Saeed, S. M. & Fine, G. (1967) Thioflavin-T for amyloid detection. *American Journal of Clinical Pathology*, **47**, 588–593.

Sagher, F. & Shanon, J. (1963) Amyloidosis cutis: familial occurrence in three generations. *Archives of Dermatology*, **87**, 171–175.

Sander, S. (1964) Whipple's disease associated with amyloidosis. *Acta pathologica et microbiologica scandinavica*, **61**, 530–536.

Scheinberg, M. A. & Cathcart, E. S. (1974) Casein induced experimental amyloidosis, III. Response to mitogens, allogeneic cells and graft versus host reactions in the murine model. *Immunology*, **27**, 953–963.

Scheinberg, M. M., Goldstein, A. L. & Cathcart, E. S. (1976) Thymosin restores T cell function and reduces the incidence of amyloid disease in casein treated mice. *Journal of Immunology*, **116**, 156–161.

Scheinberg, M. A. & Cathcart, E. S. (1976) Casein induced experimental amyloidosis VI. A pathologic role for B cells in the murine model (in press).

Schober, R. & Nelson, D. (1975) Fine structure and origin of amyloid deposits in pituitary adenoma. *Archives of Pathology*, **99**, 403–410.

Schwartz, P. (1965) Senile cerebral pancreatic insular and cardiac amyloidosis. *Transactions of New York Academy of Sciences*, **27**, 393–413.

Schwartz, P. (1970) *Amyloidosis: Cause and Manifestation of Senile Deterioration*, 1st ed. Springfield, Illinois: Thomas.

Shibolet, S., Merker, H. J., Sohar, E., Gafni, J. & Heller, H. (1967) Cellular proliferation during the development of amyloid. *British Journal of Experimental Pathology*, **48**, 244–249.

Shirahama, T. & Cohen, A. S. (1965) Structure of amyloid fibrils after negative staining and high resolution electron microscopy. *Nature, (London)*, **206**, 737–738.

Shirahama, T. & Cohen, A. S. (1967) High resolution electron microscopic analysis of the amyloid fibril. *Journal of Cell Biology*, **33**, 679–685.

Shirahama, T. & Cohen, A. S. (1973) An analysis of the close relationship of lysosomes to early deposits of amyloid. *American Journal of Pathology*, **73**, 97–107.

Shirahama, T. & Cohen, A. S. (1974) Blockage of amyloid induction by colchicine in an animal model. *Journal of Experimental Medicine*, **140**, 1102–1107.

Shirahama, T., Benson, M. D., Cohen, A. S. & Tanaka, A. (1973) Fibrillar assemblage of various segments of immunoglobulin light chains: an electron microscopic study. *Journal of Immunology*, **110**, 21–29.

Shmueli, U., Gafni, J., Sohar, E. & Ashkenazi, Y. (1969) An x-ray study of amyloid. *Journal of Molecular Biology*, **41**, 309–311.

Shuttleworth, J. S. & Ross, H. (1956) Secondary amyloidosis in leprosy. *Annals of Internal Medicine*, **45**, 23–38.

Siegal, S. (1945) Benign paroxysmal peritonitis. *Annals of Internal Medicine*, **23**, 1–21.

Skinner, M. & Cohen, A. S. (1971) N-terminal amino-acid analysis of the amyloid fibril protein. *Biochimica et biophysica acta*, **236**, 183–190.

Skinner, M., Cathcart, E. S., Cohen, A. S. & Benson, M. D. (1974a) Isolation and identification by sequence analysis of experimentally induced guinea-pig amyloid fibrils. *Journal of Experimental Medicine*, **140**, 871–876.

Skinner, M., Cohen, A. S., Shirahama, T. & Cathcart, E. S. (1974b) P-component (pentagonal unit) of amyloid: isolation, characterization and sequence analysis. *Journal of Laboratory and Clinical Medicine*, **84**, 604–614.

Sletten, K. & Husby, G. (1974) The complete amino acid sequence of non-immunoglobulin amyloid fibril protein AS in rheumatoid arthritis. *European Journal of Biochemistry*, **41**, 117–120.

Sletten, K., Westermark, P. & Natvig, J. B. (1976) Characterization of amyloid fibrillar proteins from medullary thyroid carcinoma. *Journal of Experimental Medicine*, **143**, 993–998.

Smetana, H. (1925) Experimental study of amyloid formation. *Bulletin of Johns Hopkins Hospital*, **37**, 383–391.

Sorenson, G. D. & Bari, W. A. (1968) Murine amyloid deposits and cellular relationships. In *Amyloidosis*, ed. Mandema, E., Ruinen, L., Scholten, J. H. & Cohen, A. S. Amsterdam: Excerpta Medica Foundation.

Sorenson, G. D. & Binington, H. B. (1964) Resistance of murine amyloid fibrils to proteolytic enzymes. *Federation Proceedings*, **23**, 550 (Abstract).

Sorenson, G. D. & Shimamura, T. (1964) Experimental amyloidosis, III. Light and electron microscopic observations of renal glomeruli. *Laboratory Investigation*, **13**, 1409–1417.

Spiro, D. (1959) The structural basis of proteinuria in man. Electron microscopic studies of renal biopsy specimens from patients with lipid nephrosis, amyloidosis and subacute and chronic glomerulonephritis. *American Journal of Pathology*, **35**, 47–59.

Sterba, J. (1968) Metastasierendes Bronchialkarzinoid mit Amyloid in Stroma. *Zeitblatt allergische Pathologie, pathologische Anatomie*, **111**, 555–561.

Symmers, W. St C. (1956) Primary amyloidosis: a review. *Journal of Clinical Pathology*, **9**, 187–211.

Tan, M. & Epstein, W. (1972) Polymer formation during degradation of human light chains and Bence Jones proteins by an extract of the lysosomal fraction of normal human kidney. *Immunochemistry*, **9**, 9–16.

Tashjian, A. H., Wolfe, H. J. & Voelkel, E. F. (1974) Human calcitonin. *American Journal of Medicine*, **56**, 840–849.

Taylor, D. L., Allen, R. D. & Benditt, E. P. (1974) Determination of the polarization optical properties of the amyloid–congo red complex by phase modulation microspectrophotometry. *Journal of Histochemistry and Cytochemistry*, **22**, 1105–1112.

Teilum, G. (1952) Cortisone–ascorbic acid interaction and the pathogenesis of amyloid mechanism of cortisone on mesenchimal tissue. *Annals of Rheumatic Diseases*, **11**, 119–136.

Teilum, G. (1956) Periodic acid Schiff-positive reticuloendothelial cells producing glycoprotein: functional significance during formation of amyloid. *American Journal of Pathology*, **32**, 945–959.

Teilum, G. (1964) Amyloidosis secondary to agammaglobulinemia. *Journal of Pathology and Bacteriology*, **88**, 317–320.

Teilum, G. (1968) In *Amyloidosis*, ed. Mandema, E., Ruinen, L., Scholten, J H. & Cohen, A. S., pp. 37–44. Amsterdam: Excerpta Medica Foundation.

Teilum, G. & Lindahl, A. (1954) Frequency and significance of amyloid changes in rheumatoid arthritis. *Acta medica scandinavica*, **149**, 449–455.

Terry, R. D., Gonatas, N. K. & Weiss, M. (1964) Ultrastructural studies in Alzheimer's pre-senile dementia. *American Journal of Pathology*, **44**, 269–297.

Terry, W. D., Page, D. L., Kimura, S., Isobe, I., Osserman, E. F. & Glenner, G. G. (1973) Structural identity of Bence Jones and amyloid fibril proteins in a patient with plasma cell cyscrasia and amyloidosis. *Journal of Clinical Investigation*, **52**, 1276–1281.

Thung, P. J. (1957) Senile amyloidosis in mice. *Gerontologia*, **1**, 259–279.

Vazquez, J. J. & Dixon, F. J. (1956) Immunochemical analysis of amyloid by the fluorescent technique. *Journal of Experimental Medicine*, **104**, 727–734.

Vickers, R. A., Dahlin, D. C. & Gorlin, R. J. (1965) Amyloid-containing odontogenic tumors. *Oral Surgery, Oral Medicine and Oral Pathology*, **20**, 476–480.

Virchow, R. (1854) Ueber eine im Gehirn und Rückenmark des Menschen aufgefundene substanz mit der chemischen Reaction der Cellulose. *Virchows Archiv (Pathologische Anatomie)*, **6**, 135–151.

Von Rokitansky, C. F. (1846) *Handbuch der pathologischen Anatomie*, Vol. 3. Vienna: Braumuller U. Seidel.

Wald, M. H. (1955) Clinical studies of secondary amyloidosis in tuberculosis. *Annals of Internal Medicine*, **43**, 383–395.

Waldenstrom, H. (1928) On formation and disappearance of amyloid in man. *Acta chirurgica scandinavica*, **63**, 479–530.

Wallace, S. L., Fedeinam, D. J., Berlin, I., Harris, C. & Glass, A. G. (1950) Amyloidosis in Hodgkin's disease. *American Journal of Medicine*, **8**, 552–557.

Waugh, D. F. (1946) A fibrous modification of insulin. I. The heat precipitate of insulin. *Journal of American Chemical Society*, **68**, 247–250.

Westermark, P. (1974) On the nature of amyloid in human islets of Langerhans. *Histochemistry*, **38**, 27–33.

Westermark, P., Skinner, M. & Cohen, A. S. (1975) The P-component of amyloid human islets of Langerhans. *Scandinavian Journal of Immunology*, **4**, 95–97.

Westermark, P., Natvig, J. B., Anders, R. F., Sletten, K. & Husby, G. (1976) Coexistence of protein AA and immunoglobulin light chain fragments in amyloid fibrils. *Scandinavian Journal of Immunology*, **5**, 31–36.

White, G. C., II, Jacobson, R. J., Binder, R. A., Linke, R. P. & Glenner, G. G. (1975) Immunoglobulin D myeloma and amyloidosis. Immunochemical and structural studies of Bence Jones and amyloid fibrillar proteins. *Blood*, **46**, 713–722.

Williams, R. C., Jr & Law, D. H. (1960) Serum complement in amyloidosis. *Journal of Laboratory and Clinical Medicine*, **56**, 629–633.

Wilks, S. (1856) Cases of lardaceous disease and some allied affections: with remarks. *Guy's Hospital Report Series*, **3** (2), 103–109.

Wisnievski, H. M. & Terry, R. D. (1975) Reexamination of the pathogenesis of the senile plaque. *Progress in Neuropathology*, **2**, 1–25.

Wolman, M. & Bubis, J. J. (1965) The cause of the green polarization color of amyloid stained with Congo red. *Histochemie*, **4**, 351–359.

Wolman, M. (1971) Amyloid, its nature and molecular structure; comparison of a new toluidine blue polarized light method. *Laboratory Investigation*, **25**, 104–110.

Zucker-Franklin, D. (1970) Immunophagocytosis of human amyloid fibrils by leukocytes. *Journal of Ultrastructural Research*, **32**, 247–257.

Zucker-Franklin, D. & Franklin, E. C. (1970) Intracellular localization of human amyloid by fluorescence and electron microscopy. *American Journal of Pathology*, **59**, 23–42.

Zucker-Franklin, D. (1976) Study on the cellular origin of the AA protein. *Conference on Amyloidosis*, Helsinki, August 1974, ed. Wigelius, O. & Pasternak, A. New York and London: Academic Press.

4

AGEING AND IMMUNE FUNCTION

William H. Adler   Kenneth H. Jones   Hideo Nariuchi

The study of immune function in ageing mammals is currently attracting a great deal of interest. The findings that, in some instances, certain functional characteristics of the immune system decrease with age have spurred these studies. One reason that these studies are pursued with enthusiasm is the belief that an age-associated immune deficiency may have a causative role to play in the pathogenesis of age-related diseases, and the correction of this immunodeficiency may result in the modulation of ageing phenomena so that some of the manifestations of ageing can be changed.

There are many difficulties with this manipulative approach to age-associated disorders of immune function, the primary one being the nature of the ageing process itself. Ageing must be viewed as a normal, pathogenetic process; but when does the process start? At what point can you assay an immune response and say that it represents an ageing effect —or a lack of an ageing effect? If one must wait until the appearance of an age-related disease to show a decrease in immune function, then one must deal with pathogenetic factors in addition to ageing which might affect declining functions of the immune system. Therefore, from the very basic problems in deciding what constitutes an age-related immunodeficiency, there must be further consideration of what assay to use, what to infer from the results of the assay, what to predict in terms of function in other systems and what a deficiency might mean in terms of disease susceptibility.

In this chapter, the manifestations of an age-related immunodeficiency will be examined. The assays used in animal and human experimental models will be compared in order to arrive at an appreciation of the whole organism's functional capability. The possible effects of the deficiency will also be considered. At present the knowledge of normal immunological function remains, to a large extent, inadequate. As such, the appreciation of the mechanism of age-associated immune deficiency must be severely limited and definite conclusions would be premature. Table 4.1 summarises the clinical and experimental findings in age-associated changes of immunological function. These are general findings in the species studied, mainly humans and mice. Not all of the assays listed have been used universally and, therefore, some findings only apply to certain species.

T- AND B-LYMPHOCYTES

The lymphoreticular system can be defined as those tissues normally containing accumulations of lymphocytes within the interstices of a reticular meshwork. The system is, understandably, diffuse throughout the body since it includes both the formed encapsulated lymphoid organs (spleen, thymus, lymph nodes) and the unencapsulated, often transient lymphoid follicles (e.g. follicles found in the lamina propria of the gastrointestinal and respiratory tracts).

Although it is convenient to collect all of the tissues of the lymphoid system together

Table 4.1   Summary of age-associated changes in immunological parameters

I.	Stem cells	
	Generally sufficient in number and functional capability	
II.	Thymic influence	
	Morphological involution of thymus gland	
	Possible decrease in thymic hormonal effects	
III.	'T' lymphocytes—responsible for cellular immunity which provides host defence against fungi, mycobacteria, intracellular parasites, some viruses and bacteria, and probably tumours	
	In vivo findings:	
	Allograft rejection	
	Graft-versus-host reaction	All decreased
	Delayed hypersensitivity	
	Lymphocyte proliferation in peripheral T-dependent areas	
	In vitro findings:	
	Cell-mediated cytotoxicity	
	Mixed lymphocyte culture	All decreased
	Mitogen stimulation by Con A and PHA	
	Rosette formation with sheep erythrocytes (humans)	Possibly decreased
	Interferon production by splenic T cells (mice)	Increased
IV.	'B' Lymphocytes—antibody synthesizing cells which provide humoral immunity against some bacteria and viruses, bacterial products/toxins, and probably tumours	
	In vivo findings:	
	Normal to increased numbers of 'B' cells	
	Increased numbers of spontaneous 'errors' (autoantibodies and excess homogeneous antibody)	
	Serum immunoglobulin levels	No change
	Antibody production in response to specific antigens—	
	(a) Thymus-dependent antigens	Decreased
	(b) Thymus-independent antigens	Increased
	Germinal centre formation in peripheral lymphoid tissue	Decreased
	In vitro findings:	
	Membrane immunoglobulin-positive fluorescence	No change
	LPS[a] stimulation (mice)	Increased
	Plaque-forming cells—	
	(a) Thymus-dependent	
	(b) Thymus-independent	Decreased
V.	Interaction between cells	
	Helper T-cell functions (mice)	Decreased
	Suppressor T-cell functions (mice)	Increased
	Macrophage functions	Probably unchanged

[a] Bacterial lipo-polysaccharide

on the basis of their most common morphological feature, the lymphocyte, such a single criterion obscures the functional identity of the various components. Indeed, investigations of the last 15 years have revealed that the homogeneous appearing lymphocytes are physiologically heterogeneous subpopulations of cells specialised to interact with each other and/or mediate specific host-immune responses.

Lymphocytes are ultimately derived from the multipotential haematopoietic stem cells, the origin of which has been traced to the embryonic yolk sac. Such cells migrate to the fetal liver and eventually to the bone marrow where they are found in the adult. It is from the multipotential stem cells of the bone marrow that the lymphoid progenitor cells arise and whose progeny colonise the thymus and peripheral lymphoid organs (Ford et al, 1966; Owen and Ritter, 1969; Owen and Raff, 1970). Further differentiation of lymphoid precursor cells into immunocompetent lymphocytes depends on the microenvironment in which such development takes place (Trentin, Wolf and Curry, 1969).

It has been determined by studying human immune-deficiency diseases and by animal experiments involving extirpation of the thymus and bursa of Fabricius that there exists at least two functionally different main classes of lymphocytes referred to as 'T' cells and 'B' cells (Gitlin et al, 1959; Roitt et al, 1969). Lymphoid precursor cells which lodge in the thymic subcapsular cortex differentiate into thymocytes. Some of these thymocytes migrate from the thymus to the peripheral lymphoid tissues (Weissman, 1967), where they are called 'T' cells, and selectively occupy the periarteriolar sheath of the splenic white pulp, the paracortical areas of lymph nodes and the interfollicular areas of the un-encapsulated lymphoid follicles; these anatomical sites are collectively referred to as *thymus-dependent* areas (Parrott, DeSousa and East, 1966). The B-cell differentiates under the influence of the bursa of Fabricius in birds (Warner et al, 1969) and a bursal equivalent, possibly the bone marrow, in mammals (Unanue et al, 1971). B-cells are found histologically in the *thymus-independent* areas: the follicles and medullary cords of lymph nodes, and the lymphoid follicles of the spleen and gastrointestinal tract (Parrott and DeSousa, 1971). Both T- and B-cells recirculate through their respective lymphoid compartments although it is likely that proportionately fewer B-cells recirculate and at a slower rate than do T-cells (Howard, Hunt and Gowans, 1972).

Morphologically murine T-cells can be identified by the presence of a specific antigenic membrane marker called *theta*, 'θ' (Raff, 1969), and human T-cells are able to form rosettes with sheep erythrocytes. Physiologically T-cells initiate *cell-mediated immunity*, those immunological reactions which can be transferred by cells and not by serum. Such immunity is important in host defence against viruses, fungi, and mycobacteria (Mackaness, 1971; Alder and Rabinowitz, 1973). In addition T-cells play an active role in delayed hypersensitivity, graft rejection, graft-versus-host reactions, antitumour immunity, and also elaborate lymphokines.

It is now known that B-cells can be distinguished from T-cells by the presence of membrane immunoglobulins and Fc and complement receptors on their surfaces. Functionally, B-cells differentiate into cells which synthesise and secrete antibody and, therefore, are responsible for *humoral immunity*, immunological responses which can be transferred by serum. Such immunity includes immediate hypersensitivity, Arthus reactions and specific antibody production. Although B-cells may be stimulated directly by some antigens with a large number of repeating identical determinants, T-cells are usually required to perform some *helper function* in initiating antibody production by B-cells.

Recent careful study of the normal physiology of lymphocytes reveals a more complex system than just outlined. Investigations have only just begun to describe the subpopulations which exist within T- and B-cell classes. The study of the interactions between the various subpopulations of T- and B-cells, and between lymphocytes and such cells as macrophages, granulocytes, and mast cells must be pursued in order to better understand the mechanisms of the immune system.

NORMAL MORPHOLOGICAL CHANGES WITH AGEING

It has been well established that lymphoid tissues undergo morphological changes with age. Andrew (1952) has reviewed much of the older literature on the gross and micro-anatomical changes associated with the ageing of the lymphoid system. He noted that the accumulated evidence, in general, indicates a maximum size for lymphoid organs immediately after puberty, and there is a reduction in absolute size with advancing age. The involution witnessed is an atrophic process involving a decrease in the number of cellular elements present.

In mice, the maximum relative thymic weight is reached at 15 days of age. A sharp exponential decrease in thymic weight relative to body weight occurs throughout the remainder of the lifespan (Pepper, 1961). The principal microanatomical change seen in the thymus with advancing age is atrophy of the lymphoid tissue, chiefly in the cortex, and its replacement by connective tissue.

Similar but less dramatic atrophic changes are seen in the spleen and lymph nodes of ageing mammals. Spleen and lymph node weights decrease very gradually with advancing age. In the spleen, there is a decrease in the amount of white pulp and a relative increase in the amount of red pulp. Accompanying the decrease in the amount of follicular tissue is a loss of the distinctness in the two zones of the splenic follicle, as well as in the de-marcation between the red and white pulps. Splenic germinal centres are not normally seen in older individuals. Although there is only a slight decrease in lymph node weights during ageing, histological changes are striking. The lymph nodes of older individuals show a decrease in the thickness of the cortical areas with germinal centres greatly reduced in number, if present at all. In addition the boundary between cortex and medulla becomes obscured by diffusely distributed plasma cells, and there is an increased number of macrophages in the medulla. The lymph nodes of old animals are also characterised by dilated medullary sinuses.

Although the organised lymphoid organs undergo more or less regressive changes with advancing age of the individual, there is good evidence for an actual increase in the amount of diffuse lymphoid tissues throughout the body. Thus, in ageing mammals there is a striking increase in the number of lymphoid follicles found in the bone marrow, salivary glands, portal triads, and lung parenchyma (Andrew, 1952; Walford, 1969).

ASSESSMENT OF IMMUNOLOGICAL FUNCTIONS

Stem cells

In the consideration of age-associated defects in immune function an obvious starting point is stem cell function. If an immune system is to continue to deal with different anti-genic challenges throughout life, a supply of immunocompetent cells must be available. Studies on stem cell function in ageing mice indicate that there are more than enough cells available, but that there may be a defect in differentiation of these cells in an ageing host (Price and Makinodan, 1972a; Harrison and Doubleday, 1975). However, a problem in studying murine stem cells is that the results show great variation between genetically defined strains (Farrar, Loughman and Nordin, 1974). Therefore, if genetic factors have a strong influence, then stem cell functions in ageing humans may vary greatly and be very difficult to predict. Other factors which may account for the disparity in results could be the greater susceptibility of some strains of mice to certain age-related diseases or tumours which could affect the stem cell assay. It could also be that although sufficient numbers of these precursor cells are generated, many might be defective and be responsible for altered functions, such as the production of auto- or monoclonal immunoprotein.

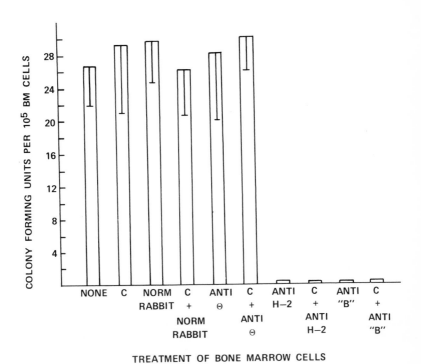

Figure 4.1   C57 Bl/6 bone marrow cells were treated with complement (C) with or without various sera (normal rabbit, anti-θ, anti-H-2, anti-'B' cell). The antisera in the absence of C did not cause cytotoxicity. After treatment the bone marrow cells were administered intravenously into lethally irradiated C57 Bl/6 recipients and the number of spleen colonies (CFU) were determined nine days later

Another difficulty in measuring stem cell function is that morphological criteria for stem cell identification are vague, and without such identification one must rely on a functional assay such as colony-forming units. In this assay each colony represents the progeny of a single stem cell. Recent experiments show that antiserum prepared in rabbits against lymph nodes from athymic mice (an anti-B-cell serum) completely abrogates the colony-forming capacity of stem cells from young adults without killing the stem cells (Figure 4.1). Therefore, it cannot be assumed that the reduced number of colony-forming units from the bone marrow of aged mice indicates a deficiency in the number of stem cells, since stem cells might be present but altered to the point of not performing in the assay system. Failure to perform in the CFU assay might be explained by a possible change in the homing-pattern of the stem cells to the spleen, or the possibility that old mice could have an autoantibody against their own stem cells.

T-cells

It appears fairly clear that although the number of T-cells may be decreased in aged individuals, as measured by morphological criteria such as a decreased sheep red cell rosetting population in the peripheral blood from humans and a decrease in θ-positive cells in the lymphoid tissue of mice, the decrease is not dramatic. The range of values in all age groups overlaps a great deal. In some cases the number of T-cells are the same in all age groups studied; and in other cases the proportion of T-cells may decrease, but the absolute number of T-cells remains the same (Augener et al, 1974; Stutman, 1974b; Weksler and Hutteroth, 1974; Diaz-Jouanen, Williams and Strickland, 1975; Alexopoulous and Babitis, 1976). When a variety of assays based on functional criteria are used, it is found consistently that T-cell function is quite deficient in older humans and animals. However, the assay employed can determine the nature of the results obtained. For example, in assaying T-cell helper function by measuring antibody formation in response to antigens which require T-cell cooperation with B-cells, the results could possibly be misleading since adequate B-cell function is also necessary for the response. Even if one uses a purely T-cell functional assay, in the final analysis it is necessary to determine a relevance in terms of overall immune function.

PHA MITOGENIC ASSAY

In animals and humans several assays for a T-cell function do exist. These are usually in vitro assays, for instance, the short-term lymphocyte culture system in which phyto-haemmagglutinin (PHA) is added. The observation has been made that a response to PHA in terms of lymphocytic proliferation with attendant morphological changes and DNA synthesis requires the presence of a thymus in the cell donor (Takiguchi, Adler and Smith, 1971). Neonatal thymectomy in mice, or the absence of thymic development in humans, can result in a failure of lymphocyte response to PHA. The results of the assay in both of the above conditions are easy to interpret and to assign to an abnormal group when compared to a 'normal' lymphocytic PHA response of lymphocytes. The difficulties arise when the human or animal lymphocytes display a 'lower than normal response'. The interpretation of such a result is difficult: (1) because of wide variation in the response of different individuals' lymphocytes to PHA, (2) because no one knows at what level of a decreased response one will begin to detect a causative effect in terms of disease, (3) because the cellular proliferation kinetics of an in vitro assay can be influenced by technical problems inherent in the culture system, and (4) because the cells being assayed represent only one tissue, organ, or in the case of humans, the peripheral blood which is not a lymphoid organ. Each of these difficulties must be considered before making the diagnosis of an immune deficiency, or T-cell functional loss.

In a study of healthy young adults, McIntyre and Cole (1969) found tremendous variation in the response of each person's peripheral blood lymphocytes to PHA. No reason for this daily or weekly variation could be determined. Other studies show that not only does an individual's response vary from day to day (White, Adler and McGann, 1974; Golub, Sulit and Morton, 1975) but the variation within a human population is such as to establish a very wide range of normal responses in terms of the levels of PHA-stimulated DNA synthesis. The variation in the spleen cell response to PHA in an inbred strain of young mice is not as marked as in the human. If, however, the data from mice of several different strains are pooled, wide variation is found (Adler et al, 1970). In addition, one can find variation in a mouse lymphocyte response to PHA, conconavalin A (Con A) and bacterial lipopolysaccharide (LPS) which follows a cyclical pattern (Brock, unpublished). The variability of results not only makes the assay of questionable value, but it complicates any experiment that seeks to improve a low responding system by use of cell transfers or thymic transplant. In an outbred, closed colony of rats, the variation in PHA response of spleen cells is again very marked (Fig. 4.2) so that it is truly difficult to define an abnormally low response, that is, anything higher than no response. Therefore, the identification of such a low responder in prospect is difficult and cannot be made on age criteria alone.

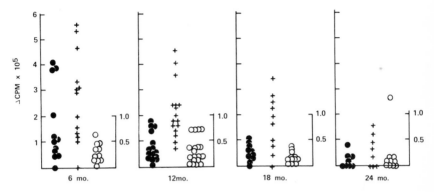

Figure 4.2   Spleen cells from Wistar rats of varying ages were cultured in RPMI-1640 with 2 per cent heat inactivated human serum. 2×10^5 cells in 0.2 ml media were cultured for three days with PHA (●), Con A (+), or LPS (○) with tritiated thymidine (1 μCi) present for the final 6 h. The results are expressed as the mean CPM in the TCA precipitated material from five replicate stimulated cultures minus the mean CPM of non-stimulated cultures. The expanded CPM scale on the right of each age group refers only to LPS stimulated cultures

The attempt to correlate a level of a PHA response and a level of immune deficiency which could lead to disease is difficult, as demonstrated by the study of inbred strains of mice. In mice a great difference can be seen even within an H-2 genotype. Although DBA/2 (H-2^d) mice are poor responders to PHA, BALB/c (H-2^d) mice are among the best responders. Therefore, the number of T-cells responding to PHA is greater in the spleens from BALB/c than it is in DBA/2 mice, and yet there is no evidence of specific disorders in DBA/2 mice which could be accounted for by this deficit. In humans and animals many infectious disorders may be dealt with efficiently by other mechanisms, such as granulocytes, so that a relatively T-cell deficient animal or human may have few problems over an extended period of time.

The difficulties with the kinetics of the culture system can be demonstrated easily. In any culture system, there is a medium which supplies the cells with vital factors. Also, the media has a buffer system to deal with the incubation atmosphere and the hydrogen ion production of the metabolically active cells. Changes in the medium's ability to support vital functions will be more extensive in cultures with a greater number of metabolising, dividing and growing cells. Therefore an active culture will deplete medium of both nutrients and buffering capacity more quickly than will a slower culture containing fewer stimulated cells. Using x-irradiation as a damaging agent and then comparing the kinetics of cultures containing damaged cells to cultures with normal cells, it is evident that the normal cells reach maximum DNA synthesis earlier than do damaged cells (Fig. 4.3A); then DNA synthesis in normal cell cultures declines during the time when DNA synthesis in the damaged cells cultures is still increasing. When assayed after two or three days, the normal cells perform better than the damaged cells; after four or five days the damaged cells show greater DNA synthesis compared to the normal cells. However, if the overall

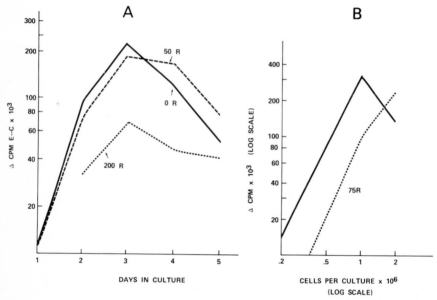

Figure 4.3   (A) C57 B1/6 spleen cells, normal or irradiated with 50 to 200 rad, were cultivated at 5 × 10⁵ cells per 0.2 ml in RPMI-1640 plus 5 per cent inactivated human serum. The cultures were stimulated with Con A and at varying periods tritiated thymidine was added for the final 6 h of culture. Results are expressed as the mean CPM value of five replicate Con A stimulated samples minus the mean CPM of the non-stimulated background control cultures. (B) C57 B1/6 spleen cells, normal or irradiated with 75 rad, were distributed into 0.2 ml cultures in varying concentrations and stimulated with LPS. The cultures were maintained as usual, with tritiated thymidine present for the final 6 h of a three-day culture period

amount of DNA synthesis is determined for a full five-day period, there is no difference between normal and damaged cells.

Another variation of this same problem can be demonstrated by culturing the normal and the damaged cells at varying densities (Fig. 4.3B). At lower densities, 1 × 10⁵ to 5 × 10⁵ lymphocytes per culture, the normal cells will outperform the damaged cells in terms of DNA synthesis in a three-day culture assay. However, at a higher density, 1 × 10⁶ to 2 × 10⁶ cells per culture, the damaged cells will now perform better than the normal because at higher cell densities the media cannot support the level of metabolic activity in the normal cell cultures. These are only two examples of factors in a cell culture system which can markedly influence the results and make things appear to be what they are not.

An additional consideration in the possible problems associated with even a single assay system, like a mitogen response, is the variability seen in each tissue studied and what this might mean in terms of immune function in the whole animal or human. If there is no response to PHA by lymphocytes from the spleen or other lymphoid tissue or by peripheral blood lymphocytes, one can make the case that the individual human or animal is T-cell deficient in terms of this assay. However, in mice where all lymphoid tissues can be examined it can be found that lymphocytes from some lymphoid tissues respond to PHA while cells from other lymphoid organs from the same animal may not (Fig. 4.4). Further-

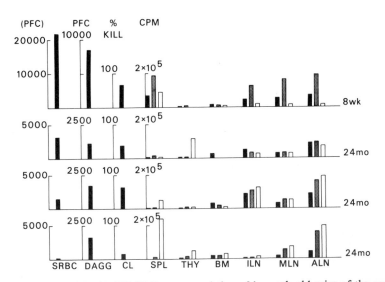

Figure 4.4 One eight-week old C57 Bl/6 mouse and three 24-month old mice of the same strain were examined using a variety of assay systems. Sheep red blood cell (SRBC) antibody producing spleen cells generated in an in vitro Mishell Dutton culture system were assayed in the plaque forming cell system (PFC/spleen). Cells producing antibody to a T independent antigen (DAGG-Ficoll) were assayed in the same type system after a five-day in vitro culture (PFC/spleen). Cytotoxic lymphocytes (CL) were generated in an allogeneic mixed lymphocyte culture (MLC) versus DBA/2 spleen cells and assayed on P-815 mastocytoma cells labelled with chromium-51. Results are expressed as percentage target cells (P-815) killed in a 1.5 h incubation with cultured lymphocytes derived from 2×10^6 cells. Mitogen assays were conducted as described in Figure 4.3 using PHA (■) Con A (▨) and LPS (□) to stimulate spleen cell cultures (SPL), thymic cell cultures (THY), bone marrow cells (BM), inguinal (ILN), mesenteric (MLN) and axillary (ALN) lymph node cell cultures. Results demonstrate individual variability of the old mice in terms of the level of performance in each assay and the level of performance of each tissue

more, there may be variation within a group of mice as to which lymphoid organs contain cells which will or will not respond. In humans, it is certainly more convenient to assay blood lymphocytes, but it might be erroneous to say that the results of such an assay truly reflect the state of the entire immune system.

The shortcomings of PHA reactivity as an assay of T-cell function lead to the conclusion that as a test its use is limited and only general statements of a predictive nature in terms of other functional assays or of overall immune status can be made. This is true in the mouse, where the PHA reactivity of spleen cells from relatively middle-aged mice of many different strains can effectively be zero before other immune assays can be seen to decrease (Hori, Perkins and Halsall, 1973; Walters and Claman, 1975). In humans, the PHA reactivity rarely reaches zero (Pisciotta et al, 1967; Hallgren et al, 1973; Weksler and

Hutteroth, 1974) so the problems in interpretation are even greater. For this reason, there has been a great deal of attention to other assays of T-cell function in ageing although in humans the assays available are limited.

DELAYED HYPERSENSITIVITY REACTIONS

An in vivo, non-mitogenic assay for T-cell function is the type of skin test which elicits a delayed hypersensitivity response (Najarian and Feldman, 1963). It has been reported that the skin test reaction to tuberculin does diminish or disappear with age in humans (Giannini and Sloan, 1967; Waldorf, Wilkins and Decker, 1968) while in mice no decrease is seen (Walters and Claman, 1975). The problems with this assay are that a negative reaction may reflect a lack of a previous sensitisation with the antigen or there may be a selection favouring non-reactors in an ageing population. Additionally, the development of anergy resulting from the presence of certain diseases may cause the lack of reactivity. Finally, there may be changes in the ageing skin which are less conducive to the elicitation of the test response.

Using mice as the experimental model more assays for T-cell function can be performed. Three areas have been examined in detail, and in all these assays the T-cells from aged mice perform poorly. In general, the difficulty in interpreting the results remains in the variability one finds in the response of the old mice, even within an inbred strain, and in correlating the performances found among the different assays. Antigens which require a T-cell–B-cell interaction, such as sheep red blood cells, have been shown to elicit a poor antibody forming response in old mice, either when the antigen is given in vivo or when the antigen is added to an in vitro culture system (Makinodan and Peterson, 1964; Wigzell and Stjernswärd, 1966; Nordin and Makinodan, 1974). The poor response could be attributable to a variety of possible causes which involve either an absence of a functional T-cell or the presence of a cell population which inhibits the development of an antibody-forming cell population. The mechanism of such suppression is not at all clear (Folch and Waksman, 1974; Segre and Segre, 1976b; Hirano and Nordin, 1975). There is evidence that B-cells in the old mice are also at fault in a poor antibody response (Kishimoto, Takahama and Mizumachi, 1976).

MIXED LYMPHOCYTE REACTIONS

Mixed lymphocyte cultures (MLC) and T-cell dependent cytotoxicity are both T-cell assays which supposedly measure the ability of T-cells to proliferate (MLC) and to differentiate into cytotoxic killer cells (CTL). In the MLC, the reacting lymphoid cells from one strain of mouse are mixed in culture with a second, stimulating cell population from a different strain of mouse. The stimulator cells differ from the reactor cells by crucial genetic and antigenic factors, and therefore induce a proliferative response by the reactor cells. Generally in the MLC assay the proliferative capacity of T-cells decreases with advancing age (Weksler and Hutteroth, 1974; Adler, Takiguchi and Smith, 1971a). A major finding in this area is that much of the decrease in T-cell proliferation occurs at a relatively young age although this is not true in all mouse strains tested—again an indication of possible genetic considerations (Walters and Claman, 1975). Another feature of the MLC is that some of the cells in the reactor population can develop into CTL capable of killing target cells which are syngeneic to the stimulatory cells in the original MLC (Häyry and Defendi, 1970). However, results of the MLC and CTL assays do not always correlate. For example it has been found that although spleen cells from 18-month old

C57 Bl/6 mice respond poorly in an MLC, the cells develop only slightly lower than normal cytotoxic ability when compared to the cells from three-month old mice (Fig. 4.5). This may reflect a sensitivity difference between the two assay systems, but it may also indicate that the assays are actually measuring a function of two different T-cell sub-populations. By 30 months, however, the cytotoxic response also is greatly diminished so that at this age both the MLC and CTL show low response levels.

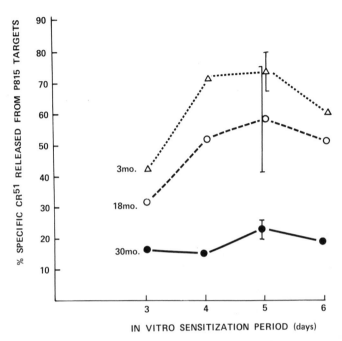

Figure 4.5 In these experiments spleen cells from various age C57 Bl/6 mice (- - - - - - 3 months) (– – – – 18 months) (——— 30 months) were incubated with mitomycin-C treated DBA/2 spleen cells for three, four, five, or six days, then assayed on each day for a cytotoxic effect on chromium-labelled P-815 mastocytoma cells. Results are expressed as the mean ($\pm$s.d.) of chromium release from the P-815 cells after incubation for 3 h with a lymphocyte to target cell ratio of 50:1

Further inconsistencies in MLC and the development of cytotoxic effectors can be mirrored in various experiments conducted on immunodeficient chimeric mice (Fig. 4.6). C3H mice, x-irradiated and repopulated with DBA/2 spleen cells, develop into adults with lymphoid tissue populated with cells carrying the H-2^d antigen of the DBA/2 strain (Dauphinee and Nordin, 1974). These mice have spleen cells which contain only one-fourth the number of θ-positive cells, have a poor reactivity to T-cell mitogens, but have excellent reactivity to alloantigen-carrying target cells in MLCs. The level is above that found with either DBA/2 or C3H mouse spleen cells. However, in spite of the increased level of MLC reactivity, the generation of cytotoxic lymphocytes is negligible. It may be, as stated before, that these assays are testing subpopulations or combinations of sub-populations of T-cells and, as such, cannot be correlated.

It is also possible that some of these assays may not be measuring a T-cell function at all (Fig. 4.7). It has been shown that athymic, nude mice, a congenitally T-cell deficient mouse, lack θ-positive cells, show no response to T-cell mitogens, and do not generate cytotoxic T-lymphocytes. Yet spleen cells from nude mice can respond normally in MLC. These experimental results using immunodeficient mice cast some doubt on the interpretation of the mixed cell culture as a T-cell assay procedure.

If one considers the ability of bone marrow from young or old mice to induce fatal graft versus host disease, a T-cell function in immunocrippled allogeneic recipients, no differ-

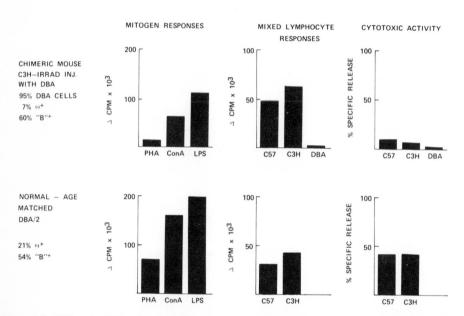

Figure 4.6   Chimeric C3H mice irradiated and then injected with DBA/2 cells at three months of age were tested at 20 months of age using several assays. Their responses were compared to the responses of spleen cells from 20-month old DBA/2 mice. The mitogenic responses were tested as detailed above (Fig. 4.3) in an in vitro culture system. The mixed lymphocyte responses were tested against mitomycin-C treated C57 B1/6, C3H, or DBA/2 cells and thymidine incorporation determined for the final 6 h of a three-day culture period. Results are presented as the mean CPMs in the allogenic cultures less the mean CPMs in syngeneic cultures. Cytotoxic lymphocytic responses generated in MLCs were determined as detailed in Figure 4.5.

ences can be seen in some of the strains tested while in other strains a deficiency can be seen (Peterson et al, 1972; Stutman, 1974b; Walters and Claman, 1975; Nariuchi, unpublished). In some of the strains tested there is obviously an adequate number of immunoprecursor cells in the bone marrow from the old mice since sufficient cells differentiate to kill the host. Furthermore the graft versus host disease progresses in exactly the same time interval in the recipients of old or young allogeneic marrow. Therefore, in this assay some of the old mice have normal MLC reactivity (T-cell function ?) while others have a deficiency.

THYMIC HORMONAL INFLUENCE

There is an age-related morphological and, apparently, a physiological involution of the thymus. How the thymus influences lymphocytes is not known, but precursor cells must physically journey through thymic tissue in order to develop into T-lymphocytes. It is hypothesised that the thymus can then further influence T-lymphocyte development by elaboration of a thymic hormone. If the differentiation of a precursor cell into an immunocompetent T-cell requires thymic influence, it follows that there would be a decrease in the number of immunocompetent T-cells in an aged host. Experiments have shown

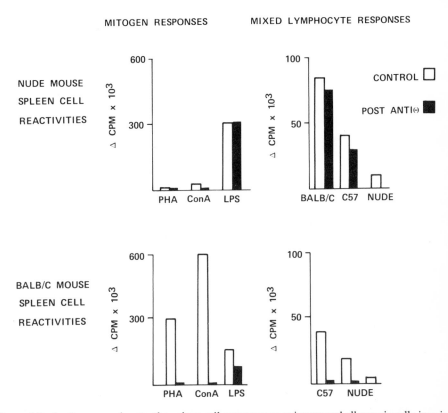

Figure 4.7   In these experiments the spleen cell responses to mitogen and allogeneic cells in mixed lymphocyte cultures were determined for nude mice and normal or heterozygous BALB/c littermates. The responsive cell populations were investigated using an anti-θ plus C treatment prior to culture. The mitogen and MLC cultures were performed as detailed in Figures 4.3 and 4.5

that thymic hormone can increase the number of T-cells in human peripheral blood as determined by the sheep erythrocyte rosetting technique; and thymic hormone can cause an increase of θ-bearing cells in a T-cell deficient mouse (nude mouse). However, thymic hormone has been less successful in engendering the appearance of cells which will respond in assays designed to measure T-cell function. Therefore, thymic hormone has as yet an undecided role to play in reconstituting T-cell deficient humans or mice. There are indications, however, that in humans the level of circulating thymic hormone does decrease with age. Perhaps this reflects a decline in one form of thymic influence, and this results in a decrease of functional T-cells (for a review of this subject see van Bekkum, 1975).

Thymus grafts from different aged mice show a progressive decrease in ability to reconstitute syngeneic, thymectomised mice as judged by a variety of assays. In these experiments thymic influence decreases rapidly with age, far in advance of the appearance of other age-related phenomena (Hirokawa and Makinodan, 1975). Interestingly, the MLC assay is not an assay which is able to detect diminished thymic influence.

B-lymphocytes

In humans and animals there are morphological criteria for identification of B-cells and for determining their presence in the mouse or human (see Ch. 7). The studies are extensive and the results show some discrepancies. It has been reported that the number of Ig-bearing cells in human peripheral blood decreases, increases, or remains constant with age (Weksler and Hutteroth, 1974; Augener et al, 1974; Diaz-Jouanen et al, 1975). The discrepancies probably reflect the considerable variability among individuals and techniques used to identify B-cells or Ig-positive cells (Kunkel, 1975; Vossen and Hijmans, 1975). Furthermore, cells bearing an Fc receptor may complex an anti-immunoglobulin reagent and appear as Ig-positive cells. It is also possible that in an autoimmune disease, there could be a variable percentage of Ig-positive lymphocytes which are actually lymphoid cells with autoantibody on their surfaces. In mice, there are several other B-cell antigens which can be identified using appropriate antisera, and we will consider them next in discussing B-cell functional criteria.

Assays of B-cell functions rely on methods using both mitogens and antigens. Mitogens for mouse, rat and guinea-pig B-cells are the Gram-negative endotoxin lipopolysaccharides (LPS) (Peavy et al, 1973). LPS appears to stimulate B-cells to proliferate and differentiate into immunoprotein-forming cells, and the active mitogenic part of the LPS molecule is lipid A. There is some evidence that the cells which do respond to LPS do not necessarily have to be B-cells. In humans there is no B-cell mitogen although in some cases the peripheral blood cells from some individuals can respond to LPS. Several interesting observations can be made in studying the age-related change in the response of mouse spleen and thymus cells to LPS. The LPS response of spleen cells from several strains of old mice increases with age, sometimes quite dramatically (Fig. 4.4; Makinodan and Adler, 1975). In the mouse, young thymus cell populations respond poorly, if at all, to LPS while thymus cells from older mice can respond in some cases very well to LPS stimulation. On this basis, one could predict that B-cell proliferative function in old mice is as good or better than the function in young animals.

However, a primary consideration is, are the cells responding to LPS actually B-cells? Using a B-cell antiserum it is possible to show that the LPS responsive cells in spleens from young mice are B-cells while the LPS responsive cells in the spleen and thymus from old mice might not be B-cells (Fig. 4.8). It has been shown that there are shifts in the cellular components of the spleen cell population from older mice with an increase in a larger-sized, lower density cell population in which the LPS-responsive cells are usually found (Makinodan and Adler, 1975). Therefore, there is a correlation between the appearance of a new subpopulation in the spleens from older animals and the higher degree of LPS responsiveness, but these cells might not carry the B-cell identification antigens.

Another way to examine B-cell function is to determine the immune response to an antigen that does not require the cooperation of T-cells (a 'B' antigen). In an in vitro culture system, it can be shown that the in vitro antibody-forming response of spleen cells from old C57 Bl/6 mice to B antigens is very poor, much less than the level reached by the cells from young mice (Fig. 4.4; Nordin, unpublished). Such evidence reinforces the finding that the LPS mitogen assay does not measure a B-cell function in the old mice. However, in an in vivo assay of antibody-forming ability, old mice respond to the T-independent antigens better than do young mice (Blankwater, Levert and Hijmans, 1975; Nordin, unpublished). Therefore in an in vivo assay B-cells appear to have a normal or a better than normal function while in vitro the B-cells from the old mice respond poorly.

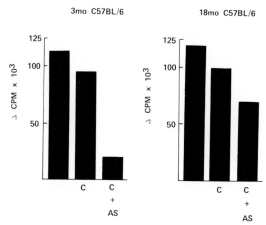

Figure 4.8   In these experiments the effects of an anti-'B'-cell antisera were determined on the mitogenic responsiveness to LPS of three-month, and 18-month old C57 B1/6 spleen cells. Cultures were performed as described in Figure 4.3. The spleen cells were treated with complement (C) or with the antisera + C prior to the initiation of the culture period. Thymidine incorporation was determined for the final 6 h of a three-day culture period and the results are expressed as the mean CPM of the LPS stimulated cultures minus the CPM of the background non-stimulated cultures.

It should be clear that the results of in vitro immunological assays must be considered carefully in light of the inherent limitations of the particular technique used and their relevance to in vivo functions (Schreier and Nordin, 1976). This is especially important in ageing research. A criticism to be always kept in mind is that in choosing a particular assay system—or even worse, relying on only one assay—the investigator may be biasing the results obtained (Pilarski and Cunningham, 1975). It could also be that physical procedures used in preparing cell suspensions could have a selective effect on the results of an assay. An example of this is the suggestion that the spleen cells from aged mice may be more fragile than those from younger mice.

CLINICAL CONSIDERATIONS

In studying an individual's ability to produce antibody as a function of age, it has been suggested that the levels of certain serum antibodies decrease with advancing age (Thompsen and Kettel, 1929). The decline is gradual, usually does not decrease to immeasurably low levels, and what this decline reflects is difficult to say. However, more recent data shows that the decline in particular antibody levels could result from a variety of factors and would not necessarily be classified as evidence of an immunodeficiency. Furthermore, the levels of serum immunoproteins do not decrease with advancing age (Buckley, Buckley and Dorsey, 1974), even after intensive immunisation (White et al, 1974). It could be that in a developing organism the response to many different antigens results in competition with varying responses to antigens during a particular time interval. It is also well documented that after immunisation the serum antibody level can rise, descend, and then repeat this cyclical pattern for an extended length of time (Wilkie, 1971; Romball and Weigle, 1973; Macario and de Macario, 1975). Therefore, the particular level of an antibody may depend on the point during such a cycle that the serum is sampled rather than on the age of the organism. Patterns of exposure to certain antigens may also change with age so that the degree of sensitisation could determine the antibody levels. It has been thought that secondary immune responsiveness remains relatively intact with age, accounting for the age-related pattern of childhood diseases. If true, this could further complicate the interpretation of low antibody levels in ageing humans. However, recent evidence disputes this and, instead, suggests a defect is present in ageing mice in their secondary response to a hapten antigen (Segre and Segre, 1976a). This could reflect the presence of suppressor mechanisms (Segre and Segre, 1976b), a deficit in immunological memory, or an age-related defect in B-cell proliferation.

There is other evidence of defects or aberrations of B-cell function which occur with age. They are the appearance of homogeneous immunoproteins in the absence of a disease such as multiple myeloma, and the appearance of autoantibody usually not associated with any particular disease state. In the first instance, in humans and in several strains of mice, there is an age-related appearance of electrophoretically homogeneous immunoprotein which usually does not have a known antibody specificity (Radl and Hollander, 1974; Radl et al, 1975). This may reflect an immunodeficiency perhaps caused by the loss of a T-cell control mechanism, or there may be the loss of control in a particular B-cell clone after which the cells undergo greater proliferation with subsequent immunoprotein synthesis. Takiguchi, Adler and Smith (1974) have demonstrated that it is possible to induce the appearance of an homogeneous, specific antibody in young mice using several different antigens without causing the mice to be immunodeficient prior to repeated sensitisation. Therefore the control mechanism for B-cell differentiation and eventual antibody synthesis may be lost prior to the B-cells being compromised by ageing effects, but it is not possible to form definite conclusions. A loss of T-cell control may account for the appearance of autoantibody (Teague et al, 1970) although other possibilities are equally open questions at this time (Allison, Denman and Barnes, 1971). If T-cell deficiencies occur prior to a decrease in antibody forming potential, a decreased delayed hypersensitivity mechanism could result in a viral infection becoming chronic (Waldorf et al, 1968; Hallgren et al, 1973). Antibody would be made against viral-associated antigens, either viral antigen itself or tissue antigens present in viral infected cells. The results would be antibody which react with self tissue (Oldstone and Dixon, 1974; Adler, 1974). Other attempts to explain the appearance of autoantibody attribute a normal functional purpose for autoantibody as a mechanism for eliminating damaged or degenerative tissue (Graber, 1974). Since the autoantibody found in older humans or mice does not seem to be associated with any disease state it may be a method of dealing with altered cells or protein (Peterson and Makinodan, 1972). Other investigators believe that the autoantibody is crucial to the development of several diseases (Mackay, 1972) and may play a role in the process of ageing itself (Walford, 1969), but these associations may not be causative.

There are many diseases which can affect the immune system, and in some of them it is difficult to ascertain which came first, an immune deficiency causing a disease or vice versa.

In age-associated diseases, the difficulties are equally complex. As an example, there are clinical reports that patients with cancer demonstrate depressed delayed hypersensitivity reactions and decreased lymphocyte mitogenic responses (Krant et al, 1968; Eilber and Morton, 1970; Pinsky, 1975). The experimental data would seem to indicate that a growing cancer may result in a general depression of immune function. These are not prospective studies, but the assumptions are made that a decrease in T-cell function has led somehow to tumour development (Garrioch, Good and Gatti, 1970). In mice, though, it is quite easy to decrease the PHA response of spleen cells by either inoculating the animals with tumour cells or by immunising the mice with a variety of antigens (Adler, Takiguchi and Smith, 1971b; Gillette and Boone, 1973). The tumour need not be antigenic to cause this effect, nor do the antigens need to be tissue associated. Furthermore, the extracts from tumours or the supernates from tumour cell cultures can cause many of the same effects on the PHA reactivity of normal spleen cells (Frost and Adler, unpublished). It is easy to see that the different assays that are used to determine immune status could be influenced by the presence in an individual of a growing tumour (Konda, Nakao and Smith, 1973). Decreased immune function may be secondary to a tumour or might reflect the fact that the host is undergoing an inflammatory response and/or an immunological response to the tumour.

CANCER

One of the major problems in trying to correlate cancer with advancing age is the fact that cancer is not a single disease. Cancer is a group of diseases which includes all varieties of malignant growths; but it must be kept in mind that each particular type of malignant tumour has biological characteristics peculiar to itself and that these characteristics may or may not be shared by other types. In addition, each tumour is not autonomous in its growth, but rather tumour growth is the resultant of a complex disease–host relationship influenced by a multitude of physiological parameters.

Although, when compared to each other, specific types of malignant diseases vary greatly in their peak incidences throughout the human lifespan, it has been shown to be generally true that frequency of cancer in man increases with the age of the population studied (Dorn and Cutler, 1959; Doll, 1971). Willis (1967) collected statistical data showing people over 50 years of age (38 per cent of the population studied) accounted for 85 per cent of the fatal carcinomas found at autopsy. Several other studies have shown that clinically unsuspected malignant tumours were found in 25 to 30 per cent of the elderly people who died of unrelated causes (Stjernswärd, 1972). Studies on the occurrence of cancer in laboratory animals, particularly extensive in mice, have supported the conclusion that increased cancer incidence is associated with advancing age (Cloudman, 1941; Russell, 1966; Cotchin and Roe, 1967).

During the past 10 years efforts have been made to try to correlate the decrease in immune function seen in advancing age with the age-related increase in cancer. Teller et al (1962, 1964) were among the first to attempt to demonstrate a correlation between old age, depressed immune function, and spontaneous tumour incidence. It was found that as the immune resistance of random-bred Swiss mice to xenogeneic tumour grafts (human HEP-3 tumour) decreased with advancing age, there was an increase in the cumulative spontaneous tumour incidence. Stjernswärd (1966) found that methylcholanthrene depressed the immune response of CBA mice to sheep red blood cells and that animals so immunologically depressed had a decreased resistance to tumour isografts. Konen et al

(1973) measured a significant decrease in cell-mediated immunity in mice 150 weeks of age. The tumour incidence for old males from this strain of mice was 48 per cent, while 92 per cent of the animals with tumours had malignant lymphomas. Clinical data also have been reported which indicates a possible correlation between an age-related waning of immune function and increased cancer incidence (Gross, 1965; Gatti and Good, 1970).

However, the assumption that a cancer developed principally as the result of an individual's weakened immune system has proven to be an oversimplification of a very complex tumour–host relationship. Prehn (1971) was the first to caution against the dogmatic interpretation that cancer resulted from the failure of immunosurveillance. More recent experiments using T-cell deficient mice have shown that such animals were no more susceptible to spontaneous or chemically induced tumours than were normal mice (Custer et al, 1973; Rygaard and Poulsen, 1974; Stutman, 1974a; Gillette and Fox, 1975). Furthermore, the high incidence of cancer, mainly malignant lymphomas, in children with primary immunodeficiency diseases (Gatti and Good, 1971) which was formerly cited in support of the immunosurveillance hypothesis, now more likely appears to be the result of chronic antigenic stimulation of the deficient immune system (Krueger, 1972). Additionally, a decrease in immunological function has been found to be only one of many changes in an ageing individual's physiology; any number of such changing physiological parameters might be involved in the proliferation and metastasis of malignant cells.

Along a similar line of reasoning, attempts were made to cite the immunodeficiencies found in certain cancer patients as additional indirect support of the correlation between ageing, weakened immune function and malignancy. However, close study of the statistical data showed that most of the cancer patients reported to have immunodeficiencies suffered from lymphoreticular malignancies. The finding of immunodeficiency was not as consistent in patients with tumours other than of the lymphoid system. It should not have been surprising to find a decrease in the immune competence of patients with lymphoid cancers; abnormal cells should not have been expected to function normally. The cause of immune deficiency in patients with other tumours was not as clear.

Studies using experimental animals have established the existence of tumour-specific immunogenicity (Prehn and Main, 1957; Klein et al, 1960); and there is little doubt that most people respond to their own cancers, but the specificity, nature, and intensity of such an immunological response is still controversial (Baldwin et al, 1973; Takasugi, Mickey and Terasaki, 1973; Hellström and Hellström, 1974; Berkelhammer et al, 1975; Jeejeebhoy, 1975). The difficulty in human tumour immunology lies in attempts to correlate in vitro immune assays, which are limited by inherent technical problems, with the in vivo tumour–host relationship. A case in point is human bladder carcinoma. A recent workshop report compiled by some of the most experienced tumour immunologists reveals that studies on normal human peripheral blood lymphocytes are subject to many variables, and in cancer patients the problem of variation is compounded. Furthermore, there is a marked variation in the percentages of the different types of lymphoid cells recovered, and of the cell-mediated cytotoxicity demonstrated by these cells among laboratories examining aliquots of the same blood sample (Bean et al, 1975).

Finally, it is increasingly apparent that the host immune response to a malignant tumour is a combination of both general and specific reactions which result from the interaction of B-cells, T-cells, macrophages and inflammatory cells. The overall immune response influences tumour growth to different extents (Shearer, Philpott and Parker, 1973) depending on other host conditions, one of which is age—a multifactorial physiological state. In turn, the immune response itself can be affected by tumour growth, usually adversely.

OTHER FACTORS

There are a variety of other age-associated conditions which can affect the immune system such as malnutrition, vitamin deficiency, diabetes and anaemia. Correcting these conditions can change immunological function in the elderly. Furthermore, the increase in infectious diseases seen among the elderly may be the result of physical factors rather than poor immune function. A bed-ridden patient with a hip fracture may develop pneumonia because of poor lung ventilation and immobility. A person with emphysema or with an occupational history of exposure to dust or other air pollution may develop pulmonary infections in spite of a normally functioning immune system. Even if the immune system were deficient in these instances, such deficiency may be the result of a suppressive insult rather than an age-associated immunodeficiency. It may be that some of the age-associated diseases may have a microbiological aetiology. Recent research has suggested that atheroscelerosis may have a viral aetiology. However, the evidence for this is only indirect: (1) atherosclerotic plaques are monoclonal (Benditt and Benditt, 1973), (2) aortic tissue can support viral growth and replication with no signs of cytopathological changes (Blacklow, Rose and Whalen, 1975) and (3) there are viral strains which can cause the formation of cholesterol crystals in infected tissue (Fabricant, Krook and Gillespie, 1973).

With the immunodeficiency of ageing, the clinician and laboratory scientist face a situation which is unique. The diagnosis of immunodeficiency in childhood is aided by a variety of factors—family history and genetic implications, history of disease and levels of immune function that are usually strikingly low rather than relatively reduced. After diagnosis, th therapy is also straightforward although inadequate for a variety of conditions in which cellular reconstitution has been the attempted therapeutic method. With the conditions which result in a secondary immunodeficiency, again the picture is quite straightforward. Determining the cause and effect and the prognosis of the deficiency is simplified, although again therapy is complicated. With ageing and the attendant decrease in immune function, however, the diagnosis is difficult. Assigning a primary cause and a secondary effect is difficult, therapy at this time non-existent, the pattern of the disorder not necessarily related to a chronologic age, and the effects of a deficiency are in large measure unappreciated at present.

There are other considerations, though, which are not seen in other types of immunodeficiency as outlined above. At this time there is no way of predicting what a long-term chronic decrease (relative) in immune function might mean in terms of life span or disease pattern. There may be different considerations of a T-cell defect as opposed to a B-cell defect over a long interval. If the early phases of a decrease are without clinical symptoms, then the onset and duration of this condition are impossible to ascertain. Another consideration is the prospect of an unbalanced immune system in which the different parts of the system are changing at different rates as the individual grows older; the effects of any immune deficiency may change as the different stages are reached.

Hypothetically, in normal young adults all parameters of immune function are at their peak. As the individual reaches middle age, T-cell functions begin to decrease, but B-cell functions would be at or near normal. During this early stage of waning immunological function viral infections may start and become chronic, tumours may grow faster because of immunostimulation by antibody in the absence of sufficient killer T-cells, and autoantibody may appear as the result of damaged tissues which express viral antigens or a loss of T-cell regulation of B-cells. The loss of B-cell function would occur late in life and would usher in senescence of immunological function. In this last stage characterised by low T- and B-cell activities, several diseases would appear or change in character. There would be a greater incidence of primary tumours with increased number of metastases, but the tumours may not grow as rapidly. Infections would be more severe. Autoantibody, although found less frequently, would have greater consequences and degenerative diseases would progress rapidly. It is on this complicated framework with the multitude of unanswered questions that the future course of ageing research in immunity will be directed.

REFERENCES

Adler, W. H. (1974) An autoimmune theory of aging. In *Theoretical Aspects of Aging*, ed. Rockstein, M, New York: Academic Press.

Adler, W. H. & Rabinowitz, S. G. (1973) Host defences during primary Venezuelan equine encephalomyelitis infection in mice. II. In vitro methods for the measurement and quantitation of the immune response. *Journal of Immunology*, 110, 1354–1362.

Adler, W. H., Takiguchi, T., Marsh, B. & Smith, R. T. (1970) Cellular recognition by mouse lymphocytes in vitro. I. Definition of a new technique and results of stimulation by phytohemagglutinin and specific antigens. *Journal of Experimental Medicine*, 131, 1049–1078.

Adler, W. H., Takiguchi, T. & Smith, R. T. (1971a) Effect of age upon primary alloantigen recognition by mouse spleen cells. *Journal of Immunology*, 107, 1357–1362.

Adler, W. H., Takiguchi, T. & Smith, R. T. (1971b) Phytohemagglutinin unresponsiveness in mouse spleen cells induced by methylcholanthrene sarcomas. *Cancer Research*, 31, 864–867.

Alexopoulous, C. & Babitis, P. (1976) Age dependence of T lymphocytes. *Lancet*, i, 426.

Allison, A. C., Denman, A. M. & Barnes, R. D. (1971) Cooperating and controlling functions of thymus-derived lymphocytes in relation to autoimmunity. *Lancet*, i, 135–140.

Andrew, W. (1952) Lymphatic tissue. In *Cowdry's Problems of Aging*, ed. Lansing, A. I., pp. 527–561. Baltimore: Williams and Wilkins.

Augener, W., Cohnen, G., Reuter, A. & Brittinger, G. (1974) Decrease of T lymphocytes during aging. *Lancet*, i, 1164.

Baldwin, R. W., Embleton, M. J., Jones, J. S. P. & Langman, M. G. S. (1973) Cell-mediated and humoral immune reactions to human tumors. *International Journal of Cancer*, 12, 73–83.

Bean, M. A., Bloom, B. R., Herberman, R. B., Old, L. J., Oettgen, H. F., Klein, G. & Terry, W. D. (1975) Cell-mediated cytotoxicity for bladder carcinoma: evaluation of a workshop. *Cancer Research*, 35, 2902–2913.

Benditt, E. P. & Benditt, J. M. (1973) Evidence for a monoclonal origin of human atherosclerotic plaques. *Proceedings of the National Academy of Sciences (U.S.A.)*, 70, 1753–1756.

Berkelhammer, J., Mastrangelo, M. J., Laucius, J. F., Bodurtha, A. J. & Prehn, R. T. (1975) Sequential in vitro reactivity of lymphocytes from melanoma patients receiving immunotherapy compared with the reactivity of lymphocytes from healthy donors. *International Journal of Cancer*, 16, 571–578.

Blacklow, N. R., Rose, F. B. & Whalen, R. A. (1975) Organ culture of human aorta: prolonged survival with support of viral replication. *Journal of Infectious Diseases*, 131, 575–578.

Blanckwater, M. J., Levert, L. A. & Hijams, W. (1975) Age related decline in the antibody response to *E. coli* lipopolysaccharide in New Zealand black mice. *Immunology*, 28, 847–854.

Buckley, C. E., III, Buckley, E. G. & Dorsey, F. C. (1974) Longitudinal changes in serum immunoglobulin levels in older humans. *Federation Proceedings*, 33, 2036–2039.

Cloudman, A. M. (1941) Spontaneous neoplasms in mice. In *Biology of the Laboratory Mouse*, ed. Snell, G. D., pp. 168–233. New York: Dover.

Cotchin, E. & Roe, F. J. (1967) *Pathology of Laboratory Rats and Mice*. London: Blackwell.

Custer, R. P., Outzen, H. C., Eaton, G. J. & Prehn, R. T. (1973) Does the absence of immunologic surveillance affect the tumor incidence in 'nude' mice? First recorded spontaneous lymphoma in a 'nude' mouse. *Journal of the National Cancer Institute*, 51, 707–711.

Dauphinee, M. J. & Nordin, A. A. (1974) Studies of the immunological capacity of germ-free mouse radiation chimeras. IV. Cell-mediated immunity. *Cellular Immunology*, 14, 394–401.

Diaz-Jouanen, E., Williams, R. C., Jr & Strickland, R. G. (1975) Age related changes in T and B cells. *Lancet*, i, 688–689.

Doll, R. (1971) The age distribution of cancer: implications for models of carcinogenesis. *Journal of the Royal Statisticsl Society*, **134**, 133–166.

Dorn, H. F. & Cutler, S. J. (1959) Morbidity from cancer. In *U.S. Public Health Monograph No. 56*. Washington D.C.: U.S. Government Printing Office.

Eilber, F. R. & Morton, D. L. (1970) Impaired immunological reactivity and recurrence following cancer surgery. *Cancer*, **25**, 362–367.

Fabricant, C. G., Krook, L. & Gillespie, J. H. (1973) Virus induced cholesterol crystals. *Science*, **181**, 566–567.

Farrar, J. J., Loughman, B. E. & Nordin, A. A. (1974) Lymphopoietic potential of bone marrow cells from aged mice: comparison of the cellular constituents of bone marrow from young and aged mice. *Journal of Immunology*, **112**, 1244–1249.

Folch, H. & Waksman, B. H. (1974) The splenic suppressor cell. I. Activity of thymus-dependent adherent cells: changes with stress. *Journal of Immunology*, **113**, 127–139.

Ford, C. E., Micklem, H. S., Evans, E. P., Gray, J. G. & Ogden, D. A. (1966) The inflow of bone marrow cells to the thymus: studies with part body irradiated mice injected with chromosome marked bone marrow and subjected to antigenic stimulation. *Annals of the New York Academy of Sciences*, **129**, 283–296.

Garrioch, D. B., Good, R. A. & Gatti, R. A. (1970) Lymphocyte response to PHA in patients with non-lymphoid tumours. *Lancet*, **i**, 618.

Gatti, R. A. & Good, R. A. (1970) Aging, immunity, and malignancy. *Geriatrics*, **25**, 158–168.

Gatti, R. A. & Good, R. A. (1971) Occurrence of malignancy in immunodeficiency diseases. *Cancer*, **28**, 89–98.

Giannini, D. & Sloan, R. S. (1957) A tuberculin survey of 1285 adults with special reference to the elderly. *Lancet*, **i**, 525–527.

Gillette, R. W. & Boone, C. W. (1973) Changes in phytohemagglutinin response due to presence of tumors. *Journal of the National Cancer Institute*, **50**, 1391–1393.

Gillette, R. W. & Fox, A. (1975) The effect to T-lymphocyte deficiency on tumor induction and growth. *Cellular Immunology*, **19**, 328–335.

Gitlin, D., Janeway, C. A., Apt, L. & Craig, J. M. (1959) Agammaglobulinemia. In *Cellular and Humoral Aspects of the Hypersensitive States*, ed. Lawrence, H. S., pp. 375–441. New York: Hoeber–Harper.

Golub, S. H., O'Connell, T. X. & Morton, D. L. (1974) Correlation of in vivo and in vitro assays of immunocompetence in cancer patients. *Cancer Research*, **34**, 1833–1837.

Golub, S. H., Sulit, H. L. & Morton, D. L. (1975) The use of viable frozen lymphocytes for studies in human tumor immunology. *Transplantation*, **19**, 195–202.

Graber, P. (1974) 'Self' and 'non-self' in immunology. *Lancet*, **ii**, 1320–1322.

Gross, L. (1965) Immunological defect in aged population and its relationship to cancer. *Cancer*, **18**, 201–204.

Hallgren, H. M., Buckley, C. E., Gilbertsen, V. A. & Yunis, E. J. (1973) Lymphocyte phytohema-glutinin responsiveness, immunoglobulins and autoantibodies in aging humans. *Journal of Immunology*, **111**, 1101–1107.

Harrison, D. E. & Doubleday, J. W. (1975) Normal function of immunologic stem cells from aged mice. *Journal of Immunology*, **114**, 1314–1317.

Häyry, P. & Defendi, V. (1970) Mixed lymphocyte cultures produce effector cells: model in vitro for allograft rejection. *Science*, **168**, 133–135.

Hellström, K. E., & Hellström, I. (1974) Lymphocyte mediated cytotoxicity and blocking serum activity to tumor antigens. *Advances in Immunology*, **18**, 209–277.

Hirano, T. & Nordin, A. A. (1975) The regulatory mechanism(s) of in vitro cell-mediated immunity in aged mice. *Gerontologist*, **15** (5II), 28.

Hirano, T. & Nordin, A. A. (1976) Age associated decline in the in vitro development of cytotoxic lymphocytes in NZB mice. *Journal of Immunology*, **117**, 1093–1098.

Hirokawa, K. & Makinodan, T. (1975) Thymic involution: effect on T cell differentiation. *Journal of Immunology*, **114**, 1659–1664.

Hori, Y., Perkins, E. H. & Halsall, M. K. (1973) Decline in phytohemagglutinin responsiveness of spleen cells from aging mice. *Proceedings of the Society for Experimental Biology and Medicine*, **144**, 48–53.

Howard, J. C., Hunt, S. V. & Gowans, J. L. (1972) Identification of marrow-derived and thymus-derived small lymphocytes in the lymphoid tissues and thoracic duct lymph of normal rats. *Journal of Experimental Medicine*, **135**, 200–219.

Jeejeebhoy, H. F. (1975) Immunological studies of women with primary breast carcinoma. *International Journal of Cancer*, **15**, 867–878.

Kishimoto, S., Takahama, T. & Mizumachi, H. (1976) In vitro immune response to the 2,4,6-trinitrophenyl determinant in aged C57B1/6J mice: changes in the humoral immune response to, avidity for the TNP determinant and responsiveness to LPS effect with aging. *Journal of Immunology*, **116**, 294–300.

Klein, G., Sjögren, H. O., Klein, E. & Hellström, K. E. (1960) Demonstration of resistance against methylcholanthrene induced sarcoma in the primary autochthonous host. *Cancer Research*, **20**, 1561–1572.

Konda, S., Nakao, Y. & Smith, R. T. (1973) The stimulatory effect of tumor bearing upon the T- and B-cell subpopulations of the mouse spleen. *Cancer Research*, **33**, 2247–2256.

Konen, T. G., Smith, G. S. & Walford, R. L. (1973) Decline in mixed lymphocyte reactivity of spleen cells from aged mice of a long-lived strain. *Journal of Immunology*, **110**, 1216–1221.

Krant, M. J., Manskopf, G., Brandrup, C. S. & Madoff, M. A. (1968) Immunologic alterations in bronchogenic cancer. *Cancer*, **21**, 623–631.

Krueger, G. R. F. (1972) Chronic immunosuppression and lymphomagenesis in man and mice. *National Cancer Institute Monograph*, **35**, 183–190.

Kunkel, H. G. (1975) Surface markers of human lymphocytes. *Johns Hopkins Medical Journal*, **137**, 216–223.

Macario, A. J. L. & de Macario, E. C. (1975) Long-lasting in vitro immune response to a distinct antigenic determinant of a bacterial protein. *Journal of Immunology*, **115**, 106–111.

Mackaness, G. B. (1971) Delayed hypersensitivity and the mechanism of cellular resistance to infection. In *Progress in Immunology*, ed. Amos, B., Vol. I, pp. 413–424. Amsterdam: North Holland Publishing.

Mackay, I. R. (1972) Ageing and immunological function in man. *Gerontologia*, **18**, 285–304.

Makinodan, T. & Adler, W. H. (1975) Effects of aging on the differentiation and proliferation potentials of cells of the immune system. *Federation Proceedings*, **34**, 153–158.

Makinodan, T. & Peterson, W. J. (1964) Growth and senescence of the primary antibody-forming potential of the spleen. *Journal of Immunology*, **93**, 886–896.

McIntyre, O. R. & Cole, A. F. (1969) Variation in the response of normal lymphocytes to PHA. *International Archives of Allergy and Applied Immunology*, **35**, 105–118.

Najarian, J. S. & Feldman, J. D. (1963) Specificity of passively transferred delayed hypersensitivity. *Journal of Experimental Medicine*, **118**, 341–352.

Nordin, A. A. & Makinodan, T. (1974) Humoral immunity in aging. *Federation Proceedings*, **33**, 2033–2035.

Oldstone, M. B. A. & Dixon, F. J. (1974) Aging and chronic virus infection: is there a relationship? *Federation Proceedings*, **33**, 2057–2060.

Owen, J. J. T. & Raff, M. C. (1970) Studies on the differentiation of thymus-derived lymphocytes. *Journal of Experimental Medicine*, **132**, 1216–1232.

Owen, J. J. T. & Ritter, M. A. (1969) Tissue interaction in the development of thymus lymphocytes. *Journal of Experimental Medicine*, **129**, 431–437.

Parrott, D. M. V. & DeSousa, M. A. B. (1971) Thymus-dependent and thymus-independent populations: origin, migratory patterns and lifespan. *Clinical and Experimental Immunology*, **8**, 663–684.

Parrott, D. M. V., DeSousa, M. & East, J. (1966) Thymus-dependent areas in the lymphoid organs of neonatally thymectomised mice. *Journal of Experimental Medicine*, **123**, 191–204.

Peavy, D. L., Shands, J. W., Adler, W. H. & Smith, R. T. (1973) Selective effects of bacterial endotoxins on various subpopulations of lymphoreticular cells. *Journal of Infectious Diseases*, **S 128**, 83–91.

Pepper, F. J. (1961) The effect of age, pregnancy and lactation on the thymus gland and lymph nodes of the mouse. *Journal of Endocrinology*, **22**, 335–340.

Peterson, W. J. & Makinodan, T. (1972) Autoimmunity in aged mice. *Clinical and Experimental Immunology*, **12**, 273–290.

Peterson, W. J., Makinodan, T., Price, G. B. & Chen, M. G. (1972) Differential aging in the capacity of spleen and bone marrow cells to induce graft vs host reactions. In *Proceedings of the 9th International Congress of Gerontology*, ed. Chebotarev, D. F., Frolkis, V. V. & Ya Mints, A., Vol. 3, p. 46. Kiev: The Congress.

Pilarski, L. M. & Cunningham, A. J. (1975) Host derived antibody-forming cells in lethally irradiated mice. *Journal of Immunology*, **114**, 138–140.

Pinsky, C. M. (1975) V. Clinical implications of tumor–host studies. In *Immunobiology of the Tumor–Host Relationship*, ed. Smith, R. T. & Landy, M., pp. 301–307. New York: Academic Press.

Pisciotta, A. V., Westring, D. W., Deprey, C. & Walsh, B. (1967) Mitogenic effect of phytohemmaglutinin at different ages. *Nature (London)*, **215**, 193–194.

Prehn, R. T. (1971) Immunosurveillance, regeneration and oncogenesis. *Progress in Experimental Tumor Research*, **14**, 1–24.

Prehn, R. T. & Main, J. M. (1957) Immunity to MCA induced sarcomas. *Journal of the National Cancer Institute*, **18**, 769–778.

Price, G. B. & Makinodan, T. (1972a) Immunologic deficiencies in senescence. I. Characterization of intrinsic deficiencies. *Journal of Immunology*, **108**, 403–412.

Price, G. B. & Makinodan, T. (1972b) Immunologic deficiencies in senescence. II. Characterization of extrinsic deficiencies. *Journal of Immunology*, **108**, 413–417.

Radl, J. & Hollander, C. F. (1974) Homogeneous immunoglobulins in sera of mice during aging. *Journal of Immunology*, **112**, 2271–2273.

Radl, J., Sepers, J. M., Skvaril, F., Morell, A. & Hijmans, W. (1975) Immunoglobulin patterns in humans over 95 years of age. *Clinical and Experimental Immunology*, **22**, 84–90.

Raff, M. C. (1969) Theta isoantigen as a marker of thymus-derived lymphocytes in mice. *Immunology*, **19**, 637–650.

Roitt, I. M., Greaves, M. F., Torrigiani, G., Brostoff, J. & Playfair, J. H. L. (1969) The cellular basis of immunological responses: a synthesis of some current views. *Lancet*, **ii**, 367–371.

Romball, C. G. & Weigle, W. O. (1973) A cyclical appearance of antibody-producing cells after a single injection of serum protein antigen. *Journal of Experimental Medicine*, **138**, 1426–1442.

Russell, E. S. (1966) Lifespan and aging patterns. In *The Biology of the Laboratory Mouse*, ed. Green, E. L., pp. 511–520. New York: McGraw-Hill.

Rygaard, J. & Poulsen, C. O. (1974) Is immunological surveillance not a cell mediated immune function? *Transplantation*, **17**, 135–136.

Schreier, M. & Nordin, A. A. (1976) Evaluation of the immune response in vitro. In *B and T Cells in Immune Recognition*, ed. Loor, F. & Roelants, G. E. London: J. Wiley (in press).

Segre, M. & Segre, D. (1976a) Humoral immunity in aged mice. I. Age related decline in the secondary response to DNP of spleen cells propagated in diffusion chambers. *Journal of Immunology*, **116**, 731–734.

Segre, M. & Segre, D. (1976b) Humoral immunity in aged mice. II. Increased suppressor T cell activity in immunologically deficient old mice. *Journal of Immunology*, **116**, 735–738.

Shearer, W. T., Philpott, G. W. & Parker, C. W. (1973) Stimulation of cells by antibody. *Science*, **182**, 1357–1359.

Stjernswärd, J. (1966) Age-dependent tumor–host barrier and effect of carcinogen-induced immunodepression on rejection of isografted methylcholanthrene-induced sarcoma cells. *Journal of the National Cancer Institute*, **37**, 505–512.

Stjernswärd, J. (1972) Modification of immunity and carcinogenesis. *National Cancer Institute Monograph*, **35**, 149–156.

Stutman, O. (1974a) Tumor development after 3-methylcholanthene in immunologically deficient athymic-nude mice. *Science*, **183**, 534–536.

Stutman, O. (1974b) Cell-mediated immunity and aging. *Federation Proceedings*, **33**, 2028–2032.

Takasugi, M., Mickey, M. R. & Terasaki, P. I. (1973) Reactivity of lymphocytes from normal persons on cultured tumor cells. *Cancer Research*, **33**, 2898–2902.

Takiguchi, T., Adler, W. H. & Smith, R. T. (1971) Cellular recognition in vitro by mouse lymphocytes: effects of neonatal thymectomy and thymus graft restoration on alloantigen and PHA stimulation of whole and gradient-separated subpopulations of spleen cells. *Journal of Experimental Medicine*, **133**, 63–80.

Takiguchi, T., Adler, W. H. & Smith, R. T. (1974) Strain specificity of monidsperse gammaglobulin appearance after immunization of inbred mice. *Proceedings of the Society for Experimental Biology and Medicine*, **145**, 868–873.

Teague, P. O., Ynis, E. J., Rodey, G., Fish, A. J., Stutman, O. & Good, R. A. (1970) Autoimmune phenomena and renal disease in mice: role of thymectomy, aging, and involution of immunologic capacity. *Laboratory Investigation*, **22**, 121–130.

Teller, M. N., Curlett, W., Rose, B., Lardis, M. P. & Stohr, G. (1962) A possible correlation between old age, depressed immune response and spontaneous tumor incidence in mice. *Proceedings of the American Association for Cancer Research*, **3**, 367.

Teller, M. N., Curlett, W., Kubisek, M. L. & Curtis, D. (1964) Aging and cancerigenesis. I. Immunity to tumor and skin grafts. *Journal of the National Cancer Institute*, **33**, 649–656.

Thompsen, O. & Kettel, K. (1929) Die starke der menschilchen isoagglutinine und entsprechenden blutkoperchenrezeptoren in verschiedenen lebensaltern. *Zeitschrift für Immunitätsforschung*, **63**, 67–93.

Trentin, J. J., Wolf, N. S. & Curry, J. L. (1969) Homing and differentiation of bone marrow stem cells. In *Cellular Recognition*, ed. Smith, R. T. & Good, R. A., pp. 91–93. New York: Appleton Century Crofts.

Unanue, E. R., Grey, H. M., Rabellino, E., Campbell, P. & Schmidtke, J. (1971) Immunoglobulins on the surface of lymphocytes. II. The bone marrow as the main source of lymphocytes with detectable surface-bound immunoglobulin. *Journal of Experimental Medicine*, **133**, 1188–1198.

van Bekkum, D. W. (ed.) (1975) *The Biological Activity of Thymic Hormones*. Rotterdam: Kooyker Scientific Publications.

Vossen, J. M. & Hijmans, W. (1975) Membrane-associated immunoglobulin determinants on bone marrow and blood lymphocytes in the pediatric age group and on fetal tissues. *Annals of the New York Academy of Sciences*, **254,** 262–279.

Waldorf, D. S., Wilkins, R. F. & Decker, J. C. (1968) Impaired delayed hypersensitivity in an aging population: association with antinuclear antibody. *Journal of the American Medical Association*, **203,** 821–834.

Walford, R. (1969) *The Immunologic Theory of Aging*. Copenhagen: Munksgaard.

Walters, C. S. & Claman, H. N. (1975) Age-related changes in cell-mediated immunity in BALB/c mice. *Journal of Immunology*, **115,** 1438–1443.

Warner, N. L., Uhr, J. W., Thorbecke, G. W. & Ovary, Z. (1969) Immunoglobulins, antibodies and the bursa of Fabricius: induction of agammaglobulinemia and the loss of all antibody-forming capacity by hormonal bursectomy. *Journal of Immunology*, **103,** 1317–1330.

Weissman, I. L. (1967) Thymus cell migration. *Journal of Experimental Medicine*, **126,** 291–304.

Weksler, M. E. & Hutteroth, T. H. (1974) Impaired lymphocyte functions in aged humans. *Journal of Clinical Investigation*, **53,** 99–104.

White, C. S., Adler, W. H. & McGann, V. G. (1974) Repeated immunization: possible adverse effects re-evaluation of human subjects at 25 years. *Annals of Internal Medicine*, **81,** 594–600.

Wigzell, H. & Stjernswärd, J. (1966) Age dependent rise and fall of immunological reactivity in the CBA mouse. *Journal of the National Cancer Institute*, **37,** 513–517.

Wilkie, M. H. (1971) Analysis of sequential humoral antibody responses. In *The Annual Report to the Armed Forces Epidemeology Board Fiscal Year 1971 Commission on Epidemeologic Survey*, pp. 11–19. Washington, D.C.

Willis, R. A. (1967) *Pathology of Tumours*, 4th edn, pp. 92–104. London: Butterworth.

5

THE IMMUNOPATHOLOGY OF SCHISTOSOMIASIS

Daniel G. Colley

The expression 'host–parasite relationship' is an euphemism used to cloak a multiplicity of sins. It refers to a range of interactions which may lead to consequences either beneficial or detrimental to the host. Ultimately, excesses of either of these effects work to the disfavour of most obligate parasites. Such organisms would much prefer an innocuous relationship, or as an alternative, a spectral relationship in which they might seek a middleground. When discussing such kaleidoscopic infections, use of the term immunopathology would indicate a shift in the clinical spectrum towards the end where the host not only fares poorly, but is also, in part, responsible for the pathogenesis of its adverse state. Chronic infection with the schistosomes provides an excellent example of such a situation. This chapter will attempt to present clinical and experimental mammalian schistosomiasis from this point of view, and to discuss some of the speculated host responses which are induced. For other current reviews of the total immunologic framework of schistosomiasis and the pathology of schistosome infections, the reader is referred to Warren (1971, 1973), WHO Memorandum (1974) and Smithers and Terry (1976).

Schistosomes are multistaged, metazoan parasites, each of which utilises specific snails as the sites of their asexual replicative phase. There are many species of these trematodes, and they infect a wide assortment of animals as their definitive hosts. Three main species, *Schistosoma mansoni*, *S. japonicum* and *S. haematobium*, complete their life cycle in man. Infection is initiated by penetration of the skin by the body of free-swimming cercariae which have issued from infected snails. These immediately transform into schistosomula, a larval stage, which migrate to the capillary bed of the lungs and eventually to the vessels of the portal or vesicular systems. The adult male and female worms, living in copula in the veins along side either the intestine or the bladder, produce embryonated eggs which are intended to exit the body by working their way to the lumen of the gut or bladder, and thus, transported by faeces or urine, enter the environment, to hatch, and infect the proper species of snail. The immunopathology of the infection will be discussed in relationship to this sequence of events which leads to the establishment of chronic infection.

Dermal Penetration by Cercariae

The process of cercarial penetration appears to be facilitated by muscular activity and the secretion of a variety of enzymes by the penetrating organism (Stirewalt and Hackey, 1956). Such penetration is not host-specific, and upon penetration of an abnormal host (for example: an avian schistosome into a human) the organisms die in the epidermis, or soon thereafter (Macfarlane, 1952), and evoke a polymorphonuclear inflammatory response (von Lichtenberg and Ritchie, 1961).

Cort (1928) observed that upon repeated exposure to the cercariae of bird or rodent schistosomes, man developed a dermatitis which consisted primarily of puritic papules. This schistosome dermatitis, or 'swimmer's itch', can be induced by a variety of schistosomes (Olivier, 1949) and is seen to intensify upon repeated exposure. Initially, immediate macules occur and fade within a few hours. They are replaced by large papules which are oedematous and contain infiltrates of round cells (Macfarlane, 1949; Malek and Armstrong 1967).

Lin and Sadun (1959) and Colley, Magalhães-Filho and Coelho (1972) have observed infiltrates in the mouse in response to repeated S. mansoni cercarial penetration. The latter group studied the response, by passive transfer, and demonstrated the participation of early humoral and subsequent cell-mediated immune components. Recently, Askenase, Hayden and Higashi (1976) have reported that secondary penetration of guinea-pigs by S. mansoni cercariae elicited a cutaneous basophil hypersensitivity response. These lesions closely resembled contact sensitivity reactions in the guinea-pig and appeared grossly similar to human cercarial dermatitis lesions. Upon exposure to S. mansoni and S. haematobium cercariae, Barlow (1936) described a swimmer's itch syndrome in Egyptians with documented schistosomiasis.

Patients with confirmed histories of schistosome dermatitis have been studied in relationship to their skin test reactivity to S. mansoni worm or cercarial extracts. Moore et al (1968) determined that prior history of schistosome dermatitis against bird schistosomes did lead to some cross-sensitisation against S. mansoni antigens, and that the degree of this cross-responsiveness was inversely related to the length of time between the last exposure to bird schistosome cercariae and the S. mansoni skin test. In a similar study, Wiedermann et al (1973) found that little, if any, cross-sensitisation was detected when swimmer's itch patients were skin tested with a S. mansoni worm extract.

Neither the antigens, nor the actual underlying immune mechanisms responsible for schistosome dermatitis have been experimentally defined. Whether this immunopathologic reactivity occurs consistently upon re-exposure to human schistosomes, and whether it is, or could be, involved in protective responses against reinfection, remains to be elucidated.

Migration of Schistosomula and Immature Worms

During successful penetration of the epidermis and dermis, cercariae transform into schistosomula. These larval forms enter the subcutaneous tissues and by venous vessels (and possibly the lymphatics) are transported to the right heart and to the lungs. This requires approximately three to six days. After a few days' sojourn in the lungs, schistosomula proceed on their migration to the portal vessels of the liver. It is here that feeding upon erythrocytes and active growth initiates. Upon maturity, estimated to occur between four and five weeks, paired worms are found in portal, mesenteric, or vesicular veins. Some evidence exists both for circulatory transport from the lungs to portal veins, and for the direct passage from lungs via pleural space–diaphragm–liver to the portal venous system.

Pulmonary lesions have been described (Smith et al, 1975) in some re-exposed hosts (mice, rhesus monkeys and golden hamsters) and the reactivity has been ascribed to combined antibody and cellular functions. Earlier studies (Vogel and Minning, 1953; Sadun and Lin, 1959; von Lichtenberg and Ritchie, 1961; Hsu, Davis and Hsu, 1965) have all observed such 'tuft-like foci' around schistosomula in the lungs of rhesus monkeys or mice (Magalhães-Filho, 1959). There is not complete agreement as to the occurrence of such pulmonary antischistosomular reactions in experimental hosts other than the rhesus monkey (von Lichtenberg, personal communication). Their immunologic basis, except as studied by Smith et al (1975), remains undefined.

Acute Schistosomiasis

Symptomatic acute schistosomiasis (Katayama fever, toxaemic form) has been observed in human infections with S. japonicum (Billings, Winkenwerder and Hunninen, 1946), and less frequently with S. mansoni (Diaz-Rivera et al, 1956; Oliveira et al, 1969). Symptomatology includes fever, urticaria, splenomegaly, lymphadenopathy, epigastric and liver tenderness, anorexia and diarrhoea, and is accompanied by eosinophilia. This syndrome is commonly associated with initial infection, often in conjunction with heavy exposure to cercariae, and occurs 3 to 11 weeks after such an exposure. In extreme cases the acute disease can be fatal, but this is extremely rare. The common sequence is spontaneous resolution of the condition. Its pathogenesis is not known. Due to circumstantial parasitological and clinical observations, it is often discussed as being based upon an immune-complex aetiology (Warren, 1971). The symptoms are compatible with those of serum sickness. Furthermore, the timing is such that most symptomatology coincides with the production and continued release of large amounts of antigens (worm excretions and secretions, and eggs) and a concomitant rise in antibody production. It has been hypothesised that these events, coupled with potential selective immunodepression, might lead to both localised (at the site of egg deposition) and systemic antigen–antibody–complement mediated lesion formation (Colley, 1974). Such theories remain conjectural in the absence of either clinical or experimental studies regarding this acute form of the disease.

Immune Complexes

Detection of circulating complexes

Soluble, circulating antigens and immune complexes have been detected in the sera from a variety of hosts, including man, infected with schistosomes (Berggren and Weller, 1967; Hillyer, 1973; Bawden and Weller, 1974). The antigens detected have included DNA (Hillyer, 1973) and a high molecular weight carbohydrate (Nash, Prescott and Neva, 1974) which appears to originate from the schistosome gut (von Lichtenberg, Bawden and Shealey, 1974; Nash, 1974). This, and other circulating antigens, may correlate with the intensity of infection in hamsters (Gold, Rosen and Weller, 1969) and in man (Carlier et al, 1975). Precipitating antibodies to denatured *Bacillus subtilis* and calf DNAs, and *S. mansoni* DNA have been observed in sera from schistosome infected hosts (Hillyer, 1973).

Sensitive assays for the detection of circulating antigen–antibody complexes have recently been employed in studies involving sera from schistosomiasis patients. Initial studies indicated that four out of ten patients sera tested displayed increased binding of radio-labelled C1q. Preliminary indirect assays aimed at analysing catabolism of complement components and complement–immune complex interactions, indicated that sera from *S. mansoni* and *S. haematobium* patients often exhibited decreased levels of C3, C4 and factor B, and eight out of nine had increased levels of the C3d fragment of C3. Immunoconglutinin levels were elevated in six of seven of these sera (P. H. Lambert, personal communication; WHO Memorandum, 1974).

It should be mentioned that the existence of soluble immune complexes may lead not only to the immunopathologic results normally considered in this situation, but could also contribute to a variety of altered immune effector mechanisms, including antibody-mediated cell-dependent cytoxicity, and cell-mediated responses. The participation of such an 'enhancing' effect, contributing to worm survival in the rat, may be inferred from the work of Phillips et al (1975).

Renal involvement in clinical schistosomiasis

Immunoglobulins, antigens and complement components have been demonstrated within antischistosome egg granulomas (to be discussed below) and associated with a variety of nephropathies which occur during clinical and experimental schistosomiasis. In a series of independent studies, several Brazilian investigators have focused attention on renal lesions in patients with the hepatosplenic form of S. mansoni infections. Lopez (1964) demonstrated a high prevalence of proteinuria in this group, as opposed to lightly infected patients, and demonstrated focal glomerulonephritis in 2 of 16 patients. Machado (1965) observed an 88 per cent prevalence of proteinuria and showed that the urines of these patients contained γ- and β-globulins and lipoproteins. At autopsy, Andrade and Queiroz (1968) described membranous glomerular alterations, fibrillar thickening and cellular proliferation of the mesangium in the kidneys of patients who had died of severe hepatosplenic schistosomiasis. Based upon a study of the S. mansoni infection prevalence of patients with chronic glomerulonephritis and a statistical post-mortem study, Lima, Brito and Rocha (1969) suggested that severe chronic S. mansoni infection may contribute greatly to chronic glomerulonephritis. Brito et al (1970) examined 11 cases of hepatosplenic-form disease, and reported intense proliferation of mesangial cells, and matrix deposition and focal thickening of basement membranes. At the ultrastructural level they observed electron-dense deposits, which, when examined by immunofluorescence, contained immunoglobulins and C3. After studying 80 necropsies of hepatosplenic cadavers, Andrade, Andrade and Sadigursky (1971) clearly indicated that this condition was associated with an increased prevalence of nephropathies, and pointed out that these alterations included mesangial cell proliferation, deposition of mesangial matrix, glomerulosclerosis and glomerulonephritis.

Until recently, no schistosomal antigens had been noted in association with these lesions in human cases. In an unusual setting, involving the transplantation of a normal kidney into a S. mansoni infected patient, Falcão and Gould (1975) have reported the glomerular localisation of schistosome antigen, immunoglobulin and complement. Whether the deposition of immune complexes resulting from chronic infection, into a virgin kidney, is a unique occurrence, or reflects a normal process, remains to be determined.

Immune complexes in experimental schistosomiasis

Experimental S. mansoni infections have also been examined in relationship to possible renal involvement. Infections in Cebus apella monkeys led to basement membrane-associated deposits of immunoglobulin (Brito et al, 1971). However, when Brack et al (1972) compared renal lesions in uninfected and S. mansoni-infected baboons, they were unable to ascribe any increase in pathologic findings to the existence of the disease. Hillyer and Lewert (1974) have observed widespread tubular and glomerular pathology associated with S. mansoni infection in hamsters. Glomerular lesions involved both mesangial and basement membrane alterations. The latter contained localised hamster immunoglobulin, showing granular, lumpy-bumpy distribution. Natali and Cioli (1974) have described the presence of immunoglobulins, C3, and heterogeneous *S. mansoni* antigens in the glomeruli of some infected mice.

Experimental schistosome infections of chimpanzees indicate that in contrast to *S. mansoni* and *S. haematobium* infections, *S. japonicum* infections are associated with a high incidence of renal pathology, and occasionally easily detectable proteinuria and elevated blood urea nitrogen levels. Severe glomerular lesions were reported in most of the chimpanzees that had developed hepatic pipe-stem fibrosis (von Lichtenberg et al, 1971b) and were histopathologically described as clearly inflammatory and classified as 'membrano-proliferative'. A subsequent study (Sadun et al, 1975) very nicely dissociated these renal lesions from the normally coincident occurrence of liver damage and pipe-stem fribosis. This was accomplished by demonstrating the nephropathies in infected chimpanzees which had surgically received portocaval shunts. Rabbits (von Lichtenberg, Sadun and Bruce, 1972) and hamsters (Hillyer, 1973) infected with *S. japonicum*, exhibited somewhat milder lesions than those observed in chimpanzees.

Perspective on role of immune complexes

While urogenital complications are often associated with clinical and experimental *S. haematobium* infections (discussed below), renal lesions, other than pyelonephritis and hydronephrosis, have not been commonly reported (Smith et al, 1974; Webbe, James and Nelson, 1974). However, recent presentations (Ezzat et al, 1974) which described nephropathies in Egyptian *S. haematobium* patients, indicated the existence of granular immunoglobulin deposits in glomeruli, and suggest that this aspect of *S. haematobium* infection might require further investigation.

It should be emphasised that several areas remain to be defined in regard to schistosome-related renal lesions. Although the initial investigations into renal involvement in schistosomiasis were made in regard to proteinuria (Lopez, 1964; Machado, 1965) and glomerulonephritis can unquestionably be shown to contribute to morbidity in individual hospitalised patients (Lima et al, 1969), the population-based clinical relevance of renal pathology in *S. mansoni* infection needs to be more clearly shown (Lehman et al, 1975). Further substantiation would also be in order in regard to *S. haematobium* and *S. japonicum* infections. In some of the lesions discussed, the involvement of immune complexes appears clear. However, the identity of the antigens responsible has not yet been satisfactorily demonstrated. In light of the anti-DNA studies reported, their identity as schistosome antigens should not be taken for granted.

Granuloma Formation

Worms

The adult worm stage of the schistosomes which infect man range from 0.25 to 2.00 mm in breadth and 7 to 28 mm in length. Although their size is not large by comparison with many other helminths, it should be remembered that these worms reside within the vascular system of the host, and not in the intestine. Furthermore, their place of residence is clearly an immunologically hostile environment, in which they are continually bathed by antibodies, and bumped by lymphoid cells which, when studied in vitro, react and respond with specificity against their antigenic components. Yet, the worms do not yield to these presumed immunologic insults in vivo, nor do they initiate such other host regulatory capabilities as the clotting system. The mechanisms which are hypothesised to be involved in the worm's evasion of the immune threats are fascinating, and include such evasion techniques as molecular mimicry (the synthesis of host, or host-like, antigens), acquisition of a 'masquerade costume' of host antigens (glycolipid blood group substances have been observed to participate), rapid membrane turnover, or sloughing, and induction of immunoregulatory mechanisms such as suppressive immune complexes or negatively regulatory cells. However, full exploration of these potential escape mechanisms comprises the sub-

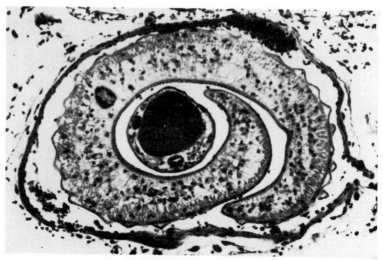

Figure 5.1 Cross-section through a male and female *S. mansoni* worm pair within a mesenteric venule from a mouse. The body of the larger male is folded over. The slender (near round in cross-section) female is held in the fold, or gynaecophoric canal. Haematoxylin and eosin, × 190

ject of another tale, which has been discussed by others (Clegg, 1974; WHO Memorandum, 1974; Smithers and Terry, 1976). Tsang and Damian (1975) are currently studying alterations in the host clotting mechanism and have recently presented evidence that at least one aspect of such interference is focused specifically at inhibiting the intrinsic pathway.

In the current discussion of immunopathologic events, it is sufficient to say that paired male and female adult worms successfully survive within the venous system of the infected host. A cross-section of such a pair of *S. mansoni* worms, within a mesenteric venule in a mouse, is shown in Figure 5.1. While the mean life-span of these worms in humans has been estimated to be 5 to 10 years (Warren et al, 1974a), individual patients have been reported to harbour, in the absence of reinfection, living schistosomes for 30 years (Berberian, Paquin and Fantauzzi, 1953).

However, when a worm does die, either naturally or under the influence of chemotherapeutic modalities, it usually forms an embolus, and is associated with an intense inflammatory reaction. These massive reactions are granulomatous in nature, and involve infiltrates of eosinophils, lymphocytes and mononuclear phagocytes. Their contribution to the morbidity associated with schistosomiasis has been debated, but in most situations this appears to be minimal. Cheever, DeWitt and Warren (1965) have demonstrated that mice subjected to three cycles of heavy infection and treatment, and therefore forced to absorb the impact of multiple dead worms three times, did not exhibit any gross manifestations of hepatosplenic disease.

Eggs

Although schistosome eggs do not multiply within the mammalian host, several hundreds to thousands are produced by each worm pair per day. These eggs either reach the environment by way of excreta, or are retained within the tissues. It has been estimated that with *S. mansoni* infections, in various host species, between 15 and 63 per cent of the eggs become lodged in the liver (Cheever, 1969). This circumstance is of no use to the parasite. During the six-day period after oviposition, the eggs embryonate and the embryo (miracidium) then lives for another 15 days. When trapped in the tissues, with no access to the external environment, this process occurs fruitlessly. This consequence usually occurs in the gut or bladder wall, or, due to their size (40–70 × 70–190 μm), in a capillary bed, the location of which is determined by the location of the worm pair, and whether collateral circulatory patterns have been established. Once eggs become stationary, they become the nidi of intense granulomatous reactions, often referred to as schistosome pseudotubercles. These anti-egg responses have been shown to be immunologic in aetiology, and have been implicated as being the primary basis of the pathogenesis of the severe forms of schistosomiasis (to be discussed below).

EXPERIMENTAL STUDIES OF EGG GRANULOMATA

Granulomas resulting from eggs of the three human schistosomes have been studied in man and a multiplicity of experimental animals ranging from chimpanzees to tree shrews, and chipmunks to chickens (von Lichtenberg, Smith and Cheever, 1966; von Lichtenberg et al, 1962; Davis, Mahmoud and Warren, 1974). Some qualitative and quantitative differences have been noted when granulomas of a single species of schistosome are compared in multiple host species (Akpom, Abdel-Wahab and Warren, 1970; Hsu et al, 1973). Such differences lessen, but are not eliminated, when only good hosts (those which support substantial, stable populations of adult worms) are compared (Cheever, 1965a, b). Likewise, comparisons between the granulomas induced by eggs of the three species, *S. mansoni*, *S. haematobium* and *S. japonicum*, are beginning to suggest considerable distinctions in regard to histopathologic appearances and mechanisms of immunopathogenesis. In a study of the characteristics of liver granulomas produced by the three species in hamsters, von Lichtenberg, Erickson and Sadun (1973) very beautifully described a set of arbitrarily defined progressive stages of granuloma formation, and correlated these with the stages of maturity, or degeneration of the central egg, the duration of infection, and the intensity of infection. In general, their observations appear to be applicable to most moderate-to-good host systems. Minimal reactions were associated with immature 'cell-ball' or 'neural' egg stages. Mature eggs were initially surrounded by an accumulation of lymphocytes, macrophages, eosinophils and/or neutrophils, and plasma cells. These reactions commonly proceeded with, or without, central neutrophilic and/or eosinophilic necrosis, to a more epithelioid cell granuloma, which was still composed of a mixed-cell infiltrate. This stage eventually involuted, becoming more fibroblastic, with the subsequent deposition of collagen and fibrosis.

The aetiology of such granulomas has been most extensively studied in relationship to *S. mansoni* eggs. Using immunofluorescence techniques, von Lichtenberg (1964) investigated these lesions in the livers of infected mice, and he also pioneered a technique using isolated eggs and tail vein injections, in which the eggs lodge in the microvasculature of the lungs. He demonstrated that mature eggs contained and elaborated antigenic material. Granuloma formation was accompanied by 'sequestration' of these antigens. Infection, sensitisation, or progression of initial reactions, was associated with the development of antibody against these antigenic components, and led to antigen–antibody complex formation within the granulomas.

The role of cell-mediated reactions

Warren and his colleagues, principally using the pulmonary localisation technique, have investigated the nature of the egg granuloma from a rich variety of points of view. The bases of, and observations gained through, this multidisciplinary approach to the immunopathogenesis of granuloma formation have been reviewed by Warren (1972). It was initially noted that a variety of immunosuppressive agents and manipulations could effectively suppress anti-egg granuloma formation, and this occurred most readily with the use of methods which most affected cell-mediated immune capabilities, rather than antibody production. It was concomitantly demonstrated that prior sensitisation to eggs accelerated and augmented granuloma formation, that the response was transferrable from infected or sensitised mice to normal mice by the use of lymphoid cells, but not sera, and that the reaction displayed specificity in regard to other parasites, the life-cycle stages of *S. mansoni*, and the eggs of the three human schistosome species (Warren, Domingo and Cowan, 1967; Warren and Domingo, 1970a, b). Subsequent studies using other hosts such as guinea-pigs (Boros et al, 1973a) and chickens (Davis et al, 1974) and other suppressive agents (Warren et al, 1974b) have continued to confirm the primary correlation between *S. mansoni* egg granuloma formation and anti-egg cell-mediated immune responsiveness, and have established that the major aetiologic mechanisms responsible for this granuloma are cell-mediated.

Active infections in immunosuppressed hosts

As cited above, the use of moderate immunosuppressive measures in the lung granuloma model resulted in the production of smaller granulomas (Warren, 1972). These measures were not generally effective in suppressing granuloma formation during active infection. In studies in which marked suppression of T-lymphocyte function was achieved (Fine, Buchanan and Colley, 1973; Buchanan, Fine and Colley, 1973), patent infection was accompanied by an altered pathogenesis. Hepatic and gut egg-focused lesions occurred, but were liquefactive necrotic in nature. Such animals also developed bacteraemia, which was probably related to their gut lesions. The hosts which were devoid of their cell-mediated mechanisms were capable of developing anti-egg agglutinating antibody, but not reaginic antibody. They died prior to animals which were infected in parallel, but which were immunologically intact. Studies are currently under way in several laboratories regarding *S. mansoni* infections in congenitally athymic (nude) mice. The data are as yet varied and anecdotal, but use of this model, in combination with selective reconstitution, may add to our understanding of granuloma formation.

The studies of Warren and his colleagues, and others, clearly show that cell-mediated responses are capable of expressing granuloma formation in response to *S. mansoni* eggs.

They do not, however, exclude a role or interaction for antibody in this lesion during complete infection. Numerous anti-egg antibodies have been shown to be induced by *S. mansoni* infection (von Lichtenberg, 1964; Boros and Warren, 1970; Colley, 1972, 1975; Boros, Pelley and Warren, 1975.

Immune Responses to a Soluble Egg Antigenic Preparation

The discovery by Boros and Warren (1970) that the soluble portion of a balanced salt homogenate of *S. mansoni* eggs, soluble egg antigens (SEA), was sufficient to induce and elicit granuloma formation, has allowed the study of many correlative humoral and cellular anti-SEA immune responses. Intradermal tests of infected mice with SEA demonstrated the existence of early (5 h) and late (24 h) reactivity, which was passively transferrable with sera and lymphoid cells respectively (Colley, 1972). Lymphoid cells from appropriately infected mice, exposed to SEA in vitro respond by lymphocyte blastogenesis (Colley, 1971) and produce the lymphokines migration inhibitory factor (MIF) (Boros et al, 1975) and eosinophil stimulation promoter (ESP) (Colley, 1973). In fact, the actual lesions, intact granulomas, isolated from infected livers have been shown to elaborate these lymphokines when maintained in tissue culture (Boros, Warren and Pelley, 1973b; James and Colley, 1975). Sera from infected mice contain agglutinating and reaginic antibody activities against SEA. On the basis of varying heat-lability patterns, two such long-latent period, reaginic antibodies have been reported (Colley, 1975).

The evidence that eggs are probably produced and destroyed continuously, in a steady-state manner, throughout chronic infection (Cheever, 1968), that eggs produce and release antigenic materials both in vivo (von Lichtenberg, 1964) and in vitro (Hang, Warren and Boros, 1974b), and that multiple types of immune responses have been demonstrated against these antigens, would suggest the existence of a complex immunologic framework, fraught with numerous possibilities of positive and negative influences, the sum total of which would be the observed granuloma formation.

Immunoregulatory control of responses to eggs and SEA

Prior to the existence of any evidence of this complexity, Andrade and Warren (1964) noticed that the massive granulomatous response observable at eight weeks of infection in the mouse (Fig. 5.2) diminished as chronic infection progressed. That is, granulomata formed late in infection, in response to recently deposited eggs, were demonstrably smaller (Fig. 5.3) in diameter and volume than those observed at the early stages of patent infection. In subsequent studies, Domingo and Warren (1968) injected eggs, which had been isolated from livers obtained during early infections, into the pulmonary microvasculature of mice at various times during chronic infection. The kinetics of granuloma formation remained the same throughout chronic infection, but the size of the granulomas induced clearly diminished over the course of 16 to 52 weeks of infection. In these experiments, there could be no question concerning any possible decrease in the antigenicity of the eliciting eggs, thus the host's immune capabilities were dampened. The occurrence of this phenomenon, originally termed 'endogenous desensitisation' has been associated with marked improvement in hepatosplenic disease of mice between 32 and 52 weeks of infection (Warren, 1966).

In attempts to understand the immunologic mechanisms which might be operative in this situation, Colley (1974, 1975) and Boros et al (1975), have followed a variety of in

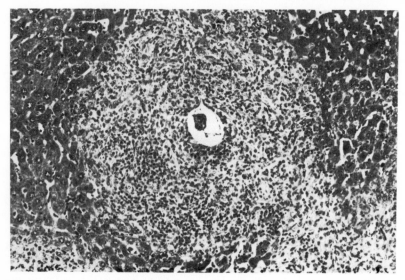

Figure 5.2   Perioval hepatic granuloma in a section from a mouse infected with *S. mansoni* for eight weeks. Liver parenchyma is intact; the lesion is large, composed of lymphocytes, eosinophils, and macrophages; the central egg was recently deposited. Haematoxylin and eosin, × 120

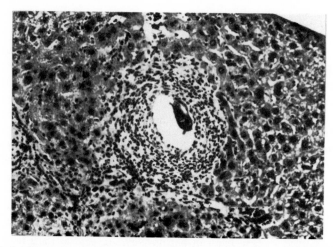

Figure 5.3   Perioval hepatic granuloma in a section from a mouse infected with *S. mansoni* for 35 weeks. Liver parenchyma is still intact; the lesion is small, but composed of cells which have recently infiltrated in response to the central egg, which was recently deposited in the tissue; the cells include lymphocytes, some eosinophils, and macrophages. Haematoxylin and eosin, × 120

vivo and in vitro anti-SEA immune responses in parallel with the diminution of granuloma formation during primary *S. mansoni* infections in mice. Both groups observed relatively low titres of anti-SEA agglutinating antibody at eight weeks, the time of maximal granuloma formation. These levels increased dramatically during chronic infection. Concomitant with the decrease in granuloma size, Colley (1974, 1975) reported a decrease in serum levels of anti-SEA, heat-labile, 72-h skin-fixing reaginic antibody, and conversely, an increase in a similar but heat-stable reaginic antibody. No further information is available concerning the class identity of these antibody activities.

Boros et al (1975) demonstrated that production of MIF by spleen cells lessens during chronic infection, and this is accompanied by an altered antigen dose–response curve. That is, as infection progressed, peak MIF production occurred with progressively decreasing doses of antigen. This was paralleled by suppression by supraoptimal doses of antigen. Anti-SEA delayed footpad swelling was also studied in this investigation. It too was seen to diminish progressively. Intriguingly, similar responses against PPD, elicited in *S. mansoni*-infected mice sensitised with complete Freund's adjuvant, remained prominent throughout the course of infection, possibly indicating a specific diminution of immune capabilities.

Colley (1974, 1975) demonstrated progressive decreased production of another lymphokine, in response to SEA, eosinophil stimulation promoter (ESP) (Colley, 1973; Greene and Colley, 1974, 1976) and a gradual lessening of the ability of lymph node cells to respond to SEA by in vitro lymphocyte blastogenesis throughout infection. This has recently been confirmed by Lewert (1975) and Lewert, Olsen and Cahill (1975) and extended by the observation that antiworm extract responsiveness was maintained, while anti-SEA reactivity declined. Anti-PPD responses also remained strong in this system.

Lewert (1975), Lewert et al (1975) and Pelley, Ruffier and Warren (1976) have observed progressively decreased responsiveness of lymphocytes from chronically infected mice upon exposure to the T-lymphocyte phytomitogens phytohaemagglutinin (PHA) and concanavalin A (Con A). The latter group again demonstrated a clear alteration in regard to dose–response analysis, which was reminiscent of those curves correlated with the activity of suppressor T-lymphocytes by Bash and Waksman (1975). To date, Colley (unpublished data) has not observed any decrease in lymphocyte responsiveness to PHA. However, the various investigators have used different strains of mice and different lymphocyte culture techniques. Recent studies (Colley et al, 1975; 1977) of the in vitro ability of human lymphocytes from patients infected with *S. mansoni* indicate that chronic infection led to diminished responsiveness to SEA, while lymphoid reactivity to cercarial and worm antigen preparations increased during long-term infection.

Thus, a variety of anti-SEA responses are altered in both positive and negative directions, concomitantly with the observed diminution of granuloma formation (Boros et al, 1975; Colley, 1975). Colley (1976) has recently employed a more direct analysis of this phenomenon. This involved passive transfer studies from chronically infected (20–30 weeks) mice into mice with recently patent infections (six weeks). At eight weeks of their infection (two weeks post-transfer) the recipients were studied in regard to the size of their hepatic granulomas. To date, the data indicate that large amounts (total of 3 ml over two weeks) of chronic sera did not appreciably affect the size of eight-week granulomas. In contrast, chronic lymph node or spleen cells markedly suppressed granuloma formation in this situation. Earlier in infection this attribute appears to be compartmentalised in the spleen. Current studies (Lewis and Colley, in progress) indicate that suppression is titratable by quantitative transfers of spleen cells, and the suppressive effects of the cells is eliminated by incubation of cells in anti-θ allosera and complement, prior to transfer. These studies imply, but do not yet establish, that suppressor T-lymphocytes contribute to the modulation of granuloma size during chronic infections.

Immunological unresponsiveness to SEA

In 1969, Lewert and Mandlowitz reported another situation which led to a diminution of anti-egg granuloma formation in mice. The offspring of female mice which had heavy, mature, *S. mansoni* infections prior to their insemination exhibited significantly smaller granulomas when eggs were injected into their pulmonary microvasculature. Further-more, following exposure to eggs, these 'tolerant-like' mice were seen to be unresponsive to SEA by both lymphocyte blastogenesis and the macrophage migration inhibition assay (Lewert, 1975). Hang, Boros and Warren (1974a) confirmed the observations regarding the offspring of infected mice and indicated that the intensity of the mother's infection was critical, in that the progeny of light or moderately infected mice did not exhibit such unresponsiveness. The administration of high doses of SEA to uninfected pregnant females resulted in the induction of a state of unresponsiveness in the offspring. When mice which had received a very high (1 mg) dose of SEA as neonates, were challenged with eggs at eight weeks of age, they responded poorly compared to control littermates. Although low-zone tolerance was not achievable, it may be critical that as little as 0.1 ng of SEA was capable of sensitising a mouse. The administration of very high doses of SEA was required to get any reduction in anti-egg responsiveness in adult mice. The effects of such manipulations were seen to be more transitory than those associated with induction in utero. When chronic infections were established in these mice, the observed un-responsiveness was shown to be ineffective in preventing hepatosplenic disease (Warren, 1974).

A perhaps related phenomenon has been observed (A. Capron, personal communication) in Bahia, Brazil. In an area where no transmission of schistosomiasis was occurring, 50 per cent of the children of heavily infected mothers were positive by a leucocyte migration assay and delayed-type hypersensitivity skin tests to a schistosomal antigen preparation. These children were seen not to be infected and antigenic exposure was presumed to have occurred from the mother.

The granulomatous process induced by *S. haematobium* eggs has been studied during experimental infections and following injection of isolated eggs into the pulmonary capillary bed of mice. The latter situation revealed the response to be relatively specific. Upon histopathologic analysis, the process appeared similar to that evoked by *S. mansoni* (Warren and Domingo, 1970a). Infection studies using *S. haematobium* (von Lichtenberg et al, 1973; Erickson, Jones and Tang, 1974; Sadun et al, 1970) have indicated similar results. However, two general properties may distinguish the conditions of *S. haematobium* granulomas from those of *S. mansoni*. These are that eggs of the former are much more commonly observed as clusters, and they more often calcify in old lesions.

The progressive diminution of granuloma size, discussed above in regard to chronic *S. mansoni* infection was not observed in hamsters infected with *S. haematobium* (Erickson et al, 1974). However, measurements of single egg granulomas are difficult to perform, due to the clustering of the eggs. Studies in chimpanzees (Sadun et al, 1970) and man (von Lichtenberg et al, 1971a) suggested that the *S. haematobium* induced granulomatous response did decrease with progressive infection. The occurrence of early observed florid lesions appeared to subside with the development of the later stage lesions, referred to as sandy patches.

S. *Japonicum* Egg Granulomata

Lesion formation in response to *S. japonicum* eggs which are also produced in clusters and which calcify readily, has recently become the subject of renewed interest and investigation. The clinical severity often observed with *S. japonicum* infection has anecdotally been ascribed to the high rate of egg production per worm pair with this species. However, in 1953, Meleney et al reported that comparisons of infections with the three schistosomes indicated that the eggs of *S. japonicum* usually produced more severe lesions than those of *S. mansoni* or *S. haematobium*. They attributed this to the fact that the eggs are usually deposited in large groups, but also noted that individual *S. japonicum* eggs seemed to exert, or evoke, a more intense reaction to themselves.

S. japonicum infections in chimpanzees (von Lichtenberg et al, 1971b) resulted in 'classical' hepatic pseudotubercles which were described as large, exudative and destructive. The disproportionate intensity of these lesions was noted, and their cellular composition was described as often containing large numbers of neutrophils or eosinophils, with plasma cells, macrophages, giant cells, fibroblasts and lymphocytes. Hsu et al (1972, 1973) have reported that in several experimental hosts, the hepatic lesions evoked by *S. japonicum* eggs appeared to involve more neutrophils than those induced by *S. mansoni* eggs. This association was also reported by von Lichtenberg et al (1973) using the hamster as host. Other traits cited for *S. japonicum* lesions were their exudative and necrotic nature, the relative increase of plasma cells within the lesions, and the frequency of the occurrence of the Hoeppli phenomenon.

The Hoeppli phenomenon (Hoeppli, 1932) which was initially reported in *S. japonicum* infections, and has been described in detail by von Lichtenberg et al (1966) is observed as an eosinophilic fringe surrounding a schistosome egg within a granuloma. This fringe appears to radiate from the egg. von Lichtenberg et al (1966) have shown that this is an antigen–antibody complex reaction involving egg antigens, and have related it to increased intensity of infection (probably related to the degree of antibody production). Amyloid deposition was also associated with *S. japonicum* infections.

In contrast to these reports of massive lesions occurring in *S. japonicum*-infected hosts, when Warren and Domingo (1970b) studied the size, development and cellular composition of lesions induced by isolated *S. japonicum* eggs injected into the pulmonary microvasculature, they observed that the reactions were small, essentially similar to foreign-body reactions and were not increased by prior exposure.

These studies have been continued by Warren et al (1975). Observations of early infections indicated egg production began by about three weeks, but for the following two weeks there were no reactions related to the eggs lodged in the liver. By three weeks postpatency, large abscesses occurred and, by special staining, essentially all the infiltrating cells were seen to be eosinophils. Prominent periportal inflammation was present and consisted primarily of plasma cells. After this time, large granulomatous lesions, now containing some macrophages and fibroblasts, occurred around egg aggregates, and hepatosplenomegaly and portal hypertension developed. Analysis by the lung injection assay revealed that isolated *S. japonicum* eggs elicited no reactions, even when injected into infected mice which were actively producing large hepatic lesions. Pre-exposure to eggs by the peritoneal route (known to be effective for anti-*S. mansoni* egg sensitisation) did not lead to secondary lesion formation upon challenge. In contrast, subcutaneous injection of either *S. japonicum* eggs or SEA from such eggs, with or without complete Freund's adjuvant, did sensitise the mice. In another set of experiments, it was shown that *S. japonicum* SEA, when injected into the footpads of mice infected with *S. japonicum*, induced massive early footpad swelling, which was histopathologically compatible with an Arthus reaction, but no delayed reactions were observed (Warren, 1975).

Thus, evidence continues to mount which indicates that the immunopathogenesis of anti-*S. japonicum* egg lesion formation is different from that reported for the other two human schistosomes. It appears that studies which focus upon antigen–antibody complex mechanisms are likely to prove interesting.

The previously discussed 'modulation' of granuloma formation has likewise been observed in mice chronically infected with *S. japonicum* (Warren and Berry, 1972). This was noted in regard to hepatosplenic disease and its associated phenomena, as well as a decrease in the granulomatous response, and occurred in spite of continued accumulation of large numbers of eggs in the livers.

Chronic Schistosomiasis

Hepatosplenic disease in man

Severe, hepatosplenic schistosomiasis mansoni and japonica in man is characterised by portal hypertension, and complications resulting from the development of collateral circulation and the dissemination of eggs. These include oesophageal varices, cor pulmonale, and a wide variety of ectopic granulomatous processes (Warren, 1973). Morphologic analysis indicates that primarily three hepatic phenomena are associated with this process. They are the granulomatous lesions previously discussed; diffuse, chronic inflammation of the portal spaces and fibrous septa which radiate from them; and severe Symmer's 'clay-pipe stem' periportal fibrosis. The hepatic parenchyma is often surprisingly well preserved. However, late in infection chronic hepatitis, seemingly unrelated to the intensity of infection, may be observed (WHO Memorandum, 1974). Thus, the actual aetiologic mechanism responsible for the severe morbidity observed in 4 to 12 per cent of the 200 to 300 million persons with schistosomiasis is not primarily that of impairment of liver function, but rather obstruction of portal blood flow.

Experimental studies of hepatosplenic schistosomiasis

The origin of this portal blockage, and the possible progressive relationships of the three phenomena mentioned, has been discussed by others (Warren, 1966, 1973; WHO Memorandum, 1974). In the mouse it is clear that egg granulomas in the presinusoidal capillaries do produce hepatosplenic disease with increased portal pressure and esophageal varices (Warren, 1966). It is perhaps not as convincing that the fibrous bands which result from sequential, row on row, coalescence of old fibrous granulomas (Fig. 5.4) can be directly equated with the pipe-stem fibrosis of man. The contribution of diffuse non-egg associated portal inflammation is also unclear. In contrast, infections in the chimpanzees lead to continuous progressive development of pipe-stem fibrosis (Sadun et al, 1966) and this observation is even more prominent in *S. japonicum* infection of chimpanzees (von Lichtenberg et al, 1971b). However, these animals, despite marked obstruction of intrahepatic portal vein branches, did not develop increased portal or intrahepatic pressures, nor did they have as extensive oesophageal varices as would have been predicted based upon the severity of their hepatic fibrosis. Whether this was due to their ability to markedly develop multiple collateral venous channels remains in question. In these chimpanzee studies and in humans (Cheever, 1968) it appears that the formation of pipe-stem fibrosis of the larger triads precedes egg localisation in these areas of fibrotic bands. Thus, as with most choices concerning model systems, evidence is conflicting, models are incomplete, and decisions

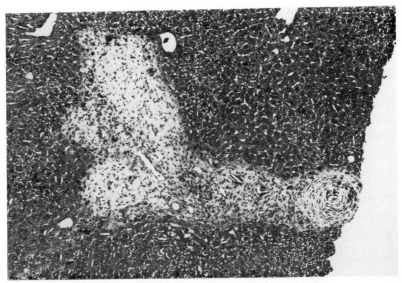

Figure 5.4   Section of a liver from a mouse infected with *S. mansoni* for 22 weeks. Liver parenchymal tissue is normal. The apparent coalescence of old, fibrotic, anti-egg granulomas resembles the appearance of classic Symmers' clay-pipe stem fibrosis. Haematoxylin and eosin, × 80

must be made in relationship to the experimental questions to be asked, and personal preferences, convictions and experience.

Chronic S. haematobium *infection*

In human schistosomiasis haematobium, because the worms primarily reside in the vesical plexuses, most symptomatology is related to the urinary tract. The bladder lesions which have been described are considered mainly egg-induced and include early, active polypoid patches, often containing diffuse exudative perioval reactions; fibrotic sandy patches containing calcified eggs; and purely fibrous lesions (von Lichtenberg et al, 1971a). Pyelonephritis and hydronephrosis have been associated with severe obstructive lesions (Smith et al, 1974; Webbe et al, 1974). It has been difficult to establish small animal models of *S. haematobium* infection which develop urinary tract involvement (Warren, 1973).

Splenomegaly

The marked splenomegaly associated with schistosomiasis is initially related to reticuloendotheial proliferation, and considerable germinal centre activity, resulting in an increased proportion of plasma cells. Passive congestion-induced alterations, resulting from portal hypertension, occur later in infection (WHO Memorandum, 1974).

The Role of Eosinophil Leucocyte Interactions

Schistosomiasis is, as are most helminthic infections, associated with prominent blood and tissue eosinophilias. Likewise, high levels of IgE antibodies, circulating and deposited immune complexes, and a high degree of T-lymphocyte sensitisation all occur during schistosomiasis. These are three immunologic responses which have been shown to influence eosinophils (WHO Memorandum, 1974; Ottesen, 1976). Peripheral blood eosinophilia has been followed in a variety of hosts with schistosomiasis (Fairley, 1920; Diaz-Rivera et al, 1956; Colley, Katz and Wikel, 1974). Upon primary infection the major episode coincides with the occurrence of strong anti-egg responses and continues throughout most of the chronic phase of infection (Colley et al, 1974; Colley, 1975). Colley and co-workers have reported a lymphokine, eosinophil stimulation (ESP), which induces enhanced migration of eosinophils (Colley, 1973), and have shown that this moiety is produced by sensitised T-lymphocytes upon exposure to SEA (Greene and Colley, 1976). The responsible factor is synthesised de novo, quite heat-stable, approximately 30 000 daltons, and a protein (Greene and Colley, 1974). This material appears to be distinct from the eosinophilotactic lymphokine ECF-p, reported by Cohn and Ward (1971) and further characterised by Torisu et al (1973). Kazura et al (1975) have recently established that lymphocytes from patients with S. mansoni also produce ESP activity in response to SEA.

While these observations presumably concern immunologic influences governing the mobility and status of eosinophils, the role of this cell in this, or any, situation remains enigmatic. It is in this area of eosinophil studies that the use of schistosomiasis as a model system may be most interesting. Two potential functional roles for eosinophils are currently being investigated in relationship to schistosomiasis. One involves interactions of eosinophils and schistosomula, both in vitro (Butterworth et al, 1974, 1975) and in vivo (Mahmoud, Warren and Peters, 1975b). These studies implicate the eosinophil as an important participant in reactions which result in resistance to reinfection. The nature of this participation, or of these mechanisms, is currently unknown. The other area deals with eosinophil–egg interactions. Eosinophils have long been prominently associated with the anti-egg granulomatous reactions. This in vivo relationship has been observed to sometimes involve actual cell-to-egg interactions with resulting discharge of cell granular enzymes (Bogitsh, 1971). However, the progression of eosinophil involvement in egg destruction has been unclear. In current in vitro studies of eosinophils cocultivated with eggs, James and Colley (1976) have reported that isolated eosinophils from S. mansoni-infected mice were capable of destroying 20 per cent of the target eggs. This activity occurred progressively over a 24-h incubation at 37°C, but did not occur during incubation at 4°C. Macrophages, neutrophils, or spleen cells were unable to effect egg destruction. Antigen-depleted eggs were less susceptible to eosinophil attack, and eosinophils from normal mice, or Trichinella spiralis-infected mice were not as effective as S. mansoni-related eosinophils. This system needs to be analysed in regard to the mechanisms of interaction responsible for these activities.

Mahmoud, Warren and Graham (1975a) have shown that injections of anti-eosinophil serum effectively reduced the size of anti-egg granulomas, by the virtual elimination of eosinophils in these lesions. It will be interesting to see whether this treatment has any effect upon disease, that is, whether it is beneficial, due to the production of smaller, less obstructive, lesions, or counter productive due to interference with the possible egg destruction–clearance role proposed above.

Summary

The predominant immunopathologic reaction in schistosomiasis appears to be the granuloma formation induced and elicited by schistosome eggs. These lesions, which occur primarily in the liver, gut and urinary tract are clearly immunologic in nature, but it appears that the actual mechanisms may be different with regard to *S. japonicum* on the one hand and *S. mansoni* and *S. haematobium* on the other. In the case of the former, the lesions are currently under study and it seems that a major role may have to be envisaged for antigen–antibody complex reactions. The latter, primarily studied with *S. mansoni*, have been shown to be largely based upon cell-mediated responses. Undoubtedly both humoral and cellular mechanisms contribute to both, especially during chronic infection. It may be that analyses of the interactions of various mechanisms, predominant and minor in nature, will be required to gain further understanding of the immunoregulatory control mechanisms active in the diminution of granuloma formation observed during chronic infection.

While granulomas may be the most striking immunologically based lesions, the possibility remains that dermal and pulmonary reactions, induced by larval forms and/or adult worms, and elicited by penetrating larvae, may be at least in part responsible for the low morbidity in schistosomiasis. This would possibly be due to their hypothetical role in resistance. This controversial subject has the benefit of a long and active history, but as yet, suffers from a lack of conclusive data. It is, however, receiving spirited attention, and may yet be resolved with a positive outcome.

The fundamental basis of acute schistosomiasis, while logically conjectured to be immunologic in nature, remains to be determined. Certainly the opportunities exist for interactions of soluble immune reactants. This is also true during chronic infection. Evidence is accumulating that such immune complex interactions exist, and their contribution to the disease state is being investigated.

It is hoped that basic information generated by studies concerning the progression and control of schistosome egg granuloma formation will be useful not only in regard to schistosomiasis, but also in designing and analysing investigations of other granulomatous disease conditions. Likewise, evidence regarding the activities of eosinophils in this system will perhaps suggest new approaches or interpretations regarding the role(s) of this cell in other situations.

ACKNOWLEDGEMENTS

The author would like to gratefully acknowledge the excellent secretarial assistance of Mrs Judith O'Connell and Mrs Lucille Grissim and to thank Dr Allen W. Cheever for his helpful suggestions and criticisms regarding the manuscript. Original research cited was supported by the Veterans Administration, US Public Health Service grant AI 11289, and grant RF 74084 from the Rockefeller Foundation and the Edna McConnell Clark Foundation.

REFERENCES

Akpom, C. A., Abdel-Wahab, M. F. & Warren, K. S. (1970) Comparison of formation of granulomata around eggs of *Schistosoma mansoni* in the mouse, guinea-pig, rat, and hamster. *American Journal of Tropical Medicine and Hygiene*, **19**, 996–1000.

Andrade, Z. A., Andrade, S. G. & Sadigursky, M. (1971) Renal changes in patients with hepatosplenic schistosomiasis. *American Journal of Tropical Medicine and Hygiene*, **20**, 77–83.

Andrade, Z. A. & Queiroz, A. C. (1968) Lesões renais na esquistossomose hepatesplenica. *Revista do Instituto de Medicina Tropical de São Paulo*, **10**, 36–40.

Andrade, Z. A. & Warren, K. S. (1964) Mild prolonged schistosomiasis in mice: alterations in host response with time and the development of portal fibrosis. *Transactions of the Royal Society of Tropical Medicine and Hygiene*, **58**, 53–57.

Askenase, P. W., Hayden, B. & Higashi, G. I. (1976) Cutaneous basophil hypersensitivity and inhibited macrophage migration in guinea-pigs with schistosomiasis. *Clinical and Experimental Immunology*, **23**, 318–327.

Barlow, C. H. (1936) Is there dermatitis in Egyptian schistosomiasis? *American Journal of Hygiene*, **24**, 587–599.

Bash, J. A. & Waksman, B. H. (1975) The suppressive effect of immunization on the proliferative responses of rat T cells *in vitro. Journal of Immunology*, **114**, 782–787.

Bawden, M. P. & Weller, T. H. (1974) *Schistosoma mansoni* circulating antigen: detection by complement fixation in sera from infected hamsters and mice. *American Journal of Tropical Medicine and Hygiene*, **23**, 1077–1084.

Berberian, D. A., Paquin, H. O., Jr & Fantauzzi, A. (1953) Longevity of *Schistosoma hematobium* and *Schistosoma mansoni*: observations based on a case. *Journal of Parasitology*, **39**, 517–519.

Berggren, W. L. & Weller, T. H. (1967) Immunoelectrophoretic demonstration of specific circulating antigen in animals infected with *Schistosoma mansoni. American Journal of Tropical Medicine and Hygiene*, **16**, 606–612.

Billings, F. T., Winkenwerder, W. L. & Hunninen, A. V. (1946) Studies on acute schistosomiasis japonica in the Philippine islands. I. A clinical study of 337 cases with a preliminary report on the results of treatment with Fuadin in 110 cases. *Bulletin of the Johns Hopkins Hospital*, **78**, 21–56.

Bogitsh, B. J. (1971) *Schistosoma mansoni*: cytochemistry of eosinophils in egg-caused early hepatic granulomas in mice. *Experimental Parasitology*, **29**, 493–500.

Boros, D. L., Pelley, R. P. & Warren, K. S. (1975) Spontaneous modulation of granulomatous hypersensitivity in schistosomiasis mansoni. *Journal of Immunology*, **114**, 1437–1441.

Boros, D. L. & Warren, K. S. (1970) Delayed hypersensitivity-type granuloma and dermal reaction induced and elicited by a soluble factor isolated from *Schistosoma mansoni* eggs. *Journal of Experimental Medicine*, **132**, 488–507.

Boros, D. L., Schwartz, H. J., Powell, A. E. & Warren, K. S. (1973a) Delayed hypersensitivity, as manifested by granuloma formation, dermal reactivity, macrophage migration inhibition, and lymphocyte transformation, induced and elicited in guinea-pigs with soluble antigens of *Schistosoma mansoni* eggs. *Journal of Immunology*, **110**, 1118–1125.

Boros, D. L., Warren, K. S. & Pelley, R. P. (1973b) The secretion of migration inhibitory factor by intact schistosome egg granuloma maintained in vitro. *Nature (London)*, **246**, 224–226.

Brack, M., McPhaul, J. J., Damian, R. T. & Kalter, S. S. (1972) Glomerular lesions in 'normal' and *Schistosoma mansoni*-infected baboons (*Papio cynocephalus*). *Journal of Medical Primatology*, **1**, 363–373.

Brito, T., Gunji, J., Camargo, M. E., Ceravolo, A. & Silva, L. C. (1971) Glomerular lesions in experimental infections of *Schistosoma mansoni* in *Cebus apella* monkeys. *Bulletin of the World Health Organization*, **45**, 419–422.

Brito, T., Gunji, J., Camargo, M. E., Penna, D. O. & Silva, L. C. (1970) Advanced kidney disease in patients with hepatosplenic Manson's schistosomiasis. *Revista do Instituto de Medicina Tropical de São Paulo*, **12**, 225–235.

Buchanan, R. D., Fine, D. P. & Colley, D. G. (1973) *Schistosoma mansoni* infection in mice depleted of thymus-dependent lymphocytes. II. Pathology and altered pathogenesis. *American Journal of Pathology*, **71**, 207–218.

Butterworth, A. E., Sturrock, R. F., Houba, V. & Rees, P. H. (1974) Antibody-dependent cell-mediated damage to schistosomula in vitro. *Nature (London)*, **252**, 503–505.

Butterworth, A. E., Sturrock, R. F., Houba, V., Mahmoud, A. A. F., Sher, A. & Rees, P. H. (1975) Eosinophils as mediators of antibody-dependent damage to schistosomula. *Nature (London)*, **256**, 727–729.

Carlier, Y., Bout, D., Bina, J. C., Camus, D., Figueiredo, J. F. M. & Capron, A. (1975) Immunologic studies in human schistosomiasis. I. Parasitic antigen in urine. *American Journal of Tropical Medicine and Hygiene*, **24**, 949–954.

Cheever, A. W. (1965a) A comparative study of *Schistosoma mansoni* infections in mice, gerbils, multimammate rats and hamsters. I. The relation of portal hypertension to size of hepatic granulomas. *American Journal of Tropical Medicine and Hygiene*, **14**, 211–226.

Cheever, A. W. (1965b) A comparative study of *Schistosoma mansoni* infections in mice, gerbils, multimammate rats, and hamsters. II. Qualitative pathological differences. *American Journal of Tropical Medicine and Hygiene*, **14**, 227–238.

Cheever, A. W. (1968) A quantitative post-mortem study of schistosomiasis mansoni in man. *American Journal of Tropical Medicine and Hygiene*, **17**, 38–64.

Cheever, A. W. (1969) Quantitative comparison of the intensity of *Schistosoma mansoni* infections in man and experimental animals. *Transactions of the Royal Society of Tropical Medicine and Hygiene*, **63**, 781–795.

Cheever, A. W., DeWitt, W. B. & Warren, K. S. (1965) Repeated infection and treatment of mice with *Schistosoma mansoni*: functional, anatomic, and immunologic observations. *American Journal of Tropical Medicine and Hygiene*, **14**, 239–253.

Clegg, J. A. (1974) Host antigens and the immune response in schistosomiasis. In *Parasites in the Immunized Host: Mechanisms of Survival. Ciba Foundation Symposium 25* (new series), pp. 161–176. Amsterdam: Elsevier–Excerpta Medica–North Holland.

Cohn, S. & Ward, P. A. (1971) In vitro and in vivo activity of a lymphocyte and immune complex-dependent chemotactic factor for eosinophils. *Journal of Experimental Medicine*, **133**, 133–146.

Colley, D. G. (1971) Schistosomal egg antigen-induced lymphocyte blastogenesis in experimental murine *Schistosoma mansoni* infection. *Journal of Immunology*, **107**, 1477–1480.

Colley, D. G. (1972) Intradermal immune responses to a schistosomal egg antigen during experimental murine *Schistosoma mansoni* infection. *Proceedings of the Society for Experimental Biology and Medicine*, **140**, 772–775.

Colley, D. G. (1973) Eosinophils and immune mechanisms. I. Eosinophil stimulation promoter (ESP): a lymphokine induced by specific antigen or phytohemagglutinin. *Journal of Immunology*, **110**, 1419–1423.

Colley, D. G. (1974) Immunologic consequences of schistosome infection. In *Progress of Immunology II*, ed. Brent, L. & Holborow, J., Vol. 4, pp. 171–179. Amsterdam: North-Holland Publishing Co.

Colley, D. G. (1975) Immune responses to a soluble schistosomal egg antigen preparation during chronic primary infection with *Schistosoma mansoni*. *Journal of Immunology*, **115**, 150–156.

Colley, D. G. (1976) Adoptive suppression of granuloma formation. *Journal of Experimental Medicine*, **143**, 696–700.

Colley, D. G., Freeman, G. L., Jr, Cook, J. A. & Jordan, P. (1975) Lymphocyte blastogenesis reactivity in patients with schistosomiasis. *Tenth Joint Parasitic Diseases Conference, US-Japan Cooperative Medical Science Program*, October 1975, Bethesda, MD.

Colley, D. G., Cook, J. A., Freeman, G. L., Bartholomew, R. K. & Jordan, P. (1977) Immune responses during human schistosomiasis Mansoni: I. In vitro lymphocyte blastogenic response to heterogeneous antigenic preparations from schistosome eggs, worms and cercariae. *International Archives of Allergy and Applied Immunology* (in press).

Colley, D. G., Katz, S. P. & Wikel, S. K. (1974) Schistosomiasis: an experimental model for the study of immunopathologic mechanisms which involve eosinophils. In *Advances in the Biosciences*, ed. Raspe, G & Bernhard, S., Vol. 12, pp. 653–665. Oxford: Pergamon Press.

Colley, D. G., Magalhães-Filho, A. & Coelho, R. B. (1972) Immunopathology of dermal reactions induced by *Schistosoma mansoni* cercariae and cercarial extract. *American Journal of Tropical Medicine and Hygiene*, **21**, 558–568.

Cort, W. W. (1928) Schistosome dermatitis in the United States (Michigan). *Journal of the American Medical Association*, **90**, 1027–1029.

Davis, B. H., Mahmoud, A. A. F. & Warren, K. S. (1974) Granulomatous hypersensitivity to *Schistosoma mansoni* eggs in thymectomized and bursectomized chickens. *Journal of Immunology*, **113**, 1064–1067.

Dias-Rivera, R. S., Rãmos-Morales, F., Koppisch, E., Garcia-Palmieri, M. R., Cintrón-Rivera, A. A., Marchand, E. J., González, O. & Torregrosa, M. V. (1956) Acute Manson's schistosomiasis. *American Journal of Medicine*, **21**, 918–943.

Domingo, E. O. & Warren, K. S. (1968) Endogenous desensitization: changing host granulomatous response to schistosome eggs at different stages of infection with *Schistosoma mansoni*. *American Journal of Pathology*, **52**, 369–379.

Erickson, D. G., Jones, C. E. & Tang, D. B. (1974) Schistosomiasis mansoni, haematobia and japonica in hamsters: liver granuloma measurements. *Experimental Parasitology*, **35**, 425–433.

Ezzat, E., Osman, R. A., Ahmet, K. Y. & Soothill, J. F. (1974) The association between *Schistosoma haematobium* infection and heavy proteinuria. *Transactions of the Royal Society of Tropical Medicine and Hygiene*, **68**, 315–318.

Fairley, N. H. (1920) A comparative study of experimental bilharziasis in monkeys contrasted with the hitherto described lesions in man. *Journal of Pathology and Bacteriology*, **23**, 289–314.

Falcão, H. A. & Gould, D. B. (1975) Immune complex nephropathy in schistosomiasis. *Annals of Internal Medicine*, **83**, 148–154.

Fine, D. P., Buchanan, R. D. & Colley, D. G. (1973) *Schistosoma mansoni* infection in mice depleted of thymus-dependent lymphocytes. I. Eosinophilia and immunologic responses to a schistosomal egg preparation. *American Journal of Pathology*, **71**, 193–206.

Gold, R., Rosen, R. S. & Weller, T. H. (1969) A specific circulating antigen in hamsters infected with *Schistosoma mansoni*. Detection of antigen in serum and urine, and correlation between antigenic concentration and worm burden. *American Journal of Tropical Medicine and Hygiene*, **18,** 545–552.

Greene, B. M. & Colley, D. G. (1974) Eosinophils and immune mechanisms. II. Partial characterization of the lymphokine eosinophil stimulation promoter. *Journal of Immunology*, **113,** 910–917.

Greene, B. M. & Colley, D. G. (1976) Eosinophils and immune mechanisms. III. Production of the lymphokine eosinophil stimulation promoter by mouse T lymphocytes. *Journal of Immunology*, **116,** 1078–1083.

Hang, L. M., Boros, D. L. & Warren, K. S. (1974a) Induction of immunological hyporesponsiveness to granulomatous hypersensitivity in *Schistosoma mansoni* infection. *Journal of Infectious Diseases*, **130,** 515–522.

Hang, L. M., Warren, K. S. & Boros, D. L. (1974b) *Schistosoma mansoni*: antigenic secretions and the etiology of egg granulomas in mice. *Experimental Parasitology*, **35,** 288–298.

Hillyer, G. V. (1973) Schistosome deoxyribonucleic acid (DNA), antibodies to DNA in schistosome infections, and their possible role in renal pathology. *Boletin Asociacion Medica de Puerto Rico*, **65,** 1–22. Supl.

Hillyer, G. V. & Lewert, R. M. (1974) Studies on renal pathology in hamsters infected with *Schistosoma mansoni* and *S. japonicum*. *American Journal of Tropical Medicine and Hygiene*, **23,** 404–411.

Hoeppli, R. (1932) Histological observations in experimental schistosomiasis japonica. *Chinese Medical Journal*, **46,** 1179–1186.

Hsu, S. Y. L., Davis, J. R. & Hsu, H. F. (1965) Histopathology in rhesus monkeys infected four times with the Formosan strain of *Schistosoma japonicum*. *Zeitshrift für Tropenmedizin und Parasitologie*, **16,** 297–304.

Hsu, S. Y. L., Hsu, H. F., Davis, J. R. & Lust, G. L. (1972) Comparative studies on the lesions caused by eggs of *Schistosoma japonicum* and *Schistosoma mansoni* in livers of albino mice and rhesus monkeys. *Annals of Tropical Medicine and Parasitology*, **66,** 89–97.

Hsu, S. Y. L., Hsu, H. F., Lust, G. L., Davis, J. R. & Eveland, L. K. (1973) Comparative studies on the lesions caused by eggs of *Schistosoma japonicum* and *Schistosoma mansoni* in the liver of hamsters, guinea-pigs, and albino rats. *Annals of Tropical Medicine and Parasitology*, **67,** 349–356.

James, S. L. & Colley, D. G. (1975) Eosinophils and immune mechanisms: production of the lymphokine eosinophil stimulation promoter (ESP) in vitro by isolated intact granulomas. *Journal of the Reticuloendothelial Society*, **18,** 283–293.

James, S. L. & Colley, D. G. (1976) Eosinophil-mediated destruction of *Schistosoma mansoni* eggs. *Journal of the Reticuloendothelial Society*, **20,** 359–374.

Kazura, J. W., Mahmoud, A. A. F., Karbs, K. S. & Warren, K. S. (1975) The lymphokine eosinophil stimulation promoter and human schistosomiasis mansoni. *Journal of Infectious Diseases*, **132,** 702–706.

Lehman, J. S., Jr, Mott, K. E., DeSousa, C. A. M., Leboreiro, O. & Muniz, T. M. (1975) The association of schistosomiasis mansoni and proteinuria in an endemic area. A preliminary report. *American Journal of Tropical Medicine and Hygiene*, **24,** 616–618.

Lewert, R. M. (1975) Hypersensitivity, tolerance, and immunopathology in schistosomiasis: some current concepts and speculations. In *Schistosomiasis in Southeast Asia and the Far East, Proceedings of the 14th SEAMO–Tropical Medicine Seminar*, Bangkok.

Lewert, R. M., Olsen, N. J. & Cahill, J. (1975) Development of tolerance to antigens in schistosome infected mice. Presented at the *24th Annual Meeting of the American Society of Tropical Medicine and Hygiene*, November 1975, New Orleans.

Lewert, R. M. & Mandlowitz, S. (1969) Schistosomiasis: prenatal induction of tolerance to antigens. *Nature (London)*, **224,** 1029–1030.

Lichtenberg, F. von (1964) Studies on granuloma formation. III. Antigen sequestration and destruction in the schistosome pseudotubercle. *American Journal of Pathology*, **45,** 75–93.

Lichtenberg, F. von & Ritchie, L. S. (1961) Cellular resistance against schistosomula of *Schistosoma mansoni* in *Macaca mulatta* monkeys following prolonged infections. *American Journal of Tropical Medicine and Hygiene*, **10,** 859–869.

Lichtenberg, F. von, Sadun, E. H. & Bruce, J. I. (1962) Tissue responses and mechanisms of resistance in schistosomiasis mansoni in abnormal hosts. *American Journal of Tropical Medicine and Hygiene*, **11,** 347–356.

Lichtenberg, F. von, Smith, J. H. & Cheever, A. W. (1966) The Hoeppli phenomenon in schistosomiasis. Comparative pathology and immunopathology. *American Journal of Tropical Medicine and Hygiene*, **15,** 886–895.

Lichtenberg, F. von, Edington, G. M., Nwabuebo, I., Taylor, J. R. & Smith, J. H. (1971a) Pathologic effects of schistosomiasis in Ibadan, Western State of Nigeria. II. Pathogenesis of lesions of the bladder and ureters. *American Journal of Tropical Medicine and Hygiene*, 20, 244–254.

Lichtenberg, F. von, Sadun, E. H., Cheever, A. W., Erickson, D. G., Johnson, A. J. & Boyce, H. W. (1971b) Experimental infection with *Schistosoma japonicum* in chimpanzees. Parasitologic, clinical, serologic, and pathologic observations. *American Journal of Tropical Medicine and Hygiene*, 20, 850–893.

Lichtenberg, F. von, Sadun, E. H. & Bruce, J. I. (1972) Renal lesions in *Schistosoma japonicum* infected rabbits. *Transactions of the Royal Society of Tropical Medicine and Hygiene*, 66, 505–507.

Lichtenberg, F. von, Erikson, D. G. & Sadun, E. H. (1973) Comparative histopathology of schistosome granulomas in the hamster. *American Journal of Pathology*, 72, 149–178.

Lichtenberg, F. von, Bawden, M. P. & Shealey, S. H. (1974) Origin of circulating antigen from the schistosome gut. An immunofluorescent study. *American Journal of Tropical Medicine and Hygiene*, 23, 1088–1091.

Lima, R. R., Brito, E. & Rocha, H. (1969) Glomerulonefrite crônica associada à hepatoesplenomegalia esquistossomotica. *Gazeta Medical de Bahia*, 69, 43–50.

Lin, S. S. & Sadun, E. H. (1959) Studies of the host–parasite relationships to *Schistosoma japonicum*. V. Reactions in the skin, lungs, and liver of normal and immune animals following infection with *Schistosoma japonicum*. *Journal of Parasitology*, 45, 549–559.

Lopez, M. (1964) *Aspectos renais da sindrome hepato-esplénica da esquistossomose mansoni*. Tese, Belo Horizonte, Faculdade de Medicina da Universidade Federal de Minas Gerais.

Macfarlane, W. V. (1949) Schistosome dermatitis in New Zealand. Part II. Pathology and immunology of cercarial lesions. *American Journal of Hygiene*, 50, 152–167.

Macfarlane, W. V. (1952) Scistosome dermatitis in Australia. *Medical Journal of Australia*, 1, 669–672.

Machado, E. (1965) *Proteinuria na esquistossomose mansonica hepato-esplenica (Estudo electroforetico de urina e do soro sanguineo)*. Tese, Recife, Faculdade de Medicina da Universidade Federal de Pernambuco.

Magalhães-Filho, A. (1959) Pulmonary lesions in mice experimentally infected with *Schistosoma mansoni*. *American Journal of Tropical Medicine and Hygiene*, 8, 527–535.

Mahmoud, A. A. F., Warren, K. S. & Graham, R. C., Jr (1975a) Anti-eosinophil serum and the kinetics of eosinophilia in schistosomiasis mansoni. *Journal of Experimental Medicine*, 142, 560–574.

Mahmoud, A. A. F., Warren, K. S. & Peters, P. A. (1975b) A role for the eosinophil in acquired resistance to *Schistosoma mansoni* infection as determined by antieosinophil serum. *Journal of Experimental Medicine*, 142, 805–813.

Malek, E. A. & Armstrong, J. C. (1967) Infection with *Heterobilharzia americana* in primates. *American Journal of Tropical Medicine and Hygiene*, 16, 708–714.

Meleney, H. E., Sandground, J. H., Moore, D. V., Most, H. & Carney, B. H. (1953) The histopathology of experimental schistosomiasis. II. Bisexual infections with *S. mansoni*, *S. japonicum*, and *S. haematonium*. *American Journal of Tropical Medicine and Hygiene*, 2, 883–913.

Moore, G. T., Kaiser, R. L., Lawrence, R. S., Putnam, S. M. & Kagan, I. G. (1968) Intradermal and serologic reactions to antigens from *Schistosoma mansoni* in schistosome dermatitis. *American Journal of Tropical Medicine and Hygiene*, 17, 86–91.

Nash, T. E. (1974) Localization of the circulating antigen within the gut of *Schistosoma mansoni*. *American Journal of Tropical Medicine and Hygiene*, 23, 1085–1087.

Nash, T. E., Prescott, B. & Neva, F. A. (1974) The characteristics of a circulating antigen in schistosomiasis. *Journal of Immunology*, 112, 1500–1507.

Natali, P. G. & Cioli, D. (1974) Immune complex nephritis in mice infected with *Schistosoma mansoni*. *Federation Proceedings*, 33, 757.

Oliveira, C. A., Bicalho, D. M., Pimenta-Filho, R., Katz, N., Ferreira, H., Bittencourt, D., Dias, R. P., Alvarenga, R. J. & Dias, C. B. (1969) A fase aguda da esquistossomose mansoni. Estude laparoscópico da disseminacao de granulomas esquistossomoticos. *GEN: Organo de la Sociedad Venezolana de Gastroenterologia*, 23, 369–383.

Olivier, L. (1949) Schistosome dermatitis: a sensitization phenomenon. *American Journal of Hygiene*, 49, 290–302.

Ottesen, E. A. (1976) Eosinophilia and the lung. In *Immunologic and Infectious Reactions in the Lungs*, ed. Kirkpatrick, C. & Reynolds, H., pp. 289–332. New York: Marcel Dekker Inc.

Pelley, R. P., Ruffier, J. J. & Warren, K. S. (1976) The suppressive effect of a chronic helminth infection, schistosomiasis mansoni, on the in vitro responses of spleen and lymph node cells to the T cell mitogens PHA and Con A. *Infection and Immunity*, 13, 1176–1183.

Phillips, S. M., Reid, W. A., Bruce, J. I., Hedlung, K., Colvin, R. C., Campbell, R., Diggs, C. L. & Sadun, E. H. (1975) The cellular and humoral immune response to *Schistosoma mansoni* infections in inbred rats. I. Mechanisms during initial exposure. *Cellular Immunology*, **19**, 99–116.

Sadun, E. H., von Lichtenberg, F., Cheever, A. W., Erickson, D. G. & Hickman, R. L. (1970) Experimental infection with *Schistosoma haematobium* in chimpanzees. Parasitologic, clinical, serologic, and pathological observations. *American Journal of Tropical Medicine and Hygiene*, **19**, 427–458.

Sadun, E. H., von Lichtenberg, F., Hickman, R. L., Bruce, J. I., Smith, J. H. & Schoenbechler, M. J. (1966) Schistosomiasis mansoni in the chimpanzee: parasitologic, clinical, serologic, pathologic, and radiologic observations. *American Journal of Tropical Medicine and Hygiene*, **15**, 496–506.

Sadun, E. H. & Lin, S. S. (1959) Studies on the host–parasite relationship to *Schistosoma japonicum*. IV. Reistance acquired by infection, by vaccination, and by injection of immune serum, in monkeys, rabbits, and mice. *Journal of Parasitology*, **45**, 543–548.

Sadun, E. H., Reid, W. A., Cheever, A. W., Duvall, R. H., Swan, K. G., Kent, K. M., Bruce, J. I. & von Lichtenberg, F. (1975) Effects of portocaval shunting on *Schistosoma japonicum* infection in chimpanzees: dissociation of pipe-stem fibrosis and glomerulopathy. *American Journal of Tropical Medicine and Hygiene*, **24**, 619–631.

Smith, M. A., Clegg, J. A., Kusel, J. R. & Webbe, G. (1975) Lung inflammation in immunity to *Schistosoma mansoni*. *Experientia*, **31**, 595–596.

Smith, J. H., Kamel, I. A., Elwi, A. & von Lichtenberg, F. (1974) A quantitative post mortem analysis of urinary schistosomiasis in Egypt. I. Pathology and pathogenesis. *American Journal of Tropical Medicine and Hygiene*, **23**, 1054–1071.

Smithers, R. S. & Terry, R. J. (1976) The immunology of schistosomiasis. *Advances in Parasitology*, **14**, 399–422.

Stirewalt, M. A. & Hackey, J. R. (1956) Penetration of host skin by cercariae of *Schistosoma mansoni*. I. Observed entry into skin of mouse, hamster, rat, monkey and man. *Journal of Parasitology*, **42**, 565-580.

Torisu, M., Yoshida, T., Ward, P. A. & Cohn, S. (1973) Lymphocyte-derived eosinophil chemotactic factor. II. Studies on the mechanisms of activation of the precursor substance by immune complexes. *Journal of Immunology*, **111**, 1450–1458.

Tsang, V. C. W. & Damian, R. T. (1975) Demonstration and mode of action of an inhibitor of the intrinsic pathway of blood coagulation from adult *Schistosoma mansoni*. *Tenth Joint Parasitic Diseases Conference, U.S.–Japan Cooperative Medical Science Program*, October 1975, Bethesda, MD.

Vogel, H. & Minning, W. (1953) Über die erworbene Resi Resistenz von *Macacus rhesus* gegenüber *Schistosoma japonicum*. *Zeitschrift für Tropenmedizin und Parasitologie*, **4**, 418–505.

Warren, K. S. (1966) The pathogenesis of 'clay-pipe stem cirrhosis' in mice with chronic schistosomiasis mansoni, with a note on the longevity of the schistosomes. *American Journal of Pathology*, **49**, 477–489.

Warren, K. S. (1971) Worms. In *Immunological Diseases*, 2nd edn, ed. Samter, M., pp. 668–686. Boston: Little, Brown & Co.

Warren, K. S. (1972) The immunopathogenesis of schistosomiasis: a multidisciplinary approach. *Transactions of the Royal Society of Tropical Medicine and Hygiene*, **66**, 417–434.

Warren, K. S. (1973) The pathology of schistosome infections. *Helminthological Abstracts, Series A, Animal and Human Helminthology*, **42**, 591–633.

Warren, K. S. (1974) Modulation of immunopathology in schistosomiasis. In *Parasites in the Immunized Host: Mechanisms of Survival. Ciba Foundation Symposium 25* (new series), pp. 243–252. Amsterdam: Elsevier–Excerpta Medicine–North Holland.

Warren, K. S. (1975) The variety of inflammatory responses in tropical parasitic infections. Presented at the 24th Annual Meeting of the American Society of Tropical Medicine and Hygiene, November 1975, New Orleans.

Warren, K. S. & Berry, E. G. (1972) Induction of hepatosplenic disease by single pairs of the Philippine, Formosan, Japanese, and Chinese strains of *Schistosoma japonicum*. *Journal of Infectious Diseases*, **126**, 482–491.

Warren, K. S., Boros, D. L., Hang, L. M. & Mahmoud, A. A. F. (1975) The *Schistosoma japonicum* egg granuloma. *American Journal of Pathology*, **80**, 279–294.

Warren, K. S. & Domingo, E. O. (1970a) *Schistosoma mansoni*: stage specificity of granuloma formation around eggs after exposure to irradiated cercariae, unisexual infections, or dead worms. *Experimental Parasitology*, **27**, 60–66.

Warren, K. S. & Domingo, E. O. (1970b) Granuloma formation around *Schistosoma mansoni*, *S. haematobium* and *S. japonicum* eggs: size and rate of development, cellular composition, cross-reactivity, and rate of egg destruction. *American Journal of Tropical Medicine and Hygiene*, **19**, 292–304.

Warren, K. S., Domingo, E. O. & Cowan, R. B. T. (1967) Granuloma formation around schistosome eggs as a manifestation of delayed hypersensitivity. *American Journal of Pathology*, **51**, 735–756.

Warren, K. S., Mahmoud, A. A. F., Cummings, P., Murphy, D. J. & Houser, H. B. (1974a) Schistosomiasis mansoni in Yemeni in California: duration of infection, presence of disease, therapeutic management. *American Journal of Tropical Medicine and Hygiene*, **23**, 902–909.

Warren, K. S., Mahmoud, A. A. F., Boros, D. L., Rall, T. W., Mandel, M. A. & Carpenter, C. C. J., Jr (1974b) In vivo suppression by cholera toxin of cell-mediated and foreign body inflammatory responses. *Journal of Immunology*, **112**, 996–1007.

Webbe, G., James, C. & Nelson, G. S. (1974) *Schistosoma haematobium* in the baboon (*Papio anubis*). *Annals of Tropical Medicine and Parasitology*, **68**, 187–203.

WHO Memorandum (1974) Immunology of schistosomiasis. *Bulletin of the World Health Organization*, **51**, 553–595.

Wiedermann, G., Aspöck, H., Graefe, G., Picher, O. & Pelham, P. (1973) Hauttests mit *Schistosoma mansoni* Antigen bei Fällen von Cercarien-Dermatitis. *Zentralblatt für Bakteriologie, Parasitenkunde, Infektionskrankheiten und Hygiene; I Abteilung: Originale, Reihe A*, **224**, 128–132.

6

IMMUNE COMPLEXES IN CLINICAL INVESTIGATION

Rudolph H. Zubler   Paul H. Lambert

Immune complexes occur frequently, particularly during infectious disease and in association with autoimmunity, but immune complex disease probably represents a much rarer event. One should consider that immune complexes are formed in vivo each time a humoral immune response to antigen is made when either free antigen molecules are still persisting, or are released from microorganisms, or from host cells, into the extracellular fluid. This process does not usually lead to evident pathological manifestations, but may exert a physiological role or interfere with cell functions.

The biological properties of immune complexes are largely dependent on the presentation of antigen and/or antibody molecules in an aggregated form, and therefore at a higher density as compared to the corresponding free molecules. Aggregated antigens or antibodies are bound more avidly than their isolated counterparts by cellular or humoral receptors. The biological effects of immune complexes are first determined by an interaction with these receptors (recognition step). The binding of immune complexes to the classical humoral receptor, the first component of the complement and particularly its C1q constituent, can trigger the activation of the complement system and its effector mechanisms (Müller-Eberhard, 1975). At cell surfaces, the binding of immune complexes may first occur specifically to cell receptors for antigens, possibly initiating cellular events involved in the immune response (Warner, 1974); secondly, an antigen non-specific binding occurs on many cells with receptors for the Fc part of immunoglobulin molecules or for complex-bound complement components (Spiegelberg, 1974; Nussenzweig, 1974). The cellular recognition of immune complexes may lead to the phagocytosis of complexes or to direct effects on the binding cells. Indeed, the cell function may be enhanced or depressed. For example, polymorphonuclear cells phagocytose immune complexes with a concomitant stimulation of the cell metabolism (Nydegger et al, 1974a) and release of lysosomal enzymes into the medium (Henson, 1971), but later the bactericidal activity of these cells is depressed (MacLennan et al, 1977). Some cells may be lysed or eliminated after the binding of immune complexes on their surface, e.g. erythrocytes or platelets.

In vivo the fate and the effects of immune complexes are directly dependent on the site of their formation (Fig. 6.1) and on the nature of the antigens and the antibodies as well as their relative concentrations. Most of the immune complexes appearing in circulating blood are cleared rapidly by the mononuclear phagocytic system and particularly by Kupffer cells (Weigle, 1961; Mannik and Arend, 1971). Only relatively small complexes may persist for some time. The clearance of immune complexes may represent a physio-

This work has been supported by the Swiss National Research Foundation (Grant No. 3.2600.74) and the World Health Organisation.

logical mechanism for the rapid elimination of antigens. In some instances, small amounts of these complexes would be fixed in vessel walls or filtering membranes such as in renal glomeruli or in the choroid plexus (Dixon, 1963; Cochrane and Koffler, 1973; Oldstone, 1975). Immune complexes formed in extravascular spaces are not cleared as rapidly and may induce local inflammatory foci. The pathological consequences will depend on their concentration, their persistence and on the chronicity of their formation. In some clinical conditions an exchange between the extravascular and the intravascular pool of immune

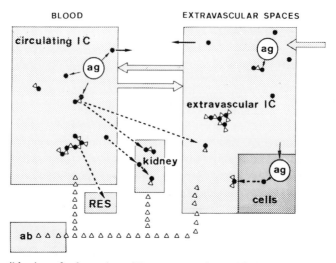

Figure 6.1   Possible sites of a formation of immune complexes (IC) in vivo: these may be formed in blood or the extravascular spaces, according to the localisation of the antigens at the time when antibodies appear (ag represents a source of antigen, e.g. a microorganism). The fate of the complexes is dependent on the site of their formation. RES represents the reticuloendothelial system, mainly the liver and spleen

complexes may be observed, but this is not a general rule and a typical immune complex disease may occur in the absence of circulating immune complexes.

Although the induction of inflammatory reactions by immune complexes is usually considered as their major pathological consequence, the interference of immune complexes with immune mechanisms and the depression of some specific cell functions may represent their most important effects in some diseases.

CLINICAL INVESTIGATIONS IN DISEASE ASSOCIATED WITH THE FORMATION OF IMMUNE COMPLEXES

Two main approaches have been used in order to demonstrate the occurrence of immune complexes in human diseases. There are, first, the analysis of tissue specimens and, secondly, the serological analysis of samples from various biological fluids.

Tissue studies by conventional histological techniques and by electron microscopy may lead to the suspicion of an involvement of immune complexes in the observed lesions on the basis of similarities with lesions induced experimentally by immune complexes. For example, typical morphological features of immune complex glomerulonephritis have been well defined through the study of animal models of this disease (Dixon, 1963).

Moreover, immunohistochemical techniques allow a more direct demonstration of immunoglobulin deposits, associated with complement components and some identified antigens in a pattern suggestive of the presence of immune complexes (Wilson and Dixon, 1974). Such techniques have been applied extensively to many tissues and to the demonstration of immune complex-like material within polymorphonuclear leucocytes in circulation (Steffelaar, De Graaff-Reitsma and Feltkamp, 1976) or at extravascular sites of inflammation (Rawson, Abelson and Hollander, 1965; Britton and Schur, 1971).

With the availability of sufficient amounts of tissue material the elution of antibodies by low pH buffers, or the destruction of a suspected antigen (e.g. DNA by the specific enzyme DNAase) allows the identification of the components of tissue-localised complexes (Koffler, Schur and Kunkel, 1967; Lambert and Dixon, 1968). However, eluted antibodies always represent a selected fraction of the complexed molecules and the elution procedures alter some antibodies more than others, particularly IgM antibodies. The amount of immunoglobulins with an identified antibody specificity must be related to the total amount of eluted immunoglobulins in order to evaluate their relative involvement in the deposited complexes.

Serological studies provide evidence for the association of immune complexes with a particular clinical condition either by the direct detection of complexes in various biological fluids or by the demonstration of serological changes which often are associated with the formation of immune complexes. Such serological methods for the study of immune complexes in disease have been considerably developed in recent years and this review will be concerned with the advances in this field.

METHODS FOR THE DETECTION OF SOLUBLE IMMUNE COMPLEXES

The methods for the detection of immune complexes may be separated into two main groups. On one hand, some methods have been devised in order to detect complexes independently of the nature of the antigen involved in the formation of these immune complexes. They represent 'antigen non-specific' methods. On the other hand, some methods allow for a selective detection of immune complexes involving one given antigen through the discrimination between free and antibody-bound antigens. They represent 'antigen-specific' methods.

Antigen Non-specific Methods

Antigen non-specific methods are based on the distinct properties of complexed immunoglobulin molecules as compared with free immunoglobulin molecules. The main properties which can be used are the physical changes due to the complex formation and the biological activities of immune complexes such as complement fixation or binding to cell membranes. All of these methods will detect non-specifically aggregated immunoglobulins as well as immune complexes.

Methods based on the physical properties of immune complexes

The formation of immune complexes leads to the occurrence of new molecular structures characterised by an increased molecular size, by changes of the surface properties, solubility and electric charge as compared with the corresponding free antigens and antibodies. The extent of these changes will depend on the nature and on the concentration of each immunological constituent of the complex and therefore will exhibit great heterogeneity.

The *analytical ultracentrifugation* has been applied to the detection of immune complexes through the demonstration in various biological fluids of an abnormal level of some material with a relatively high sedimentation velocity. Thus, very suggestive evidence of immune complexes was obtained in some well-defined clinical conditions. For instance, peaks of 22S and 9–17S material were observed in serum from patients with rheumatoid arthritis and were shown to represent IgG–IgM complexes (22S) (Franklin et al, 1957), and IgG–IgG complexes (9–17S) (Kunkel et al, 1961). However, the exclusive use of analytical ultracentrifugation does not allow one to conclude the presence of immune complexes since other material of high molecular weight may as well appear in large amounts in some biological samples. Furthermore, the sensitivity of this method is low.

The use of preparative methods such as the separation on *sucrose density gradients* or the *molecular sieving on gels* or selective *ultrafiltration* allows for the combination of the physical analysis of samples with the characterisation of various fractions by additional immunological and biological analysis. For example, in addition to 7S IgG, IgG molecules sedimenting as larger material (15S or more) were demonstrated in sucrose density gradient fractions obtained from serum (Kunkel et al, 1961) and synovial fluid (Hannestad, 1968) of patients with rheumatoid arthritis. Such heavy IgG fractions could easily be dissociated into 7S IgG at acid pH and in concentrated urea. Macromolecular aggregates containing C3 were also demonstrated by gel chromatography in sera from various patients (Soothill and Hendrickse, 1967; Amlot, Slaney and Williams, 1976). These methods can represent an important step in the purification of immune complexes. They have been successfully applied to analytical studies of many clinical conditions, such as rheumatoid arthritis (Schrohenloher, 1966; Winchester, Agnello and Kunkel, 1970), systemic lupus erythematosus (Agnello et al, 1971), measles (Myllylä, Vaheri and Penttinen, 1971), leprosy (Bjorvatn et al, 1976), cancer (Sjögren et al, 1972; Ludwig and Cusumano, 1974). One drawback of these techniques is that they are rather time-consuming and can hardly be used routinely for the detection of immune complexes.

Material with a *decreased solubility* in well-defined conditions (temperature, medium) were shown to occur frequently in serum or other biological fluid containing immune complexes. Therefore, the occurrence of an abnormal precipitation of serum proteins in a serum sample in such defined conditions may be suggestive of the presence of immune complexes. The simplest procedure is the precipitation at cold temperature. *Cryoglobulins* may frequently represent a particular type of immune complex, but monoclonal immunoglobulins or other proteins may often be involved. Extensive immunochemical analysis of the cryoprecipitates are required before considering cryoglobulins as possible immune complexes (Brouet et al, 1974).

Some media which can be used to separate serum proteins according to their physical properties can also be used to precipitate immune complexes and large serum molecules in conditions where free immunoglobulin molecules should remain soluble. The *precipitation in polyethylene glycol* (PEG, MW 6000) has been applied to clinical investigation (Creighton, Lambert and Miescher, 1973). The addition to serum of PEG, an uncharged linear polymer, results in a precipitation of proteins which is proportional to the concentration of PEG. The extent of precipitation of each protein is proportional to its molecular size (Zubler et al, 1977), so that at low concentrations of PEG, the high molecular weight proteins and immune complexes are preferentially precipitated.

An abnormal increase of the protein content of PEG precipitates was shown to be largely correlated with the level of immune complexes in some clinical conditions (Herreman et al, 1975; Mohammed, Thompson and Holborow, 1977). Such measurements of the total protein precipitation are influenced by the level of various serum proteins and should be considered as a rather non-specific screening test for the detection of immune complexes. More accurate information may be obtained through further analysis of the proteins precipitated at low PEG concentrations. For instance, an increase of the fraction of serum IgG which is precipitable in PEG is indicative of the presence of aggregated or complexed IgG in the tested serum sample. This was frequently observed in patients with systemic

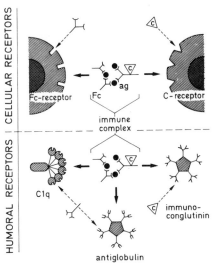

Figure 6.2 Cellular and humoral receptors which can be used for the antigen non-specific detection of immune complexes. In the aggregated form in the complex, immunoglobulins and complement components ($\triangle$) exhibit a higher avidity than the corresponding free molecules for Fc receptors and complement receptors

lupus erythematosus (Lambert et al, 1972). Furthermore, the demonstration of complement components in such PEG precipitates may be suggestive of an in vivo binding of complement to macromolecular complexes. This has been particularly done for C1q (Grangeot and Pillot, 1975; Zubler et al, 1976a).

The *electric charge* of immune complexes may differ from that of the corresponding free antibody molecules and thus complexed IgG may be found to exhibit an abnormally increased affinity for anion-exchange resins (DEAE-cellulose) (Kunkel et al, 1961; Fox, Plescia and Mellors, 1974) or an altered mobility by electrophoretic techniques (Grubb, 1975). This property is highly dependent on the nature of the antigen involved and has been more used for antigen-specific methods than for the antigen non-specific detection of immune complexes. Surface changes characterising immune complexes have also been related to the observed agglutination of uncoated latex particles in presence of serum containing complexed IgG (Heimer and Abruzzo, 1972).

Methods based on the biological properties of immune complexes

A large group of methods are based on the reactivity of immune complexes with specific receptors either on free molecules or on cell surface structures (Fig. 6.2). The presentation of immunoglobulins in aggregated form, or the presence of immune complex-bound complement components, are responsible for the recognition by Fc-receptors and by complement receptors respectively. The receptors on free molecules which are used for the detection of immune complexes are complement, particularly C1q, antiglobulins, immunoconglutinins and conglutinin. The receptors on cell surfaces include Fc-receptors and C3-receptors on isolated or cultured blood and tissue cells.

Interaction with complement

The interaction of immune complexes with the complement system as a whole or with identified complement components has been used extensively in various methods devised to detect such complexes. Two main groups of methods should be considered. The first group involves techniques based on the competitive inhibition by complexes of the whole complement haemolytic activity or of that of the C1q recognition unit. The second group represents methods in which the direct interaction of C1q with complexes is demonstrated. The main limitation of this technological approach is the reactivity with the complement system or C1q of substances other than immune complexes. This is particularly known for highly charged substances including various cellular components and microbial products (Agnello et al, 1971; Müller-Eberhard, 1974; Siegel, Rent and Gewurz, 1975; Pinckard et al, 1975). This drawback has been partially avoided in some methods through the use of particular physicochemical test conditions or by combining with an additional immunochemical characterisation.

COMPLEMENT AND C1q DEVIATION TESTS

The measurement of the *anticomplementary activity* in various biological samples is usually performed as in a classical complement fixation test (Shulman and Barker, 1969; Mowbray et al, 1973). The tested sample is first incubated with a standardised amount of serum as a source of complement, then the residual complement activity is measured. It is clear that in this method all substances which interefere with the complement reaction sequence at any level can lead to falsely positive results. Any type of activator of the alternative pathway, such as natural polysaccharides, will also result in an apparent anticomplementary activity. Often the serum is heat inactivated before the performance of the complement deviation test and this may change the structure of some immune complexes (Zubler et al, 1976a). An increased anticomplementary activity has been described in many diseases such as rheumatoid arthritis (Winchester et al, 1970), systemic lupus erythematosus (Johnson, Mowbray and Porter, 1975), dermatitis herpetiformis (Mowbray et al, 1973) and viral hepatitis-B (Shulman and Barker, 1969). At the present time, the demonstration of an anticomplementary activity in a biological sample does not appear to be sufficient by itself to prove the presence of immune complexes.

The *C1q deviation test* (Sobel, Bokisch and Müller-Eberhard, 1975) is a radioassay in which the measurement of the anticomplementary activity is restricted to C1q. The method is based on the competitive inhibition by immune complexes in a tested sample of the binding of radiolabelled C1q to sensitised red blood cells. Serum to be tested is incubated first with labelled C1q alone, after some time sensitised sheep red blood cells are added to the incubation mixture. Finally, the cells are separated from this mixture by centrifugation of aliquots on concentrated sucrose solution, and the radioactivity on the cell pellet is measured. The results are expressed as percentage inhibition of the radioactivity uptake as compared to the uptake in a test control. As compared to the measurement of the anticomplementary activity this test offers several advantages. It is extremely sensitive and is not influenced by substances activating exclusively the alternative pathway or interfering with complement components other than C1q. However, this test is performed in buffer conditions at which there is also high sensitivity for DNA or various bacterial products reacting with C1q (Sobel et al, 1975). This has to be considered when the test is done in order to detect immune complexes. The C1q deviation test has usually been done after heat inactivation of the serum sample to be tested, and therefore may be influenced by the alteration of some immune complexes or by the generation of immunoglobulin aggregates. Increased inhibition of C1q uptake was observed to occur in sera from patients with Dengue haemorrhagic fever (Sobel et al, 1975) and glomerulonephritis (Sobel, Gabay and Lagrue, 1976).

Recently C1q deviation tests using IgG-coated latex (Medof and Sukhupunyaraksa, 1975) or sepharose (Gabriel, Tai and Agnello, 1975) particles rather than sensitised red blood cells as a binding substratum for C1q have been devised.

The *inhibition of the agglutination of Ig-coated latex particles by C1q* has also been used (Lurhuma et al, 1976) as an alternative to the binding of labelled C1q to such particles. The limitations and requirement of heat inactivation are similar to those described for the C1q deviation test. This method offers the advantage of simplicity but is strongly subject to interference by rheumatoid factors. It has been applied to various clinical conditions, such as Crohn's disease and idiopathic thrombocytopenia.

DIRECT MEASUREMENT OF C1q-IMMUNE COMPLEX INTERACTION

Immune complexes in relatively large amounts in serum samples may be qualitatively detected by using the *C1q agarose precipitation test* (Agnello, Winchester and Kunkel, 1970). This test is based on the decreased solubility of immune complexes in the presence of a high concentration of C1q. Opposite holes on agarose plates are filled respectively with purified C1q and tested serum under optimal buffer conditions. A precipitation line may appear when the serum contains immune complexes. This test is simple but unfortunately quite sensitive to DNA and other polyanions. It was applied for the detection and characterisation of immune complexes in various diseases, such as systemic lupus erythematosus (Agnello et al, 1971), rheumatoid arthritis (Winchester, Kunkel and Agnello, 1971), Crohn's disease (Doe, Booth and Brown, 1973), Wegener's granulomatosis (Howell and Epstein, 1976) and leprosy (Moran et al, 1972).

More sensitive and quantitative techniques have been devised using radiolabelled C1q. The principle of the *C1q binding test* (Nydegger et al, 1974b) is to incubate patients' serum or other fluid with radiolabelled C1q and then to separate free C1q from C1q bound to immune complexes by differential precipitation with polyethylene glycol. The percentage of labelled C1q precipitated indicates the presence and the amount of complexes. The initial requirement for heat inactivation was avoided by pretreatment of the tested sample with EDTA in order to prevent the incorporation of labelled C1q into the high molecular weight C1qrs complex (Zubler et al, 1976a; Zubler and Lambert, 1976a). This pretreatment also avoids the possible reactivity of C1q with C-reactive protein complexes.

In the condition of the test the C1q present in tested serum interferes slightly with the binding of radiolabelled C1q, but this phenomenon does not appear to influence strikingly the results of the test. It is of interest that C1q reacting with low molecular weight substances or substances which are quite soluble in polyethylene glycol, such as DNA, will rarely precipitate in this test. The C1q binding test was used for detection and further analysis of immune complexes in various clinical conditions, such as systemic lupus erythematosus (Nydegger et al, 1974b; Zubler and Lambert, 1977; Zuber et al, 1976a), rheumatoid arthritis (Zubler et al, 1976b; Mohammed et al, 1977), leprosy (Bjorvatn et al, 1976), leukaemia (Carpentier et al, 1976), amyotrophic lateral sclerosis (Oldstone et al, 1976) and glomerulonephritis (Rossen et al, 1976).

Recently, *solid phase C1q binding tests* have been developed. In a first step, tested serum can be incubated in C1q-coated polystyrene tubes, in a second step, the amount of immune complexes which reacted with this C1q is measured after a further incubation with radio-labelled (Hay, Nineham and Roitt, 1976) or enzyme-linked (Ahlstedt, Hanson and Wadsworth, 1976) antiglobulins. For clinical application of this type of technique the tested sample has been heat inactivated prior to the testing in order to avoid a competition with the C1q present in the sample. This heat treatment deserves the same criticism as previously mentioned. Immune complexes were detected in patients with systemic lupus erythematosus (Hay et al, 1976). Similar techniques were described using protein A-rich staphylococci instead of antiglobulins (Farrell, Sogaard and Svehag, 1975). The inhibition of the binding of radiolabelled immunoglobulin aggregates to C1q-coated tubes in the presence of immune complexes has also been proposed for their detection. This method suffers from the interference of rheumatoid factors and was not proposed for clinical application (Svehag, 1975). C1q on solid phase has been used in order to isolate immune complexes from biological fluids (Svehag and Burger, 1976).

Interaction with rheumatoid factor

The interaction between rheumatoid factor and immune complexes, particularly those occurring in the synovial fluid and serum from patients with rheumatoid arthritis, has been demonstrated by ultracentrifugation techniques, by direct precipitation in free solution or on agarose plates and by inhibition of red cell agglutination or latex agglutination (Kunkel et al, 1961; Hannestad, 1968; Winchester et al, 1970).

The *direct precipitation in agarose gel of immune complexes by rheumatoid factor* has been used for their detection (Winchester et al, 1971), monoclonal rheumatoid factors obtained from patients with lymphoproliferative disease being more efficient than 'polyclonal rheumatoid factors' from patients with rheumatoid disease in this test. Positive results were observed in a majority of sera from patients with rheumatoid arthritis, but only rarely in systemic lupus erythematosus sera, suggesting a better reactivity of rheumatoid factor for the complexes occurring in rheumatoid arthritis (Winchester et al, 1971).

Other techniques are based on the *inhibition by immune complexes of the interaction between rheumatoid factor and aggregated immunoglobulin*. In one radioimmunoassay (Luthra et al, 1975) monoclonal rheumatoid factor was insolubilised through coupling to microcristalline cellulose. Immune complexes in sera from patients were shown to inhibit the binding to the cellulose of radio-actively labelled aggregated immunoglobulins. A similar radioassay was devised using soluble polyclonal rheumatoid factor combined with a final step of coprecipitation with an antihuman IgM antiserum (Cowdery, Treadwell and Fritz, 1975). This last method could not be applied for sera containing rheumatoid factor. The inhibition by immune complexes of the binding of labelled monoclonal rheumatoid factor to IgG-coated sepharose was also used for their detection (Gabriel et al, 1975). In a simpler technique the property of immune complexes to inhibit the agglutination of Ig-coated latex particles by rheumatoid factor has been used (Lurhuma et al, (1976).

One limitation is the fact that the presence of rheumatoid factor in patients' sera may mask the detection of complexes. Such a method also requires heat inactivation of samples before testing. One should note that free, monomeric immunoglobulin can react with rheumatoid factor, and therefore the Ig-concentration in a sample influences all tests based on the interaction of immune complexes with rheumatoid factor.

Interaction with immunoconglutinins and conglutinin

Immunoglobulins exhibiting an immunoconglutinin activity and bovine conglutinin are molecules which can react with complement components and particularly C3 when they are bound to immune complexes. Therefore they represent a potential tool for the detection of immune complexes as indicated by current investigations (Eisenberg and Theofilopoulos, 1975; Casali, Bossus and Lambert, unpublished results).

Methods based on the reactivity with cellular receptors for immune complexes

The analysis of the specific interaction of immune complexes with cells may provide information directly relevant to important biological effects of such complexes. Unfortunately the use of living cells for routine diagnostic methods renders standardisation difficult and is limited by the possible interference of various factors related to cell metabolism as well as of antibodies reacting with cell surface antigens.

INTERACTION WITH Fc-RECEPTORS ON CELLS

A wide variety of cells exhibit receptors for the Fc part of certain immunoglobulin molecules. Although these cells bind more avidly aggregated immunoglobulins or immune complexes than monomeric immunoglobulins, all methods using this property for the detection of immune complexes will be influenced to some extent by the concentration of immunoglobulin in the tested samples. Most of these methods involve active cellular processes and require intact cells and clearly defined conditions.

The platelet aggregation test is based on the aggregation of fresh human blood platelets in presence of immune complexes. The aggregation is estimated visually by reading on microtitre plates (Penttinen, Vaheri and Myllylä, 1971). Under the conditions of the test platelets may be aggregated in presence of immunoglobulin aggregates, but also of free immunoglobulin at high concentration, antibodies reacting with platelet surface antigens and other substances such as charged molecules, proteolytic enzymes and some myxoviruses (Myllylä, 1973). It was found that IgM rheumatoid factor can inhibit the aggregation of platelets induced by immune complexes (Penttinen et al, 1973; Wager et al, 1973). Suggestive evidence for the occurrence of immune complexes was obtained using this method in various diseases such as viral infections (Myllylä et al, 1971), hepatitis (Penttinen, 1972), chronic liver disease (Penttinen et al, 1973), mycoplasma pneumoniae infection (Biberfeld and Norberg, 1974), sarcoidosis (Hedfors and Norberg, 1974) and rheumatoid arthritis (Norberg, 1974). After kidney transplantation patients sera have been found to contain platelet aggregating activity associated with 7S material which may represent alloantibodies reacting with platelets (Palosuo et al, 1976).

The inhibition of antibody-dependent cell-mediated cytoxicity in presence of immune complexes has been used for their detection. Freshly isolated human blood lymphocytes are incubated with ^{51}Cr-labelled Chang liver cells (Jewell and MacLennan, 1973) or other target cells (Hallberg, 1972) sensitised with corresponding rabbit antibodies. The cell lysis is inhibited by immune complexes (MacLennan, 1972), but also to some extent by serum immunoglobulins (Barkas et al, 1976) and probably antilymphocyte antibodies (Feldmann et al, 1976). An inhibition of antibody-dependent cell-mediated cytotoxicity was observed with sera from patients with ulcerative colitis or Crohn's disease (Jewell and MacLennan,

1973), rheumatoid arthritis (Barnett and MacLennan, 1972; Hallberg, 1972), systemic lupus erythematosus (Feldman et al, 1976) and Hashimoto's thyroiditis (Barkas et al, 1976).

The inhibition of macrophage uptake test is another radioisotope assay using macrophages, based on the interference of immune complexes with the phagocytosis of labelled immunoglobulin aggregates (Onyewotu, Holborow and Johnson, 1974). Patient's serum, labelled aggregates and fresh guinea-pig peritoneal exudate cells are incubated together, the cells are then washed and the uptake of labelled aggregates is measured. A significant inhibition of the uptake of aggregates was observed with most sera from patients with systemic lupus erythematosus (Onyewotu et al, 1974) and certain types of glomerulonephritis (Stühlinger, Verroust and Morel-Maroger, 1976). In contrast, an increased uptake was found in presence of sera from patients with seropositive rheumatoid arthritis (Onyewotu et al, 1975, Mohammed, et al, 1976).

INTERACTION WITH COMPLEMENT RECEPTORS ON CELLS

Various cells exhibit a high affinity for complement-coated immune complexes due to the presence of receptors for complement components on the cell membrane. Most of these receptors interact preferentially with C3 or its breakdown products C3b and C3d. Some human lymphocyte cell lines are characterised by a high density of such receptors, and one of them, the Raji cell line, has been used in a method devised for the detection of immune complexes.

The Raji cell radioimmunoassay (Theofilopoulos, Wilson and Dixon, 1976; Theofilopoulos and Dixon, 1976) is a test in which serum is incubated with the cells, which are then washed and mixed with the radioisotope-labelled immunoglobulin fraction of a rabbit antihuman immunoglobulin antiserum. The uptake of labelled rabbit antibodies on the cells indicates the amount of human immunoglobulin bound to the cell surface under the condition of the test. Although Raji cells exhibit Fc receptors, the binding of immune complexes in tested serum is mostly dependent on the reactivity with complement (Theofilopoulos et al, 1976).

This method has been initially developed using a fluorescent rabbit antihuman immunoglobulin antiserum (Theofilopoulos et al, 1974). The presence in the tested sample of antibodies reacting at 37°C with lymphocyte surface antigens may lead to false positive results. The competition for the cell receptors of free C3 or C3b with complex-bound C3 does not appear as a limiting factor. The Raji cell radioimmunoassay has been used for the detection and further characterisation of immune complexes in various clinical conditions, such as systemic lupus erythematosus, vasculitis, B-virus hepatitis, Dengue haemorrhagic fever and cancer. Evidence for the involvement of HB_s-antigen in the immune complexes in patients with hepatitis was obtained by showing a binding of anti-HB_s-antigen fluorescent antibodies to Raji cells after the incubation with patients' sera (Theofilopoulos et al, 1976).

The inhibition of complement-dependent lymphocyte rosette formation has also been applied to clinical investigation (Ezer and Hayward, 1974). Activated complement components inhibit the rosette formation between lymphocytes bearing complement receptors and complement-coated erythrocytes. Such inhibition may be caused by complement-coated immune complexes, as well as by free complement breakdown products, and therefore is not specific for immune complexes (Ezer and Hayward, 1974), Inhibitory activity was observed in patients with various diseases, such as Crohn's disease (Ezer and Hayward, 1974), schistosomiasis (Smith et al, 1975a) and glomerulonephritis (Smith et al, 1975b).

General comments on antigen non-specific methods for the detection of immune complexes

Because of the number of methods for the detection of immune complexes (Table 6.1) the selection of techniques suitable for clinical investigation is difficult. Optimally such methods should be highly specific for immune complexes and sensitive for the large

Table 6.1   Antigen non-specific methods for the detection of soluble immune complexes based on the biological properties of the complexes

Biological activity measured	Reactants used in the test
1. Reactivity with receptors on free molecules	
(a) Interaction with complement	
Complement and C1q deviation tests	
Measurement of anticomplementary activity	Fresh serum complement, sensitised sheep red cells
C1q deviation test	^{125}I-C1q, sensitised sheep red cells (or IgG-coated particles)
Inhibition of latex agglutination by C1q	Purified C1q, IgG-coated latex particles
Direct measurement of C1q–immune complex interaction	
C1q agarose precipitation test	Purified C1q
C1q binding test	^{125}I-C1q, polyethylene glycol
Solid-phase C1q binding test	C1q-coated polystyrene tubes, ^{125}I-anti-globulin or enzyme-linked antiglobulin is used in a second step
(b) Interaction with rheumatoid factor (RF)	
RF agarose precipitation test	Monoclonal RF
Radioassay using insolubilised monoclonal RF	Monoclonal RF coupled to microcristalline cellulose, ^{125}I-IgG aggregates
Radioisotope assay using soluble polyclonal RF	Polyclonal RF, ^{125}I-IgG aggregates, purified carrier human IgM, sheep antiserum anti-human IgM
Inhibition of latex agglutination by RF	Polyclonal RF, IgG-coated latex particles
2. Reactivity with cellular receptors	
(a) Interaction with Fc receptors on cells	
Platelet aggregation test	Human blood platelets
Inhibition of antibody-dependent cell-mediated cytotoxicity	Human blood lymphocytes, ^{51}Cr-labelled sensitised Chang liver cells
Radioassay using macrophages	Guinea-pig peritoneal exudate cells, ^{125}I-aggregates
(b) Interaction with complement receptors on cells	
Raji cell radioimmune assay	Cultured lymphoblastoid (Raji) cells, ^{125}I-antiglobulin
Inhibition of complement-dependent lymphocyte rosette formation	Lymphocytes from human adenoid, complement-coated sheep red cells

variety which may occur in clinical situations. It is also clear, that they should be easily reproducible and relatively simple to perform.

PROBLEM OF SPECIFICITY

All methods proposed for the detection of immune complexes do not differentiate non-specifically aggregated immunoglobulins from true immune complexes. Therefore, all procedures which can generate such non-specific aggregates during the analysis are potential sources of error. This is particularly known for repetitive freezing–thawing and for heating of samples at more than 56°C prior to testing.

In addition immune complexes have to be differentiated from other substances which may interfere with their detection. The appropriate control experiments will differ according to the method which is used. The following analyses are usually necessary in the evaluation of any test used to detect complexes in sera:

1. Characterisation of the size of the detected immune complex-like material, since immune complexes are larger than monomeric immunoglobulins.
2. Fractionation in physicochemical conditions known to dissociate complexes and to decrease their size and biological activity, e.g. Figure 6.3.

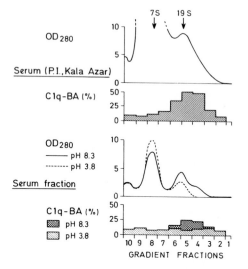

Figure 6.3 Characterisation of immune complex-like material by sucrose density gradient ultra-centrifugation. The upper part of the figure shows the optical density (OD) pattern after the sucrose gradient separation of the serum obtained from a patient with kala azar (note positions of the 7S and 19S markers), and the immune complex-like activity (percentage ^{125}I-C1q binding activity, C1q-BA) measured by the C1q binding test on individual gradient fractions. The three fractions exhibiting the highest activity were pooled and subjected to a second sucrose gradient centrifugation at either pH 8.3 or 3.8. The lower part of the figure shows the corresponding results. The findings that the complex-like material exhibited a high molecular weight and was acid-dissociable support the hypothesis that true immune complexes were present in the serum

3. Confirmation that the test is negative after removal of immunoglobulins from the tested sample, e.g. by immunoabsorption, or after alteration of some of the biological properties of complexes, e.g. inhibition of the complement binding activity after reduction-alkylation (Wiedermann, Miescher and Franklin, 1963).

For some groups of tests further controls of specificity are useful, such as in tests based on the interaction with complement, the treatment with DNase, in order to exclude the intereference of DNA; or the testing in presence of EDTA, in order to exclude the interference of C-reactive protein (Kaplan and Volanakis, 1974). When cells are used for the detection of complexes, absorption experiments should be done in order to exclude the interference of antibodies reacting with cell surface structures. However, once a method has been applied extensively in combination with the proper controls to the study of a particular disease, the frequency and the nature of interfering substances may be predicted.

At a different level of specificity one has to consider the nature of the immunoglobulins involved in the complexes, since the sensitivity of each method based on biological properties will depend on the particular reactivity of the various classes and subclasses of immunoglobulins. With regard to this criterion a multispecific method would be preferable. From this short review it appears, that at the present time none of the described methods fulfils all the criteria of specificity and the combined use of some methods may be most useful.

PROBLEM OF SENSITIVITY

At the present time it is difficult to assess the sensitivity of all the different tests proposed for the detection of immune complexes. Indeed, this sensitivity is generally expressed in relation to preparations of heat-aggregated immunoglobulins which are not standardised. According to the size of the aggregates considerable variation of the observed sensitivity may occur. The choice of aggregated immunoglobulin as a standard is also relatively misleading, since such aggregates do not represent true immune complexes. In particular, they are more stable at dissociating conditions or during heat-inactivation. Therefore we think that the assessment of the sensitivity should rely upon comparative studies involving the testing by various methods of a panel of samples including (1) standardised reference preparations of aggregated immunoglobulins, (2) several types of preformed immune complexes, and (3) sera from patients with physicochemically well-characterised immune complexes. According to our own experience it would appear, that methods which are very sensitive for aggregated immunoglobulin do not *ipso facto* exhibit a similar sensitivity for immune complexes in patients' sera. Although a minimal sensitivity is requested we consider that this is less critical than the dispersion of the results obtained within a normal population and the reproducibility of a method. Usually when the data of a clinical investigation are submitted to proper statistical analysis, the low levels of immune complexes which may be detected in some patients' sera using very sensitive methods do not exceed the upper limit of the normal range observed in a control population. Therefore the significance of such results is limited.

IDENTIFICATION OF IMMUNE COMPLEXES

The methods described do not allow for a direct identification of the antigen or the antibody component in the complexes. However, if one particular antigen is suspected to be involved, this can be confirmed by a specific modification of the size or of the properties of the complex after mixing of the sample or purified complexes with a large excess of this antigen. The latter can also be searched for in native or dissociated immune complexes. The monomeric immunoglobulin molecules which can be obtained by fractionation at dissociating conditions can be analysed for their specificities versus various suspected antigens.

Antigen-specific Methods

In particular clinical conditions it may be useful to study whether a known antigen appears in the form of immune complexes. By using a proper methodology one can distinguish between free antigen molecules and those specifically bound to immunoglobulins. In the case of particulate antigen morphological analysis has been applied, e.g. the electron microscopic detection of aggregated particles of HB_s-antigen seems suggestive of their involvement in immune complexes (Almeida and Waterson, 1969). Physico-chemical methods have been applied to this problem in combination with the detection of known antigens, e.g. neuroblastoma-specific immune complexes have been detected in patients' sera by radioimmuno-counterelectrophoresis (Jose and Seshadri, 1974). The differentiation between free and complex-bound antigen can also be achieved by measuring the amount of antigen which is removed from a biological sample when the host immuno-globulins are specifically precipitated or absorbed, e.g. the infectivity of sera from mice infected with lactic dehydrogenase virus was shown to decrease strikingly after the specific precipitation of immunoglobulins (Notkins et al, 1966).

An alternative approach consisted of measuring specific antibody levels before and after removal of the corresponding antigen. This has been applied to the detection of DNA–anti-DNA (Harbeck et al, 1973) and insulin–anti-insulin (Jayarao et al, 1973) com-plexes in patients. With respect to the multiplicity of antigen–antibody systems possibly involved in the in vivo formation of immune complexes it is unlikely that such antigen-specific methods would be routinely used in clinical situations. Their use would probably be restricted to the assessment of the immune status in well-defined conditions.

Indirect Serological Evidence for the Presence of Immune Complexes

Most immune complexes which are formed in vivo can activate the complement system and particularly the classical pathway. When large amounts of such complexes occur, significant alterations of the complement profile may be observed. This is the case in systemic lupus erythematosus. In most other clinical conditions this activation may be masked by an increased synthesis of complement components and therefore the analysis of the complement profile is not conclusive (Ruddy, Gigli and Austen, 1972). The demon-stration of a hypercatabolism of some complement components by metabolic studies (Charlesworth et al, 1974) or, more practically, by demonstration and quantitation of complement breakdown products (Perrin, Lambert and Miescher, 1975) is suggestive of the presence of immune complexes and represents useful information in clinical investiga-tion.

For example, the level of the free C3d breakdown product of C3 in the plasma from patients with systemic lupus erythematosus has been shown to correlate with the level of immune complexes in serum (Fig. 6.4). The C3d concentration has been measured by an immunochemical method (Perrin et al, 1975). Briefly: in a first step, EDTA-plasma was mixed with an equal volume of a 22 per cent (w/v) polyethylene glycol solution, was left at $4°C$ for 3 h and then centrifuged at 1200 g for 30 min, in order to precipitate the native C3 and its high molecular weight fragments C3b and C3c. In a second step, the C3d was measured in the supernatant by single radial immunodiffusion using specific anti-C3d-antigen antiserum. A limitation of this approach is that the complement system may be activated by substances unrelated to immune complexes.

CLINICAL RELEVANCE OF THE DETECTION OF IMMUNE COMPLEXES IN PATHOLOGICAL CONDITIONS

Whenever immune complex-like material is detected in samples obtained from patients with a particular disease, one should wonder about the relevance of this finding in relation to the clinical manifestations, the evolution and the pathogenesis of this disease. It is clear that in some clinical conditions such as systemic lupus erythematosus (SLE) immune complexes circulate in large amounts (Fig. 6.5) and that their presence seems to be directly related to the main pathological manifestations. They trigger an important activation of the complement system which is manifested by a decrease in the levels of the principal components and the appearance of breakdown products in the plasma. There is a significant correlation between the levels of the complexes and the concentration of the C3d breakdown product of C3 (Fig. 6.4).

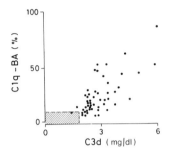

Figure 6.4   Correlation between the level of circulating immune complexes (percentage ^{125}I-C1q binding activity, C1q-BA, in serum) and the plasma C3d concentration in patients with systemic lupus erythematosus. The shadowed area represents the normal range (mean ± 2 s.d.) of the values found in healthy blood donors

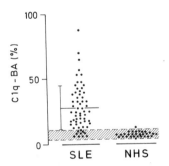

Figure 6.5   Circulating immune complex levels (percentage ^{125}I-C1q binding activity, C1q-BA) in patients with systemic lupus erythematosus (SLE). The shadowed area represents the normal range (mean ± 2 s.d.) of the C1q-BA, found in sera from healthy blood donors (NHS)

A pathogenetic role for the immune complexes is suggested by the findings of deposits of immunoglobulins and complement in many tissues and particularly in the kidney glomeruli. It is possible that particular mechanisms are involved in the tissue localisation of some complexes (Izui, Lambert and Miescher, 1976). Indeed, while DNA–anti-DNA complexes represent an important fraction of the glomerular deposits (Koffler et al, 1967) such complexes constitute only a small minority of the circulating complexes (Zubler and Lambert, 1977). However, the data presently available suggest that the quantitation of immune complexes or their indirect evaluation has a practical importance for the follow-up of patients with SLE. There is an excellent correlation between the levels of complexes and C3d and the overall clinical activity of the disease. Two possible patterns of serological parameters which may be observed during the follow-up studies are shown on Figure 6.6. In the case of patient K.S. these data reflected and objectivated a slow but continuing clinical involvement of SLE under therapy during an eight-month period from April to November 1975. In patient H.S. the serological studies reflected very closely the variable but severe course of the disease despite immunosuppressive medications, with deterioration in July–August 1975, followed by an improvement in January 1976 and a relapse three months later. In our own experience a rise of the level of immune complexes may precede a relapse of the disease.

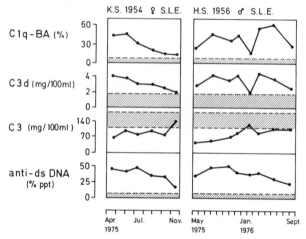

Figure 6.6   Follow-up studies in two patients with systemic lupus erythematosus of the immune complex levels in serum (percentage ^{125}I-C1q binding activity, C1q-BA), the plasma concentrations of C3d and total C3, and the levels of antidouble-stranded DNA antibodies (percentage ^{3}H-DNA precipitated in the radioimmunoassay). The shadowed areas represent the normal ranges (means ± 2 s.d.) of the values. C1q-BA and C3d values correlated directly with the overall clinical activity of the disease.

Similar observations have been made in rheumatoid arthritis (Zubler et al, 1976b; Nydegger et al, 1977). On one hand there is an excellent correlation of the levels of circulating immune complexes and C3d with the development of vasculitis (Fig. 6.7), and the overall clinical activity, on the other hand the similar analysis of the synovial fluid reflects very well the severity of the local inflammatory process in the joint spaces. This type of clinical investigation in rheumatoid arthritis should be considered as a useful adjunct to the evaluation of therapeutic trials. In some cases it may also help in the diagnosis of rheumatoid arthritis. Indeed, a high level of immune complexes in serum is rather characteristic for rheumatoid arthritis as compared to various other inflammatory joint diseases (Fig. 6.8).

In various infectious diseases immune complexes have been found. The relevance of such complexes appears mostly in diseases caused by infectious agents of relatively low pathogenicity and in which the immune response of the host plays a major role in determining the pathological manifestations. The formation of immune complexes may be involved in the pathogenesis when large numbers of infectious agents are chronically persisting. Therefore the detection of immune complexes may be particularly relevant to the clinical condition in diseases such as chronic hepatitis-B (Oldstone, 1975) or leprosy. In leprosy

(Bjorvatn et al, 1976) moderate levels of circulating immune complexes have been detected in patients with the tuberculoid as well as the lepromatous form of the disease and the levels were not significantly higher in patients with the erythema nodosum complication of lepromatous leprosy, while it is known that immunohistological studies suggested a participation of immune complexes in the pathogenesis particularly of erythema nodosum. However, when the plasma C3d concentrations were measured in these patients, a rather

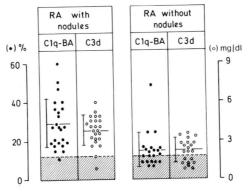

Figure 6.7 Correlation of the immune complex levels in serum (percentage ^{125}I-C1q binding activity, C1q-BA) and the C3d concentrations in plasma with the occurrence of subcutaneous nodules in patients with rheumatoid arthritis. The means of the values (± 2 s.d.) from each group are indicated. The shadowed areas represent the normal ranges (means ± 2 s.d.) of the values observed in healthy blood donors

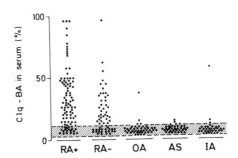

Figure 6.8 Immune complex levels in serum samples (percentage ^{125}I-C1q binding activity, C1q-BA) from patients with various joint diseases: sero-positive (RA+) and sero-negative (RA−) rheumatoid arthritis, osteoarthritis (OA), ankylosing spondylitis (AS) and various other inflammatory arthritis (IA) (gout, chondrocalcinosis, infectious monoarthritis). The shadowed area represents the normal range (mean ± 2 s.d.) of the values found in healthy blood donors

striking correlation of high C3d levels with the occurrence of erythema nodosum was observed (Fig. 6.9). In contrast, there was only a poor correlation between the C3d levels and that of the circulating immune complexes. Extravascular immune complexes may have triggered the complement activation in tissues with secondary diffusion of C3d fragments into the circulation.

In Dengue fever the acute haemorrhagic shock is probably related to the formation of immune complexes in massive amounts, and their detection may be of practical importance in clinical care as well as for studies of the pathogenesis of the disease (Sobel et al, 1975; Theofilopoulos et al, 1976). Parasitic diseases are generally characterised by a chronic release of parasite antigens in blood or in tissues and are often associated with the occurrence of immune complexes. In malaria this phenomenon is probably relevant to the development of renal and cerebral complications (Lambert and Houba, 1974; WHO Report, 1975). In schistosomiasis immune complexes may be involved in the mechanisms by which parasites escape the effects of the immune response (Butterworth et al, 1976).

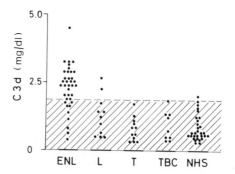

Figure 6.9 Plasma C3d levels in patients with erytheme nodosum leprosum (ENL), uncomplicated lepromatous leprosy (L), tuberculoid leprosy (T), active pulmonary tuberculosis (TBC) and in healthy blood donors (NHS). The shadowed area represents the normal range (mean ±2 s.d.) of the values found in healthy blood donors (from Bjorvatn et al, 1976; published by permission of the Editor and Publishers of *Clinical and Experimental Immunology*).

It is also possible that the detection of immune complexes will provide relevant information with regard to the immune status and the clinical prognosis in some other clinical conditions such as in certain types of neoplasia. Circulating immune complexes of tumour antigens and antibody have been detected in experimental and clinical neoplastic disease, and may possibly have an effect on the host's ability to resist cancer, by blocking cell mediated immune responses (e.g. cytotoxicity—see p. 133) to the antigens on the surface of the tumour. This is suggested by experimental animal studies (Baldwin et al, 1974) and from investigations in human leukaemia currently performed in our laboratory (Carpentier et al, 1976). It has been suggested that plasmaphaeresis, by removing circulating immune complexes, may have a therapeutic effect (Hersey et al, 1976) in patients with neoplastic disease, and such therapy would require adequate monitoring by reliable in vitro methods for immune complex detection.

CONCLUSION

The recent development of methods for the detection of immune complexes in biological fluids should allow for a better understanding of the role of immune complexes in human pathology. Some diseases are apparently directly related to the formation of such complexes and their localisation in various tissues. In these conditions, the quantitation of circulating or extravascular immune complexes and the estimation of complement catabolism may provide useful indices to follow the therapy. Frequently, the formation of immune complexes may represent a secondary event during the course of a disease, such as infection, but may account for some of the pathological manifestations. Finally, immune complexes may occur in some diseases without obvious direct pathological consequences. However, such complexes may interfere with important cell functions and possibly modulate the immune response of the patient in a more subtle fashion.

The direct investigation of immune complexes in clinical conditions should lead to the development of new concepts in the pathogenesis of a wide range of diseases. One can expect that this new methodology will in the near future be transferred from research to routine clinical laboratories.

REFERENCES

Agnello, V., Winchester, R. J. & Kunkel, H. G. (1970) Precipitin reactions of the C1q component of complement with aggregated γ-globulin and immune complexes in gel diffusion. *Immunology*, **19**, 909–919.

Agnello, V., Koffler, D., Eisenberg, J. W., Winchester, R. J. & Kunkel, H. G. (1971) C1q precipitins in the sera of patients with systemic lupus erythematosus and other hypocomplementemic states: characterization of high and low molecular types. *Journal of Experimental Medicine*, **134**, 228s–241s.

Ahlstedt, S., Hanson, L. Å. & Wadsworth, C. (1976) A C1q immunosorbent assay compared with thin-layer gel filtration for measuring IgG aggregates. *Scandinavian Journal of Immunology*, **5**, 293–298.

Almeida, J. D. & Waterson, Å. P. (1969) Immune complexes in hepatitis. *Lancet*, **ii**, 983–986.

Amlot, P. L., Slaney, J. M. & Williams, B. D. (1976) Circulating immune complexes and symptoms in Hodgkin's disease. *Lancet*, **i**, 449–451.

Baldwin, R. W., Bowen, J. G., Embleton, M. J., Price, R. A. & Robins, R. A. (1974) Cellular and humoral immune responses to neoantigens associated with chemically induced tumors. *Progress in Immunology*, **II**/3, 239–248.

Barkas, T., Al-Khateeb, S. F., Irvine, W. J., Davidson, N. McD. & Roscoe, P. (1976) Inhibition of cell-mediated cytotoxicity (ADCC) as a means of detection of immune complexes in the sera of patients with thyroid disorders and bronchogenic carcinoma. *Clinical and Experimental Immunology*, **25**, 270–279.

Barnett, I. G. & MacLennan, I. C. M. (1972) Inhibitory effect of rheumatoid sera on cell damage by lymphocytes. *Annals of the Rheumatic diseases*, **31**, 425 (abstract).

Biberfeld, G. & Norberg, R. (1974) Circulating immune complexes in mycoplasma pneumoniae infection. *Journal of Immunology*, **112**, 413–415.

Bjorvatn, B., Barnetson, R. S., Kronvall, G., Zubler, R. H. & Lambert, P. H. (1976) Immune complexes and complement hypercatabolism in patients with leprosy. *Clinical and Experimental Immunology*, **26**, 388–396.

Britton, M. C. & Schur, P. H. (1971) The complement system in rheumatoid synovitis. II. Intra-cytoplasmic inclusions of immunoglobulins and complement. *Arthritis and Rheumatism*, **14**, 87–95.

Brouet, J. C., Clauvel, J. P., Danon, F., Klein, M. & Seligmann, M. (1974) Biologic and clinical significance of cryoglobulins. *American Journal of Medicine*, **57**, 775–788.

Butterworth, A. E., Sturrock, R. F., Houba, V. & Taylor, R. (1976) *Schistosoma mansoni* in baboons. Antibody-dependent cell-mediated damage to ^{51}Cr-labelled schistosomula. *Clinical and Experimental Immunology*, **25**, 95–102.

Carpentier, N. A., Zubler, R. H., Lange, G. T., Lambert, P. H. & Miescher, P. A. (1976) Complexes immuns circulants dans les leucémies humaines. *Schweizerische medizinische Wochenschrift*, **106**, 1363–1364.

Charlesworth, J. A., Williams, D. G., Sherington, E., Lachmann, P. J. & Peters, D. K. (1974) Metabolic studies of the third component of complement and the glycine-rich beta glycoprotein in patients with hypocomplementemia. *Journal of Clinical Investigation*, **53**, 1578–1587.

Cochrane, C. G. & Koffler, D. (1973) Immune complex disease in experimental animals and man. *Advances in Immunology*, **16**, 185–264.

Cowdery, J. S., Jr, Treadwell, P. E. & Fritz, R. B. (1975) A radioimmunoassay for human antigen–antibody complexes in clinical material. *Journal of Immunology*, **114**, 5–9.

Creighton, W. D., Lambert, P. H. & Miescher, P. A. (1973) Detection of antibodies and soluble antigen–antibody complexes by precipitation with polyethylene glycol. *Journal of Immunology*, **111**, 1219–1227.

Dixon, F. J. (1963) The role of antigen–antibody complexes in disease. *The Harvey Lectures*, **58,** 21–52.

Doe, W. F., Booth, C. C. & Brown, D. L. (1973) Evidence for complement binding immune complexes in adult coeliac disease, Crohn's disease, and ulcerative colitis. *Lancet*, **i,** 402–403.

Eisenberg, R. & Theofilopoulos, A. N. (1975) Use of bovine conglutinin for the assay and isolation of complement-fixing immune complexes. *Federation Proceedings*, **36,** 670 (abstract).

Ezer, G. & Hayward, A. R. (1974) Inhibition of complement-dependent lymphocyte rosette formation: a possible test for activated complement products. *European Journal of Immunology*, **4,** 148–150.

Farrell, C., Søgaard, H. & Svehag, S. E. (1975) Detection of IgG aggregate or immune complexes using solid-phase C1q and protein A-rich *Staphylococcus aureus* as an indicator system. *Scandinavian Journal of Immunology*, **4,** 673–680.

Feldmann, J. L., Becker, M. J., Moutsopoulos, H., Fye, K., Blackman, M., Epstein, W. & Talal, N. (1976) Antibody-dependent cell-mediated cytotoxicity in selected autoimmune diseases. *Journal of Clinical Investigation*, **58,** 173–179.

Fox, A. E., Plescia, O. J. & Mellors, R. C. (1974) Assay and characterization of polyanion–immunoglobulin complexes in sera of New Zealand Black mice. *Immunology*, **26,** 367–374.

Frankland, E. C., Holman, H. R., Müller-Eberhard, H. J. & Kunkel, H. G. (1957) An unusual protein component of high molecular weight in the serum of certain patients with rheumatoid arthritis. *Journal of Experimental Medicine*, **105,** 425–438.

Gabriel, A., Tai, M. & Agnello, V. (1975) Two new radioimmunoassays for detection of immune complexes. *Federation Proceedings*, **36,** 670 (abstract).

Grangeot, L. & Pillot, M. J. (1975) Mise en évidence d'immuncomplexes circulants chez l'homme; précipitation des immuncomplexes par le polyéthylène glycol et leur charactérisation par le C1q lié aux immunoglobulines. *Comptes rendus hebdomadaire des siances de l'Académie des sciences, Série D, Sciences Naturelles*, **280,** 1201–1203.

Grubb, A. O. (1975) Demonstration of circulating IgG-lactate dehydrogenase immune complexes by crossed immunoelectrophoresis. *Scandinavian Journal of Immunology*, **4,** Suppl. 2, 53–57.

Hallberg, T. (1972) In vitro cytotoxicity of human lymphocytes for sensitized chicken erythrocytes is inhibited by sera from rheumatoid arthritis patients. *Scandinavian Journal of Immunology*, **1,** 329–338.

Hannestad, K. (1968) Rheumatoid factors reacting with autologous native γ-G-globulin and joint fluid γ-G-aggregates. *Clinical and Experimental Immunology*, **3,** 671–690.

Harbeck, R. J., Bardana, E. J., Kohler, P. F. & Carr, R. I. (1973) DNA:anti-DNA complexes: their detection in sytemic lupus erythematosus sera. *Journal of Clinical Investigation*, **52,** 789–795.

Hay, F. C., Nineham, L. J. & Roitt, I. M. (1976) Routine assay for the detection of immune complexes of known immunoglobulin class using solid phase C1q. *Clinical and Experimental Immunology*, **24,** 396–400.

Hedfors, E. & Horberg, R. (1974) Evidence for circulating immune complexes in sarcoidosis. *Clinical and Experimental Immunology*, **16,** 493–496.

Heimer, R. & Abruzzo, J. L. (1972) A latex test for the detection of IgG aggregates and IgG–anti-IgG antibody. *Immunochemistry*, **9,** 921–931.

Henson, P. M. (1971) Interaction of cells with immune complexes: adherence, release of constituents, and tissue injury. *Journal of Experimental Medicine*, **134,** 114s–135s.

Herreman, G., Godeau, P., Cabane, J., Digeon, M., Laver, M. & Bach, J. F. (1975) Etude immunologique des endocardites infectieuses subaigës par recherches de complexes immuns circulants. *La Nouvelle Presse médicale*, **4,** 2311–2314.

Hersey, P., Isbister, J., Edwards, A., Murray, E., Adams, E., Biggs, J. & Milton, G. W. (1976) Antibody-dependent cell-mediated cytotoxicity against melanoma cells induced by plasmapheresis. *Lancet*, **i,** 825–827.

Howell, S. B. & Epstein, W. V. (1976) Circulating immunoglobulin complexes in Wegener's granulomatosis. *American Journal of Medicine*, **60,** 259–268.

Izui, S., Lambert, P. H. & Miescher, P. A. (1976) In vitro demonstration of a particular affinity of glomerular basement membrane and collagen for DNA. A possible basis for a local formation of DNA–anti-DNA complexes in systemic lupus erythematosus. *Journal of Experimental Medicine*, **144,** 428–443.

Jayarao, K. S., Faulk, W. P., Karam, J. H., Grodsky, G. M. & Forsham, P. H. (1973) Measurement of immune complexes in insulin-treated diabetics. *Journal of Immunological Methods*, **3,** 337–346.

Jewell, D. P. & MacLennan, I. C. M. (1973) Circulating immune complexes in inflammatory bowel disease. *Clinical and Experimental Immunology*, **14,** 219–226.

Johnson, A. H., Mowbray, J. F. & Porter, K. A. (1975) Detection of circulating immune complexes in pathological human sera. *Lancet*, **i**, 762–765.

Jose, D. G. & Seshadri, R. (1974) Circulating immune complexes in human neuroblastoma: direct assay and role in blocking specific cellular immunity. *International Journal of Cancer*, **13**, 824–838.

Kaplan, M. H. & Volanakis, J. E. (1974) Interaction of C-reactive protein complexes with the complement system. I. Consumption of human complement associated with the reaction of C-reactive protein with pneumococcal C-polysaccharide and with the cholin phosphatides, lecithin and sphingomyelin. *Journal of Immunology*, **112**, 2135–2147.

Koffler, D., Schur, P. H. & Kunkel, H. G. (1967) Immunological studies concerning the nephritis of systemic lupus erythematosus. *Journal of Experimental Medicine*, **126**, 607–623.

Kunkel, H. G., Müller-Eberhard, H. J., Fudenberg, H. H. & Tomasi, T. B. (1961) Gamma-globulin complexes in rheumatoid arthritis and certain other conditions. *Journal of Clinical Investigation*, **40**, 117–129.

Lambert, P. H. & Dixon, F. J. (1968) Pathogenesis of the glomerulonephritis of NZB/W mice. *Journal of Experimental Medicine*, **127**, 507–522.

Lambert, P. H. & Houba, V. (1974) Immune complexes in parasitic diseases. *Progress in Immunology*, **II/5**, 57–67.

Lambert, P. H., Creighton, D., Goodman, R., Bankhurst, A. & Miescher, P. A. (1972) Approche expérimentale de la pathogénie du lupus érythémateux. *Journal d'Urologie et Néphrologie*, **78**, 973–1003.

Ludwig, F. J. & Cusumano, C. L. (1974) Detection of immune complexes using ^{125}I-goat anti-(human IgG) monovalent (Fab) antibody fragments. *Journal of the National Cancer Institute*, **52**, 1529–1536.

Lurhuma, A. Z., Cambiaso, C. L., Masson, P. L. & Heremans, J. F. (1976) Detection of circulating antigen–antibody complexes by their inhibitory effect on the agglutination of IgG-coated particles by rheumatoid factor or C1q. *Clinical and Experimental Immunology*, **25**, 212–226.

Luthra, H. S., McDuffie, F. C., Hunder, G. G. & Samayoa, E. A. (1975) Immune complexes in sera and synovial fluids of patients with rheumatoid arthritis. Radioimmunoassay with monoclonal rheumatoid factor. *Journal of Clinical Investigation*, **56**, 458–466.

MacLennan, I. C. M. (1972) Competition for receptors for immunoglobulins on cytotoxic lymphocytes. *Clinical and Experimental Immunology*, **10**, 275–283.

MacLennan, I. C. M., Roberts-Thompson, P. J., Clarke, J. R. & Gotch, F. M. (1977) Interaction of immune complexes with K-cells and neutrophils. *Annals of the Rheumatic Diseases* (in press).

Mannik, M. & Arend, W. P. (1971) Fate of preformed immune complexes in rabbits and rhesus monkeys. *Journal of Experimental Medicine*, **134**, 19s–31s.

Medof, M. E. & Sukhupunyaraksa, S. (1975) Detection and quantitation of immune complexes by inhibition of ^{125}I-C1q binding to IgG-coated latex particles. *Federation Proceedings*, **36**, 670 (abstract).

Mohammed, I., Thompson, B. & Holborow, E. J. (1977) Radiobioassay for immune complexes using macrophages. *Annals of the Rheumatic Diseases*, **36**, Suppl. 1, 49–54.

Moran, C. J., Ryder, G., Turk, J. L. & Waters, M. F. R. (1972) Evidence for circulating immune complexes in lepromatous leprosy. *Lancet*, **ii**, 572–573.

Mowbray, J. F., Hoffbrand, A. V., Holborow, E. J., Seah, P. P. & Fry, L. (1973) Circulating immune complexes in dermatitis herpetiformis. *Lancet*, **i**, 400–402.

Müller-Eberhard, H. J. (1974) Patterns of complement activation. *Progress in Immunology*, **II/1**, 173–182.

Müller-Eberhard, H. J. (1975) Complement. *Annual Review of Biochemistry*, **44**, 697–724.

Myllylä, G., Vaheri, A. & Penttinen, K. (1971) Detection and characterization of immune complexes by the platelet aggregation test. II. Circulating complexes. *Clinical and Experimental Immunology*, **8**, 399–408.

Myllylä, G. (1973) Aggregation of human blood platelets by immune complexes in the sedimentation pattern test. *Scandinavian Journal of Haematology*, Suppl. 19.

Norberg, R. (1974) IgG complexes in serum of rheumatoid arthritis patients. *Scandinavian Journal of Immunology*, **3**, 229–236.

Notkins, A. L., Mahar, S., Scheele, C. & Goffman, J. (1966) Infectious virus–antibody complex in the blood of chronically infected mice. *Journal of Experimental Medicine*, **124**, 81–97.

Nussenzweig, V. (1974) Receptors for immune complexes on lymphocytes. *Advances in Immunology*, **19**, 217–258.

Nydegger, U. E., Anner, R. M., Gerebtzoff, A., Lambert, P. H. & Miescher, P. A. (1974a) Polymorphonuclear leucocyte stimulation by immune complexes. Assessment by nitroblue tetrazolium dye reduction. *European Journal of Immunology*, **3**, 465–470.

Nydegger, U. E., Lambert, P. H., Gerber, H. & Miescher, P. A. (1974b) Circulating immune complexes in the serum in systemic lupus erythematosus and in carriers of hepatitis B antigen. Quantititation by binding to radiolabelled C1q. *Journal of Clinical Investigation*, **54**, 297–309.

Nydegger, U. E., Zubler, R. H., Gabay, R., Joliat, G., Karagevrekis, Ch., Lambert, P. H. & Miescher, P. A. (1977) Circulating complement breakdown products in patients with rheumatoid arthritis. Correlation between plasma C3d, circulating immune complexes and clinical activity. *Journal of Clinical Investigation* (in press).

Oldstone, M. B. A. (1975) Virus neutralization and virus-induced immune complex disease. Virus–antibody union resulting in immunoprotection or immunologic injury—two sides of the same coin. *Progress in Medical Virology*, **19**, 84–119.

Oldstone, M. B. A., Wilson, C. B., Perrin, L. H. & Norris, F. H., Jr (1976) Evidence for immune-complex formation in patients with amyotrophic lateral sclerosis. *Lancet*, **ii**, 169–172.

Onyewotu, I. I., Holborow, E. J. & Johnson, G. D. (1974) Detection and radioassay of soluble circulating immune complexes using guinea-pig peritoneal exudate cells. *Nature (London)*, **248**, 156–159.

Onyewotu, I. I., Johnson, P. M., Johnson, G. D. & Holborow, E. J. (1975) Enhanced uptake by guinea-pig macrophages of radio-iodinated human aggregated immunoglobulin G in the presence of sera from rheumatoid patients with cutaneous vasculitis. *Clinical and Experimental Immunology*, **19**, 267–280.

Palosuo, T., Kano, K., Anthone, S., Gerbasi, J. R. & Milgrom, F. (1976) Circulating immune complexes after kidney transplantation. *Transplantation*, **21**, 312–316.

Penttinen, K. (1972) Platelet aggregation test in the study of hepatitis. *American Journal of Diseases of Children*, **123**, 418–420.

Penttinen, K., Vaheri, A. & Myllylä, G. (1971) Detection and characterization of immune complexes by the platelet aggregation test. I. Complexes formed in vitro. *Clinical and Experimental Immunology*, **8**, 389–397.

Penttinen, K., Wager, O., Räsänen, J. A., Myllylä, G. & Haapanen, E. (1975) Platelet aggregation and cryo-IgM in the study of hepatitis and immune complex states. *Clinical and Experimental Immunology*, **15**, 409–416.

Perrin, L. H., Lambert, P. H. & Miescher, P. A. (1975) Complement breakdown products in plasma from patients with systemic lupus erythematosus and patients with membranoproliferative or other glomerulonephritis. *Journal of Clinical Investigations*, **56**, 165–176.

Pinckard, R. N., Olson, M. S., Giclas, P. C., Terry, R., Boyer, J. T. & O'Rourke, R. A. (1975) Consumption of classical complement components by heart subcellular membranes in vitro and in patients with acute myocardial infarction. *Journal of Clinical Investigation*, **56**, 740–750.

Rawson, A. J., Abelson, N. M. & Hollander, J. L. (1965) Studies on the pathogenesis of rheumatoid joint inflammation. II. Intracytoplasmic particulate complexes in rheumatoid synovial fluids. *Annals of Internal Medicine*, **62**, 281–284.

Rossen, R. D., Reisberg, M. A., Singer, D. B., Schloeder, F. X., Suki, W. N., Hill, L. L. & Eknoyan, G. (1976) Soluble immune complexes in sera of patients with nephritis. *Kidney International*, **10**, 256–263.

Ruddy, S., Gigli, I. & Austen, K. F. (1972) The complement system of man (fourth of four parts). *New England Journal of Medicine*, **287**, 642–646.

Schrohenloher, R. E. (1966) Characterization of the γ-globulin complexes present in certain sera having high titers of anti-γ-globulin activity. *Journal of Clinical Investigation*, **45**, 501–512.

Shulman, N. R. & Barker, L. F. (1969) Virus-like antigen, antibody and antigen–antibody complexes in hepatitis measured by complement fixation. *Science*, **165**, 304–306.

Siegel, J., Rent, R. & Gewurz, H. (1974) Interactions of C-reactive protein with the complement system. I. Protamine induced consumption of complement in acute phase sera. *Journal of Experimental Medicine*, **140**, 631–647.

Sjögren, H. O., Hellström, I., Bansal, S. C., Warner, G. A. & Hellström, K. E. (1972) Elution of 'blocking factors' from human tumors, capable of abrogating tumor-cell destruction by specifically immune lymphocytes. *International Journal of Cancer*, **9**, 274–283.

Smith, M. D., Verroust, P. J., Morel-Maroger, L. M., Pasticier, A. & Coulaud, J. P. (1975a) Circulating immune complexes in schistosomiasis. *British Medical Journal*, 3 May, 274 (letter).

Smith, M. D., Barratt, T. M., Hayward, A. R. & Soothill, J. F. (1975b) The inhibition of complement-dependent lymphocyte rosette formation by the sera of children with steroid-sensitive nephrotic syndrome and other renal diseases. *Clinical and Experimental Immunology*, **21**, 236–243.

Sobel, A. T., Bokisch, V. A. & Müller-Eberhard, H. J. (1975) C1q deviation test for the detection of immune complexes, aggregates of IgG, and bacterial products in human sera. *Journal of Experimental Medicine*, **142**, 139–150.

Sobel, A., Gabay, Y. & Lagrue, G. (1976) Recherche de complexes immuns circulants par le test de déviation de la fraction C1q du complément. *La Nouvelle Presse médicale*, **5**, 1465–1469.

Soothill, J. F. & Hendrickse, R. G. (1967) Some immunological studies of the nephrotic syndrome of Nigerian children. *Lancet*, **ii**, 629–632.

Spiegelberg, H. L. (1974) Biological activities of immunoglobulins of different classes and subclasses. *Advances in Immunology*, **19**, 259–294.

Steffelaar, J. W., De Graaff-Reitsma, C. B. & Feltkamp, T. M. (1976) Immune complex detection by immuno-fluorescence on peripheral blood polymorphonuclear leucocytes. *Clinical and Experimental Immunology*, **23**, 272–278.

Stühlinger, W. D., Verroust, P. J. & Morel-Maroger, L. (1976) Detection of circulating soluble immune complexes in patients with various renal diseases. *Immunology*, **30**, 43–47.

Svehag, S. E. (1975) A solid-phase radioimmunoassay for C1q-binding immune complexes. *Scandinavian Journal of Immunology*, **4**, 687–697.

Svehag, S. E. & Burder, D. (1976) Isolation of C1q binding immune complexes by affinity chromatography and desorption with a diaminoalkyl compound. *Acta pathologica et microbiologica scandinavica*, Section C, **84**, 45–52.

Theofilopoulos, A. N. & Dixon, F. J. (1976) Immune complexes in human sera detected by the Raji cell radioimmune assay. In *In Vitro Methods in Cell Mediated and Tumor Immunity*, ed. Bloom, B. R. & David, J. R. New York: Academic Press (in press).

Theofilopoulos, A. N., Wilson, C. B., Bokisch, V. A. & Dixon, F. J. (1974) Binding of soluble immune complexes to human lymphoblastoid cells. II. Use of Raji cells to detect circulating immune complexes in animal and human sera. *Journal of Experimental Medicine*, **140**, 1230–1244.

Theofilopoulos, A. N., Wilson, C. B. & Dixon, F. J. (1976) The Raji cell radioimmune assay for detecting immune complexes in human sera. *Journal of Clinical Investigation*, **57**, 169–182.

Wager, O., Penttinen, K., Räsänen, J. A. & Myllylä, G. (1973) Inhibition of IgG complex-induced platelet aggregation by antiblobulin-active cryoglobulin IgM components. *Clinical and Experimental Immunology*, **15**, 393–408.

Warner, N. L. (1974) Membrane immunoglobulins and antigen receptors on B and T lymphocytes. *Advances in Immunology*, **19**, 67–216.

Weigle, W. O. (1961) Fate and biological action of antigen–antibody complexes. *Advances in Immunology*, **1**, 283–317.

WHO Report of a Scientific Group (1975) Developments in malaria immunology. *Technical Report Series*, 579. Geneva: World Health Organization.

Wiedermann, G., Miescher, P. A. & Franklin, E. C. (1963) Effect of mercaptoethanol on complement binding ability of human 7s γ-globulin. *Proceedings of the Society for Experimental Biology and Medicine*, **113**, 609–613.

Wilson, C. B. & Dixon, F. J. (1974) Diagnosis of immunopathological renal disease. *Kidney International*, **5**, 389–401.

Winchester, R. J., Agnello, V. & Kunkel, H. G. (1970) Gamma-globulin complexes in synovial fluids of patients with rheumatoid arthritis. Partial characterization and relationship to lowered complement levels. *Clinical and Experimental Immunology*, **6**, 689–706.

Winchester, R. J., Kunkel, H. G. & Agnello, V. (1971) Occurrence of γ-globulin complexes in serum and joint fluid of rheumatoid arthritis patients: use of monoclonal rheumatoid factors as reagent for their demonstration. *Journal of Experimental Medicine*, **134**, 286s–295s.

Zubler, R. H. & Lambert, P. H. (1976a) The ^{125}I-C1q binding test for the detection of soluble immune complexes. In *In Vitro Methods in Cell Mediated and Tumor Immunity*, ed. Bloom, B. R. & David, J. R., Ch. 53. New York: Academic Press.

Zubler, R. H. & Lambert, P. H. (1977) ^{125}I-C1q binding test for the detection of soluble immune complexes. *Annals of the Rheumatic Diseases*, **36**, supplement 1, 27–30.

Zubler, R. H., Lange, G., Lambert, P. H. & Miescher, P. A. (1976a) Detection of immune complexes in unheated sera by a modified ^{125}I-C1q binding test. Effect of heating on the binding of C1q by immune complexes and application of the test to systemic lupus erythematosus. *Journal of Immunology*, **116**, 232–235.

Zubler, R. H., Nydegger, U., Perrin, L. H., Fehr, K., McCormick, J., Lambert, P. H. & Miescher, P. A. (1976b) Circulating and intra-articular immune complexes in patients with rheumatoid arthritis. Correlation of ^{125}I-C1q binding activity with clinical and biological features of the disease. *Journal of Clinical Investigation*, **57**, 1308–1319.

Zubler, R. H., Perrin, L. H., Creighton, W. D. & Lambert, P. H. (1977) The use of polyethylene glycol (PEG) to concentrate immune complexes from serum or plasma samples. *Annals of the Rheumatic Diseases*, **36**, Supplement 1, 23–25.

7
HUMAN T- AND B-LYMPHOCYTE POPULATIONS IN BLOOD

A. Hayward   M. F. Greaves

LYMPHOCYTE HETEROGENEITY

This review is concerned with tests which identify the different populations of cells involved in immune responses and their application in diagnosis and treatment of disease in man. This subject is introduced by a brief discussion of the evidence from animal and clinical studies that such separations have functional correlates.

Evidence that different populations of cells are involved in antibody and cell-mediated responses is derived from three main sources. Conceptually, the simplest are experiments in which single populations of cells are selectively eliminated. Thus Glick, Chang and Jaap (1956) showed that chickens whose bursa of Fabricius was removed in the neonatal period had depressed antibody responses to salmonella antigens. Suppression of bursal development by testosterone injections also impaired antibody responses but both these and surgically bursectomised chickens rejected foreign skin grafts normally, indicating that cell-mediated immunity was intact. The converse—selective interference with graft rejection but retaining antibody responses—was achieved in surgically thymectomised neonatal chickens (Warner and Szenberg, 1964) and mice (Miller, 1964). The latter animals showed suppression of a wider range of cell-mediated responses (including delayed hypersensitivity and increased susceptibility to graft versus host disease) than did the chickens. Both species became lymphopenic after neonatal thymectomy, suggesting that most blood lymphocytes were thymus dependent. There is no bursa of Fabricius in mammals so bursectomy experiments comparable to those performed in chickens have not been possible.

The similarities between operated animals and certain patients with selective immunodeficiencies were emphasised by Good and Cooper and their colleagues as further evidence for a two-compartment concept of immunity mechanisms. Although boys with congenital hypogammaglobulinaemia failed to make antibodies, they had normal delayed hypersensitivity skin responses and could reject foreign skin grafts. Conversely, patients with Hodgkin's disease usually had normal antibody responses but were slow to reject skin grafts and had little delayed hypersensitivity. With the subsequent recognition of patients with congenital absence of the thymus and absent cell-mediated immunity but normal immunoglobulin levels (DiGeorge, 1968) the analogy with the neonatally thymectomised mouse seemed complete. A third type of congenital severe combined immunodeficiency was characterised by lymphopenia, failure of both antibody and cell mediated immunity and by early death. The immunodeficiency in these children and in others with reticular dysgenesis was attributed to failure of a common lymphocyte stem cell to develop. As discussed later, only a small minority of immunodeficient patients belong to either of the polar groups in this classification and in most patients both T and B systems appear defective. This is consistent with the complexity of interactions between antibody and cell-mediated immunity mechanisms, the analysis of which has provided the best evidence for separate roles for T and B lymphocytes in immunity.

The availability of strains of inbred histocompatible mice facilitated experiments in which the responses of defined cell populations could be studied in irradiated recipients. Reports including those of Claman, Chaperon and Triplett (1966), Davies et al (1967)

Table 7.1 Abbreviations and glossary of terms

FACS	Fluorescence-activated cell sorter
Cells	
T cell	Thymus-derived lymphocyte
B cell	Bursa-equivalent-derived lymphocyte
ALL	Acute lymphoblastic leukaemia
CLL	Chronic lymphocytic leukaemia
Surface markers	
ALLA	Acute lymphoblastic leukaemia antigen
HuTLA	Human T-lymphocyte antigen
HuBLA	Human B-lymphocyte antigen
HuMA	Human monocyte/macrophage antigen
E rosette	Reaction of lymphocytes with sheep erythrocytes
EAhu rosette	Reaction of lymphocytes (and other cells) with human rhesus-positive red cells coated with anti-D antibody
EAC rosette	Reaction of lymphocytes and other cells with antibody (A) plus complement (C) coated erythrocytes (E)
AggIgG	Heat-aggregated immunoglobulin G
SmIg	Surface membrane immunoglobulin
EBV	Epstein–Barr virus

and Miller and Mitchell (1968) indicated that at least two populations of lymphocytes were involved in most antibody responses and these differed in their anatomical distribution. Cells of one population were the precursors of plasma cells; these were present in the bone marrow but not the thymus and they corresponded to the bursa-dependent system of chickens. Another population was dependent on and or derived from the thymus and although they had an obligatory role in most antibody responses they did not themselves turn into plasma cells. A synthesis of all these observations led to the T- (thymus derived) and B- ('bursa-equivalent' derived) cell nomenclature (Roitt et al, 1969) and a general acceptance of the central significance of the cellular dichotomy of the mammalian and avian immune systems (reviewed by Greaves, Raff and Owen, 1973). Some commonly used abbreviations are given in Table 7.1.

These various functional studies on different cell populations also led to a better appreciation of the important roles played by macrophages in immune responses. Thus in model in vitro systems macrophages appeared to be essential for T-cell activation by antigens. Macrophages have long been recognised as major cellular constituents of the cellular infiltrates seen in inflammation, delayed cutaneous reactions and in skin grafts undergoing rejection. Experiments involving selective inactivation of macrophages (selective poisoning or irradiation) have amply demonstrated that although T cells principally determine the specificity of the spectrum of cell-mediated responses the 'effector' phase usually involves a major contribution by 'aggressive' macrophages. Significantly, the activity of macrophages in these situations is regulated by soluble products of activated T cells. Experiments in which monuclear phagocyte function was depressed by loading with silica or carbon particles suggested that these cells were also necessary for antibody responses but confirmation of this was delayed until it became possible to investigate primary immune responses in vitro (Dutton and Mishell, 1967).

The recognition of T and B lymphocytes by their surface characteristics rather than their functional properties was a critical advance in cellular immunology and was aided by the different tissue distributions of these cells. Reif and Allen (1964) found that C3H mice immunised with AKR thymocytes made antibodies which bound to AKR thymus

Table 7.2   Functional activity of mouse T lymphocytes of different Ly phenotypes

	Cell type	T_H	T_{CS}	$T_E{}^a$
	Ly type[b]	1	2, 3	1, 2, 3
Helper function		+	0	
Cytotoxic activity		0	+	
Suppressor activity		0	+	

[a] T_E lymphocytes appear early in development. Their function has not yet been defined but they constitute a considerable proportion of the T-cell pool
[b] Taken from Medawar and Simpson (1975) and Beverley (1976). Another Ly phenotype, Ly 4, is a B-cell marker (Snell et al, 1973)

and brain cells. They called the antigen theta (θ) and found that it was present on some lymph node cells, possibly those derived from the thymus. This was supported by Raff and Wortis' (1970) observation that the proportion of cells lysed by anti-θ serum and complement was inversely correlated with the proportion of B lymphocytes (cells with surface immunoglobulin, see below) in preparations from a range of lymphoid tissues. Further studies have shown that T lymphocytes first express the θ-antigen while in the thymus and subsequently continue to do so, though in smaller amounts, during their re-circulating lifespan.

The θ-antigen is present on some non-lymphoid cells including brain cells, epidermal cells and fibroblasts. It is not present on B lymphocytes: nude mice which are congenitally deficient of thymus and thymus-dependent lymphocytes (and lack cell-mediated immunity) have few if any θ-positive cells but normal numbers of B cells. Neonatally thymectomised mice have a corresponding paucity of θ-positive cells so there is a functional correlation with the depletion experiments. Adult thymectomy experiments indicate that there are subsets of θ-positive lymphocytes: one of these (T_1) migrates predominantly to the spleen and the other (T_2) constitutes the recirculatory pool. There are other T-lymphocyte antigens, e.g. Ly antigens; in this system there is evidence that the separate subsets of T lymphocytes have different activities in vivo (summarised in Table 7.2).

A subpopulation of mouse lymphocytes with surface immunoglobulin staining with anti-immunoglobulin serum was observed by Möller in 1961, though its significance was not at that time fully appreciated. Raff (1970) suggested that cells with membrane immunoglobulin were B cells since they were rare in the thymus and their frequency in other lymphoid tissue correlated inversely with θ-positive cells. Experiments in chickens clearly demonstrated that surface membrane immunoglobulin-positive lymphocytes ($SmIg^+$)

developed in the bursa (in 14-day embryos) and that the initial maturation and expansion of this population was independent of the thymus.

Tests to identify human T and B lymphocytes have been extensively developed over the past three or four years. Not only do they distinguish between T and B lymphocytes, but also separate them from other free mononuclear cells in the blood and tissues, namely macrophages and cytotoxic 'lymphocytes' (K cells). The latter are a small percentage of the total blood lymphocyte-like cells. They are distinguished by their ability to produce complement independent killing or lysis of antibody-coated target cells; their role, if any, in the induction of the immune response is unknown.

Table 7.3   Membrane markers for human lymphocytes

Markers		T	B
1. *Antisera*	anti-HuTLA	+	−
	anti-HuBLA	−	+
	anti-Ig	−	+
2. *Viruses*	EBV	−	+
	Measles	+	−
3. *Erythrocyte rosettes*	Sheep	+	−
	Human	±(n)	−
	Rhesus monkey	+	−
	Japanese ape	−	+
	Mouse	−	+
4. *Lectins*	Helix pomatia	+(n)	−
5. *Complement*	C3b C3bi	−	+
	C4b	−	+
	C1q	+	+
6. *Immunoglobulin*	Agg or IgG-rbc	− or +	+
	IgM-rbc	− or +	−

n = neuraminidase-treated lymphocytes

The tests are based mainly on methods developed in laboratory animals and their evaluation has depended primarily on demonstrating a reciprocal relationship between the proportions of cells with putative specific characteristics in the blood and lymphoid tissues of healthy subjects and patients. This inevitably invites circular arguments in the interpretation of results; a cell which lacks surface immunoglobulin is not necessarily a T lymphocyte and a test which identifies all or most such cells cannot be considered specific unless it is supported by independent functional criteria. These requirements may be particularly difficult to meet in pathological states because normal function is frequently lost. Despite these limitations, tests for lymphocyte populations have become increasingly useful in the diagnosis and management of immunodeficiency and lymphoproliferative disorders. This usefulness prompts a wider clinical demand for tests and it is desirable that clinical immunologists should aim for the high standards of quality control achieved in clinical biochemistry. We have prepared our review of methodology and interpretation of results with these aims in mind.

MEMBRANE MARKERS FOR HUMAN T AND B LYMPHOCYTES

Subpopulations of human lymphocytes from blood and other lymphoid tissues can be distinguished by virtue of cell surface properties. The differences are expressed in cell surface structures which can be identified with suitably labelled antisera or other reagents and they determine the cell surface phenotype (reviewed also in Greaves, 1975; Möller, 1973; WHO/IARC Report, 1974). The list of markers reported to be specific for T and B lymphocytes is now quite extensive (Table 7.3) but comparison with the data in Table 7.4 shows that some of them are shared with monocytes. Since 5 to 25 per cent of the mononuclear cells prepared from blood by Boyum's Ficoll-isopaque method are monocytes it is important to distinguish between these cell types.

Table 7.4   Markers which identify monocytes and macrophages

Membrane markers
Complement—specific for C3d component of C3
Immunoglobulin—aggregated IgG or IgG antibody-coated erythrocytes
Antiserum—specific antihuman macrophage antiserum

Cytoplasmic markers
Enzymes (in lyzosomes), e.g. peroxidase, esterase

Functional marker
Phagocytosis

Table 7.5   General physical properties distinguishing human T and B lymphocytes

	T	B	Sample references
Adherence of polystyrene particles to lymphocyte surfaces	−	+	Jondal et al (1974)
Adherence to nylon	−/±	+/++	Greaves and Brown (1974)
Charge	(− − −) > (−)		Durandy et al (1975)
Cell surface projections (SEM)	+	< ++	Polliack and de Harven (1975)
Density		>	Yu et al (1974)

Some other physical differences between T- and B-lymphocyte populations are listed in Table 7.5. It should be emphasised that these are relative differences and none of these parameters give a complete distinction between T and B cells. These general physical properties and the better defined membrane binding sites or receptors both provide a means to separate lymphocyte populations to varying degrees of homogeneity (Table 7.6). Preliminary evidence suggests that it may also be possible to distinguish between T- and B-lymphocyte populations using relatively simple histochemical methods (see Table 7.7). It is not yet clear if this approach will have the same discriminatory capacity as membrane binding markers but it will provide a very useful parallel or corroborative technique which might be particularly useful in tissue sections.

It is likely that the T- and B-lymphocyte populations comprise a number of functionally different *subsets* and it may become possible to distinguish between these too, as has been achieved for mice with the Ly antigens. Tests in which there is already evidence of such differences in the T-cell series include the E-rosette test (Wybran and Fudenberg, 1973; Yu, 1975a), reaction with antisera raised to brain or thymus cells (Brown and Greaves, 1974a; Greaves and Janossy, 1976), autologous rosette formation (Yu, 1975b), binding of IgM or IgG (Moretta et al, 1975) and proliferative response to various mitogens (Touraine et al, 1975). Some functional correlates are emerging, for example the IgM binding T lymphocytes are those which help B cells undergo terminal differentiation in response to the pokeweed mitogen (Cooper, M. D., personal communication).

Table 7.6 Physical separation of human T and B lymphocytes

Method	Sample references
A. *Using selective membrane markers*	
1. Rosette sedimentation	Greaves and Brown (1974)
	Plum and Ringoir (1975)
2. Affinity columns or surfaces:	Chess et al (1974)
anti-Ig	Jondal, Wigzell and Aiuti (1973)
C3	
Ag-Ab	
lectin	
3. Fluorescence activated cell sorter (FACS):	Kreth and Herzenberg (1974)
fluorescent antibodies	Greaves (1975) (see also Fig. 7.1)
B. *Using general physical properties*	
1. Adherence columns, e.g. nylon	Eisen, Wedner and Parker (1972)
	Greaves & Brown (1974)
	Plum and Ringoir (1975)
2. Electrophoresis	Durandy et al (1975)

See also Möller (1975) for review of separation techniques

Table 7.7 Summary of preliminary evidence for differences between human T and B lymphocytes detectable by histochemical methods

Test	Result	Reference
1. Weak acid phosphatase + strong beta glucuronidase[1a]	T cell characteristic	Barr and Perry (1976)
2. Lactate dehydrogenase (isoenzyme pattern)	Class characteristic patterns for T and B cells	Plum and Ringoir (1975)
3. 5-Nucleotidase and adenosine triphosphatase	Selectively present in thymus-independent ($\sim$ B cell) areas of human lymph nodes	Müller-Hermelink (1974)

[a] Activated T cells (e.g. PHA-stimulated cells, T-cell lines, T-like lymphoblastic leukaemias, Sezary cell lymphoma and T lymphoblasts from infectious mononucleosis) all show strong activity of *both* acid phosphatase and β-glucuronidase. See Barr and Perry (1976) for references

T-lymphocyte Markers

E rosettes

It is now well established that the majority of the immunoglobulin negative lymphocytes (SmIg$^-$) in blood and lymphoid tissue form E rosettes with sheep erythrocytes. The variability of the percentages of E-positive lymphocytes reported in the early literature has been largely superseded as a result of some degree of standardisation of the test system itself and by the inclusion of modifications to enhance or stabilise rosette formation (e.g. pretreatment of sheep red cells with neuraminidase).

A small proportion of SmIg$^+$ cells in blood may also form E rosettes (Chiao, Pantic and Good, 1975) but these are not observed when special steps are taken to eliminate cytophilic immunoglobulin from non-B cells (see below). The approximate value for E^+ lymphocytes in blood from healthy adults is given in Figure 7.2.

Some important qualifications are needed here. We do not know if *every* E^+ cell has *functional* T-lymphocyte characteristics or that every functional T cell does indeed make an E rosette. Subtle improvements in the rosette methodology can push-up the E^- proportion to 90 per cent and thereby include effectively all SmIg$^-$ non-phagocytic mononuclear cells (in blood). The 'extra' cells enumerated by such modifications in the assay procedure are the 'unclassified' cells (Fig. 7.2); they have the membrane phenotype SmIgG labile$^-$, EAC$^+$Fc$^+$. It is unlikely that these are all bona fide T cells since this population contains cells (considered to be immature B lymphocytes) which can biosynthesise and secrete Ig in vitro and also includes cells which can lyse antibody-coated target cells (i.e. 'K cells'). It is also likely that this population contains small numbers of nonphagocytic but nevertheless monocyte-related cells (Greaves et al, 1975b).

Despite these uncertainties the E-rosette test is the best currently available for counting human T lymphocytes. Studies in selected immunodeficient patients support the view that the capacity to form E rosettes is indeed a thymus-dependent phenomenon. However, it is not necessarily a functional correlate of immunocompetence since (1) thymus lymphocytes are E^+ although they respond poorly in functional T-cell tests and (2) some patients have E^+ cells which do not respond in vitro to mitogens or allogeneic cells. In other circumstances it is possible that virus infected cells may be E^+ but immunologically suppressed.

Rosette tests using sheep erythrocytes have revealed potentially important heterogeneity of T lymphocytes both in the time required for rosetting, i.e. early versus late rosettes (Wybran and Fudenberg, 1973; Yu, 1975a) and in the number of E bound (Brown and Greaves, 1974b). Although there is no clear evidence that these data reflect different functional T-cell subsets, it has been suggested that these variably rosetting cells might be of clinical value, for example in cancer and perhaps in Crohn's disease. It is desirable that these preliminary results are extended and their prognostic value tested in carefully controlled trials.

Anti-T cell sera (anti-HuTLA or antihuman T-lymphocyte antigens)

Anti-θ sera in mice have provided important reagents for identifying and dissecting the T-cell system of mice and rats (Raff, 1971). It is likely that human T cells also possess specific differentiation antigens on their surface. However, to date this has proved difficult to establish. Some success in producing heterologous antihuman T-cell sera has been recorded using a variety of immunisation protocols (reviewed in Greaves and Janossy, 1976); however, the published works are perhaps a little misleading in two respects. Firstly, only apparent 'successes' are recorded and there is little doubt that there may be a high failure rate in such studies (i.e. most sera raised have no clear T specificity). Secondly, the evidence for T-cell specificity is in many cases circumstantial. However, it seems clear that useful anti-T lymphocyte sera can now be produced and when properly absorbed and evaluated they do seem to detect primarily the E^+, SmIg$^-$ population in blood and other tissues. No general method for producing good antisera can at present be recommended in preference to others but it does seem that rabbits immunised with *monkey* thymus often provide a reasonable titre of anti-T cell antibodies (Balch et al, 1975; Greaves and Janossy, 1976). Figure 7.1 illustrates how cell separation experiments (in this case using the

Fluorescence Activated Cell Sorter—FACS) can be used to substantiate the selectivity of membrane markers such as anti-T cell sera.

It has been known for many years that patients with a variety of diseases develop cir-

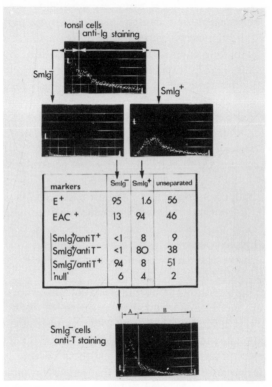

markers	SmIg⁻	SmIg⁺	unseparated
E⁺	95	1.6	56
EAC⁺	13	94	46
SmIg⁺/antiT⁺	<1	8	9
SmIg⁺/antiT⁻	<1	80	38
SmIg⁻/antiT⁺	94	8	51
'null'	6	4	2

Figure 7.1 Identification and separation of human T and B lymphocytes using the Fluorescence Activated Cell Sorter (FACS) This separates cells according to the intensity of fluorescent light they emit. The threshold for separation is adjustable, and the instrument produces a visual readout in the form of a histogram, the vertical axis of which shows the relative cell number and the horizontal axis the relative fluorescence intensity.

Viable tonsil lymphocytes were stained in suspension with fluorescein-conjugated rabbit anti-human immunoglobulin. 10^7 cells were passed through the FACS and gave the fluorescence profile shown in the upper histogram. SmIg⁺ and SmIg⁻ cells were separated using the threshold setting shown in the upper histogram. The two separated populations were reanalysed (with no further staining) and gave the lower fluorescence histograms. They were also analysed for reactivity with other markers. The results of these tests are given in the table incorporated into the figure. The reactivity of the SmIg⁻ population with fluorescein-conjugated anti-T sera is also shown in the bottom histogram.

The experiment demonstrates the existence of two major cell poulations with the membrane phenotypes SmIg⁺, EAC⁺, E⁻, HuTLA⁻, and SmIg⁻, EAC⁻, E⁺, HuTLA⁺. A small proportion of 'double' (T + B) reactive cells and 'null' (non-T, non-B) cells are also present. (Taken from Greaves and Janossy (1976), by kind permission of the editors and publishers of *In vitro Methods in Cell-mediated and Tumor Immunity*)

culating lymphocytotoxic antibodies. Patients with infectious or autoimmune diseases may have serum antibodies that are T-cell specific (Greaves and Janossy, 1976). Sera containing such antibodies usually require absorption to render them T-cell specific and at present these human sera do not appear more promising than those produced experimentally in animals.

In addition to antigen(s) shared between thymic cells, T lymphocytes and activated T lymphoblasts there are probably other T 'axis' antigens that have a more restricted expression, e.g. on thymic cells only, on T lymphoblasts or on thymic cells plus T lymphoblasts (but not on resting T lymphocytes). Although analysis of anti-T cell sera using the Fluorescence Activated Cell Sorter suggests heterogeneity of T lymphocytes and possibly the existence of two reactive subsets (Fig. 7.1) (Greaves and Janossy, 1976) there is as yet no differentially functional subset antigen marker described for man which is in principle similar to the Ly system in mice. It should be remembered in this context that both θ and Ly are alloantigens whose existence was dependent upon cross-immunisation between inbred strains of mice. It will probably be extremely difficult to produce similar reagents for human T-cell subsets.

Other T-lymphocyte markers

As listed in Table 7.2, several other membrane markers have been reported to be selective for T cells. To date these have not been sufficiently well studied for their inclusion as standard tests. However, several of them (e.g. measles virus receptor and IgM binding site) have interesting physiological implications and most of them provide further evidence for T-cell heterogeneity and possible T subsets in man.

B-Lymphocytes

Surface membrane immunoglobulin (SmIg)

The most reliable B-cell characteristic is the synthesis of immunoglobulins (Ig) and their integration or association with the cell surface membrane. This Ig comprises pairs of heavy and light chains which are restricted in idiotype, class and subclass. The molecule is presumably bound to the cell through the Fc region and in common with most other surface molecules, it is mobile in the horizontal plane of the membrane. Its distribution may change from diffuse to aggregated or a polar 'cap' form as a result of cross-linking (by antigen or anti-immunoglobulin antibodies). Immunoglobulin is probably continuously synthesised and following stripping of the surface membrane it takes 3 to 6 h to reappear. B-lymphocyte immunoglobulin is commonly identified using fluorochrome-labelled anti-immunoglobulins. Until quite recently there was a very considerable variation in the reported values of SmIg$^+$ cells in normal human blood (i.e. from an average of 10 per cent in some reports to over 30 per cent in others). These discrepancies have to a large extent been overcome or at least rationalised by an appreciation of the involvement of IgFc receptors. It is now clear that both phagocytic monocytes and a population of unclassified lymphocyte-like cells (see above) have avid cell surface binding sites for IgG. The presence of labile, non-endogenously synthesised Ig on these cells has certainly led many workers to count them as B cells. Some of the SmIg$^+$ non-B lymphocytes have monocyte characteristics and can be excluded from counts by morphological or histochemical criteria. Another approach is to reduce the amount of labile SmIg on these cells by incubation at 37° for 30 to 60 min in azide-free tissue culture medium, or by washing the cells briefly at acid pH (Kumagai et al, 1975). In either case the cell remains capable of binding the Fc region of other IgG molecules, including the fluorochrome labelled anti-immunoglobulin. This can be avoided by digesting away the Fc region of the molecule and using labelled F(ab)$_2$ fragments of the antibody.

METHODS BASED ON SmIg

Antiglobulins have been labelled either with fluorochromes, enzymes, isotopes or large particles such as red cells. There are no formal comparisons between these techniques and all are limited by the quality of the antiserum. This is relatively less of a problem with polyvalent antisera, used to identify all B cells, though these should react equally with both κ and λ chains and preferably not with heavy chains. For class-specific reagents the main problems are the nature of the antigen used to raise the antisera and the steps necessary to eliminate reaction with irrelevant substances. These are discussed only briefly here because many laboratories do not raise their own antisera. Specificity testing is discussed in more detail because this needs to be applied to both home-made and commercial antisera. Both subjects are well reviewed by Preud'homme and Labaume (1975) and WHO/IARC (1974).

PREPARATION OF ANTISERA

Ideally antiglobulins would be raised to completely pure immunoglobulins of various classes which had been isolated from healthy donors. In practice it is laborious to prepare immunoglobulin of adequate purity or amount from normal sera and myeloma proteins are commonly used. These have the disadvantage of subclass restriction and idiotype specificity, although this might be overcome by pooling several myelomas of the same class. It is easier to pool antisera from several animals each selected for high titre and reactivity with non-idiotypic determinants. Sera reacting exclusively with the Fc region may fail to bind to cells, presumably because this region is close to or buried within the cell membrane (Frøland and Natvig, 1973).

When removing unwanted antibodies from the serum it is important to use insolubilised immunoabsorbents so as to avoid making complexes since these would bind to cell Fc receptors. Isolation of the globulin fraction and removal of unwanted antibodies can be performed simultaneously by acid elution of the antibody from insolubilised antigen of the appropriate specificity.

SPECIFICITY TESTING

Specificity tests should be designed to reveal reaction of the candidate antiserum with irrelevant antigens as well as confirming reaction with the desired antigen. Their level of sensitivity should equal that of the final experimental assay. Immunofluorescence tests are more sensitive than precipitation in gel tests so while the latter can be used to confirm wanted reactions by fluorescence reagents, they are not adequate for excluding unwanted ones. Experiments involving immunoglobulin class-specific cytoplasmic immuno-fluorescence can be controlled with myeloma marrow preparations, though these will be restricted in subclass, light chain type and idiotype. Since myeloma preparations are of limited availability we have used purified IgG, IgA and IgM obtained from healthy donors and linked to cyanogen bromide activated cellulose (sigma cell 19) as a substrate for specificity testing. The particles are small enough for testing surface immunofluorescence. With any system it is essential to check that antisera to one heavy chain class do not stain myeloma cells or immunoabsorbents of other heavy chain classes, at least in the concentrations to be used. At about the same level of sensitivity are tests for separate staining; in these B lymphocytes or plasma cells are stained with mixtures of two different anti-immunoglobulins conjugated to different fluorochromes. Separate specificities for the two antisera are indicated if individual cells are stained by only one fluorochrome.

It is important to use sufficient antiglobulin to detect all the cells carrying immuno-globulin of the desired class: since optimal concentrations vary with the method, equip-ment and user this has to be done by titration.

CLASSES OF IMMUNOGLOBULIN ON HUMAN LYMPHOCYTES

IgG is lost from the surface of many blood lymphocytes following washing in tissue culture medium and incubation at 37°, so that the proportion of positive cells falls from about 10 per cent to less than 5 per cent. With the use of $F(ab)_2$ reagents the percentage falls below 1 per cent (Winchester et al, 1975a). It has been suggested that all IgG on B lymphocytes is bound by the Fc receptor but the observation of a few monoclonal IgG CLL preparations in which trypsinised cells resynthesised IgG (Preud'homme, Prouet and Seligmann, 1975) makes this unlikely. However, with the increasing efforts of most laboratories to exclude small monocytes and Fc binding of IgG from their counts the number of $SmIgG^+$ B lymphocytes generally found in the blood of healthy adults is 24 to 250×10^6/litre. Most of the 2 to 5 per cent of IgG-positive blood lymphocytes in Frøland and Natvig's (1973) series were of IgG_2 subclass. This is remarkable because most serum IgG belongs to the IgG_1 subclass: possible explanations of this discrepancy include different productivity of IgG_1 and IgG_2 plasma cells but no data is available.

IgM (and IgD) are present on most B lymphocytes; the IgM is probably present on the cell surface in monomeric form. There is no information on the subclass distribution. Most μ-positive cells also have surface IgD: both heavy chain classes are linked to the same class of light chain but the independent capping of μ and δ indicates that they move separately in the cell membrane. Idiotypic similarity of the surface IgM and IgD in CLL (Fu et al, 1975b) suggest that both classes have the same antigen-binding specificity. The high proportion of IgD-positive cells in cord blood (Rowe et al, 1973) led to speculation that IgD was a 'fetal immunoglobulin' but in both mice (Vitetta et al, 1975) and man (Vossen, 1975) surface μ is found earlier in ontogeny than δ. Perhaps the initial finding of a higher proportion of IgD cells in cord than adult blood (van Boxel et al, 1972; Piessens et al, 1973) reflects the tendency of fetal B lymphocytes to have more SmIg than adult cells (Sidman and Unanue, 1975).

IgA is present on the surface of 1 to 2 per cent of blood lymphocytes: there is no in-formation on subclass distribution. Reports of SmIgE have to be regarded as provisional because antisera to this class are particularly difficult to characterise. Cytophilic binding of IgE to blood basophils is a possible source of error.

Light chains which are present on monoclonal cell populations (e.g. CLL) are only of a single class, which can be synthesised after surface stripping. The light chain restriction to a single type on μ and δ positive cells suggests that non-malignant populations behave similarly and that the rare IgG positive cells stained for both κ and λ have bound immuno-globulin through their Fc receptors (see above). The relative proportions of κ- and λ-positive B lymphocytes is similar to the ratios of these light chains in serum immuno-globulins (i.e. about 2:1).

Membrane binding sites for complement components

Erythrocytes, granulocytes, monocytes, B lymphocytes and renal glomerular cells all have receptors for activated complement components demonstrable by the binding of erythrocytes coated with antibody and complement (Bianco, Patrick and Nussenzweig, 1970) or by indirect immunofluorescence (Ross and Polley, 1975). The receptors on B lymphocytes have specificity either for the C3c region of C3b (resembling the immune adherence receptor of erythrocytes) or for C3d, which monocytes also bind. The C3c receptor also binds C4. These are separate receptors on the cell surface because they cap independently and because of their independent inhibition by isolated complement components (Ross and Polley, 1975). Some SmIg negative cells in Ficoll-triosil preparations from blood (Ross et al, 1973a) and tonsil (Ross and Polley, 1975) make rosettes with EAC and some of these may be monocytes. The proportion of such cells in blood from healthy persons is usually less than 3 per cent but increases in some immunodeficiency (Hayward and Greaves, 1975b) and some chronic lymphatic leukaemias. EAC-rosette formation is consequently an unreliable method for identifying B lymphocytes particularly since the 'labile' IgG-positive population is EAC positive (Nussenzweig, personal communication).

Patients with Crohn's disease and some renal diseases tended to have lower than normal percentages of EAC-rosette forming cells, and their sera inhibited EAC-rosette formation by adenoid lymphocytes (Ezer and Hayward, 1974; Smith et al, 1975). These effects might be due to the presence of activated complement components in their sera or to antilymphocyte antibodies, which are also known to interfere with rosette formation (Ross et al, 1973b). Both B and T cells bind C1q (McConnell, personal communication). Although the EAC-rosette reaction has proven useful for cellular identification and physical separation the functional significance of the receptors involved (on B cells) is unclear. It has been suggested that C3 receptors could be involved in B-cell activation (Dukor et al, 1974). The influence of C3 on thymus-dependent antibody responses (Feldman and Pepys, 1974) suggests that the complement-binding sites on B lymphocytes might play a role in cell interaction and/or regulation of the B-cell response. Certainly interest in complement components and their corresponding cell-associated receptors will increase with the recent finding that several complement components are coded for by genes within the major histocompatibility locus of these species (H-2 in mice, HLA in man). A recent study suggests that the complement receptors themselves may be associated with HLA molecules (Arnaiz-Villena and Festenstein, 1975).

IgFc binding sites on lymphocytes

IgG, either aggregated and fluorescence labelled or attached to indicator red cells, is bound by up to 20 per cent of blood lymphocytes as well as by monocytes and neutrophils. In mice this receptor has specificity for the Fc region of the molecule since $F(ab)_2$ fragments are not bound. However, with respect to human lymphocytes, there is currently some dispute as to whether the receptor is specific for the Fc region of IgG. In most studies of human lymphocytes the IgG-binding population has overlapped largely with the SmIg+ population and T lymphocytes were unreactive (Dickler and Kunkel, 1972). However, some of the SmIg+, IgG binding cells lose their SmIg following acid washing or incubation at 37° (Abo et al, 1976). These 'labile' SmIg+ cells bear IgG and C3 receptors and therefore belong to the currently unclassified category.

There is separate evidence that under some circumstances T lymphocytes can bind immunoglobulin. This was first detected in populations of activated mouse T lymphocytes (Yoshida and Anderson, 1972) and more recently by human T lymphocytes (Moretta et al, 1975). In the latter studies two separate populations of T lymphocytes were found, one binding IgG and the other IgM (subsets designated Tμ and Tγ). Capacity to bind the immunoglobulin developed after 24 h in culture, but was not present on freshly prepared cells, perhaps because their receptors were saturated with serum Ig. Preliminary results suggest that the IgM binding subset of T lymphocytes can help B lymphocytes differentiate in the PWM stimulation assay while those binding IgG are ineffective (Cooper, M. D. and colleagues, personal communication).

B-cell membrane antigens

In the mouse B lymphocytes can be characterised by the expression of the alloantigen Ly-4 which is undetectable on T cells (McKenzie and Snell, 1975). Polymorphic cell membrane antigens coded for by the immune response gene region or I region are also predominantly expressed on B cells in the mouse (Hämmerling et al, 1974) although there is evidence that they may also be found in macrophages, epithelial cells, sperm and perhaps on some activated T cells. It is very likely that analogous (and homologous) gene products exist in man. Earlier attempts to define human B-lymphocyte differentiation antigens employed heteroantisera and successful anti-B cell sera were produced by immunising rabbits with either chronic lymphocytic leukaemia cells (Greaves and Brown, 1973) or tonsil lymphocytes (Ishii et al, 1975). More recently, Schlossman et al (1976) have produced very high titre B-cell specific heteroantisera by immunising with a purified B-cell glycoprotein of molecular weight 30 000 daltons. T cells appear to lack these B-cell antigens, but it remains to be established whether or not they are present on other cells (e.g. monocytes, early myeloid cells or activated T cells).

Although anti-HLA sera were commonly supposed to detect antigens present on all lymphocytes (and other cells except erythrocytes), recent work has clearly identified the existence of cytotoxic antibodies in such sera which are B-cell specific or rather which kill $SmIg^+$ cells and not $SmIg^- E^+$ cells! Absorption of anti-HLA sera (i.e. from multiparous females or transplant recipients) with platelets removes all antibodies to the A, B and C locus antigens, but leaves intact the anti-B cell antibodies (Winchester et al, 1975b). Such absorbed sera block the stimulatory capacity of B cells in the mixed lymphocyte reaction and it appears quite likely that some or all of the alloantigens being detected are products of the fourth or D locus and are closely related if not identical to the LD (lymphocyte-activating) determinants. If this is correct, then these antigens are very similar to the I-region products in the mouse and their further study could have an important impact on our capacity to 'type' for disease resistance or susceptibility as well as for closer matching in transplantation.

Epstein–Barr virus receptors

Many viruses have selective effects of different lymphocyte populations (reviewed by Greaves, 1976). Epstein–Barr virus is of particular interest as the causative agent of infectious mononucleosis and as a probable oncogenic virus, i.e. its ubiquitous presence in Burkitt's lymphoma and its ability to transform human and New World monkey lymphocytes in vitro. All lymphoid cell lines (LCL) containing the EBV genome (with or without active expression of viral antigens) have a B-cell membrane phenotype as do lymphoblasts from biopsies of Burkitt's lymphoma; it was therefore not altogether surprising to find that EBV-binding sites were exclusive to B lymphocytes (Jondal and Klein, 1973; Greaves et al, 1975a). Within the limit of the sensitivity of the 'rosette' and indirect immunofluorescence assays used no EBV receptors could be detected on thymocytes, T cells or monocytes. Virtually every B cell (i.e. $SmIg^+ E^-$ cell) in blood and tonsil was found to bind EBV (Greaves et al, 1975a). EBV receptors may not be completely exclusive to B cells since nasopharyngeal carcinoma appears to involve an EBV-associated malignant transformation of epithelial cells.

Recent studies by Jondal and colleagues have revealed an important relationship between EBV-binding sites on B cells and C3 receptors (Jondal et al, 1976). Only those lymphoblasts from CLL expressing C3 receptors have EBV receptors (and can therefore be superinfected by the virus) and more significantly, the binding sites for EBV and C3 move together on the cell surface. The binding sites do not appear to be identical but rather they are associated with the same molecular structure (or complexes).

These observations are particularly intriguing in the light of the finding that C3 receptors may express the HLA B-locus antigens 4^a and 4^b. This certainly implies that the EBV receptor itself is a product of HLA region genes (Arnaiz-Villena and Festenstein, 1975).

Interrelationship of Different Membrane Marker Binding Sites

The apparent exclusive expression of many different antigens, binding sites and receptors on T cells, B cells and their subsets raises the question of whether all of these structures are independent of each other. We have already mentioned the close relationship and probably physical association of EBV receptors, C3 binding sites and HLA antigens on B cells. In the mouse, SmIg Fc receptors and C3 receptors appear, by blocking and capping experiments, to be physically separate entities. It is interesting to note, however, that capping of the surface immunoglobulin of mouse B lymphocytes leads to concurrent redistribution of all Fc receptors (Forni and Pernis, 1975; Abbas and Unanue, 1975). This suggests that non-cross-linked aggregated membrane IgM (and/or IgD) has an affinity for the Fc receptor and might have important implications for B cell triggering. Fc receptors themselves, like the C3 receptors, may well be products of the major histocompatibility locus; thus anti-I region antisera in the mouse and analogous anti-HLA sera in man (see above) are able to block the Fc receptors (Sachs and Dickler, 1975).

Table 7.8 Functional capacity of human T and B lymphocytes in vitro

In vitro parameter	Response of T and B cells ?
1. Response to polyclonal mitogens	In blood and tonsil the proliferative response to lectins (e.g. Con A, PHA, pokeweed) is largely if not entirely T-cell dependent. In the presence of T cells a variable proportion of B cells may also be activated (particularly with certain preparations of pokeweed). Spleen cells may give a different picture (perhaps a T independent pokeweed response). Human B cells respond very poorly to LPS. They have recently been reported to respond specifically to the protein A component of Staphylococcal bacteria (Forsgren, Svedjelund and Wigzell, 1976) but others[a] find this to be a T-cell mitogen!
2. Mixed lymphocyte response	T cells are the predominant responding cells (i.e. proliferation and cytotoxic activity); B cells and perhaps monocytes the predominant stimulators.
3. MIF production	Both T and B cells are active
4. Mitogenic factor production	T cells only active
5. K-cell activity	No consensus of opinion at present

[a] Grosse-Wilde, H., Leibold, W. and colleagues, personal communication

These observations emphasise that most of the B-cell associated membrane structures are closely interrelated either physically or functionally. It is intriguing to know that the only such structure which is clearly not a product of H-2 (or HLA) genes—the immunoglobulin—nevertheless has amino acid sequence homology with β_2-microglobulin (a component of H-2 and HLA structures) which implies an evolutionary association (or derivation) with this critically important genetic region (Cunningham et al, 1973).

We have far less information on T-lymphocyte structures but it is of interest that most anti-T cell sera block E-rosette formation and at least one T-cell heteroantigen moves together on the cell surface with the sheep red cell receptor (Owen and Fanger, 1975).

Functional Correlates

The availability of multiple membrane markers and physical fractionation techniques permits an attack on the functional competence and repertoire of different cell populations (Chess et al, 1974). However, there is as yet no clear picture or general agreement as to the precise immunological or non-specific potential of T- and B-cell populations and their subsets. In Table 7.8 we have attempted to give a simplified summary of the current status of this important problem. A more detailed and critical appraisal is published elsewhere (Bloom and David, 1976).

THE CURRENT PICTURE OF 'NORMAL' HUMAN BLOOD LYMPHOCYTE POPULATIONS

Figure 7.2 summarises the general picture of human blood lymphocyte populations which has emerged as a result of the studies referred to above. The figure encorporates data on only the four most extensively studied markers and attempts to summarise the relationship of the three major groups of 'lymphoid' cells involved—the T cells, B cells and a third group referred to as unclassified cells. This picture ignores heterogeneity of T and B lymphocytes which will certainly become of more interest as the appropriate marker systems become available.

'Whole blood' tests?

When values of human blood T and B lymphocytes are sought an extrapolation is essential between the results of these tests which give proportions (percentage) to absolute values of cell types, i.e. numbers of T or B cells/mm³. Proportions of T or B cells can be very misleading (for example, if the patient is lymphophenic). Extrapolation from proportional data to absolute counts depends upon the assumption being made that no bias in T–B proportions occurs during the lymphocyte separation procedures. Unfortunately, such bias may occur particularly with pathological samples and will deviate T–B ratios inversely with lymphocyte yield. If yields are greater than 70 per cent (e.g. Ficoll-isopaque) then straight extrapolation to blood counts is possible.

An alternative approach for enumerating human T and B cells is to use membrane markers on unseparated whole blood. This has the advantage that no selective loss of populations can occur. Brown and Greaves (1974b) recently published one such method using immunofluorescent markers. The test was, however, laborious and difficult to read. A modified method developed by Pepys and colleagues (1976) incorporates peroxidase

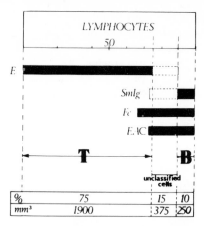

Figure 7.2   Human blood lymphocyte populations

staining of monocytes and using anti-Ig reagents gives excellent discrimination between T cells, B cells and monocytes (Fig. 7.3). The test procedure, however, is still rather time consuming and our ultimate aim is to distinguish between lymphocyte classes in a simple blood smear. Routinely, we still separate lymphocytes by the Ficoll-isopaque method; however, we have found that the centrifugation time can be shortened from 40 to 1 min simply by increasing the *g* force to 14 000 (Rapson and Greaves, unpublished observations).

Physiological Variability

T lymphocytes and B lymphocytes of the various immunoglobulin classes became detectable in tissues between the seventh and fifteenth week of fetal life (Lawton et al, 1972; Stites et al, 1972; Hayward and Ezer, 1974) and their proportion in cord blood is similar to adult blood (Frøland and Natvig, 1972). With increasing age the thymus becomes smaller and the number of blood E-RFC falls in parallel with responsiveness in other tests of cell-mediated immunity. Consequently studies on diseased elderly patients should employ age-matched controls. Little is known about physiological variations in childhood and adolescence. Normal results were found in women in the third trimester of pregnancy (Gergely et al, 1974) but a remarkable inversion in the proportion of blood T and B lymphocytes between the seventh and nineteenth week of pregnancy was reported by Strelkauskas et al (1975), which was not associated with changes in the blood lymphocyte count. They suggested that these alterations might result from a physiological depletion of suppressor T cells occurring as part of the mechanism by which the fetal homograft is tolerated.

Steel and colleagues (1974) reported a transient decrease in T lymphocyte numbers following vigorous exercise. It is likely that T- and B-cell numbers and perhaps ratios will vary in response to stress (i.e. adrenocortical hormone increases) and perhaps show diurnal or other cyclical rhythms.

cell. Antigen, macrophages and T cells all contribute to the inductive environment: current evidence suggests that the defect is in the latter since their number in the blood of affected patients was low (Schiff et al, 1974) and they made less interferon than normal in response to mitogens (Epstein and Ammann, 1974).

Other variable forms of hypogammaglobulinaemia

This is a poorly defined group of disorders ranging from deficiencies of two or more immunoglobulin classes or subclasses to undetectable levels of any class. There is frequently a familial trend and an excess of affected males suggests that there may be X-linked forms of the disorder. Sometimes transmission has been autosomal recessive. Immunopathological disorders which are common in the relatives of patients with juvenile or adult onset hypogammaglobulinaemia may be other forms of expression of the same disease, perhaps dominantly inherited.

The majority of patients with any of these variable forms of hypogammaglobulinaemia have had normal or only moderately reduced numbers of blood B lymphocytes: in about a quarter B cells were undetected. A proportion of the latter may be sporadic cases of congenital X-linked panhypogammaglobulinaemia but for the rest it seems likely that either their B cells have an intrinsic defect or that the inductive environment fails. B lymphocytes from a few patients have synthesised immunoglobulin in their cytoplasm when cultured in vitro but have failed to release it into the medium (Geha et al, 1973): presumably this is an intrinsic defect. Lymphocytes from a few patients have both synthesised and released immunoglobulin following PWM stimulation (Wu et al, 1973), which suggests a failure in the inductive environment. Low numbers of blood T lymphocytes in some and diminished proliferative responses to PHA (Douglas, Kamin and Fudenberg, 1969) in many cases are compatible with T-cell defects such as insufficient helper function or excessive suppression. No phenotypic differences have yet been defined between human helper and suppressor T cells so blood lymphocyte population studies are unhelpful. Synthesis of immunoglobulin by normal blood lymphocytes stimulated with PWM was suppressed when T lymphocytes from some variable hypogammaglobulinaemia patients were added, so there is functional evidence of suppression (Waldmann et al, 1974).

Transient hypogammaglobulinaemia

Infants are born with IgG derived from the mother, the concentration of which falls as it is diluted and catabolised in the succeeding months. The lowest levels are normally reached between four and six months, after which they rise as the infant's own IgG takes over. Some babies who present with frequent or severe infections at around this trough period are found to have very low IgG levels, and provided that these subsequently rise, a retrospective diagnosis of transient hypogammaglobulinaemia can be made. In most cases the affected infants were probably at the lower end of a normal distribution, but in some special mechanisms may operate. These include the possibility of excessive T-cell suppressor activity similar to that which limits antibody responses by some strains of young mice (Mosier and Johnson, 1975). Some others have had approximately half normal numbers of blood B lymphocytes (Moscatelli et al, 1973) though in the few (unpublished) cases we have studied the numbers have been normal.

Primary immunodeficiency affecting predominantly cell-mediated immunity: DiGeorge's syndrome

Infants with the complete form of the disease present in the neonatal period with hypocalcaemic tetany due to hypoparathyroidism and with major cardiovascular abnormalities, often a right-sided aortic arch (DiGeorge, 1968). Some of those who survive these problems have developed candidiasis or other infections suggestive of defective cell-mediated immunity. In many the thymus shadow was absent from chest x-rays, but this is not specific since the thymus involutes during severe illnesses. Failure to detect a thymus during cardiac surgery or necropsy is better evidence to support the diagnosis.

The disorder is extremely rare and in only a few cases have blood lymphocytes been studied. Their number was normal and remarkably almost all had surface immunoglobulin, suggesting that the absolute number of B cells was raised (reviewed by Lischner and Huff, 1975). In several cases the blood lymphocyte response to PHA became positive shortly after grafting the patient with a fetal thymus, even when the latter was enclosed in a millipore diffusion chamber. This effect was interpreted as evidence for the induction of T-cell responsiveness by thymic humoral factors but the location of such precursor cells is uncertain. Presumably they were not in the blood, unless human T-cell precursors have surface immunoglobulin.

Some infants with congenital hypoparathyroidism and great vessel abnormalities who died had, at necropsy, small ectopic thymuses. Their living counterparts may be those infants born with some of the features of DiGeorge's syndrome (which also include micrognathia, cleft palate and small low-set ears) who gradually acquired normal T-lymphocyte dependent responses. Considerable variation in the severity of hypocalcaemia in DiGeorge's syndrome is described: perhaps there are comparable variations in thymus hormone activity. Two infants in this group have had their blood lymphocytes studied (Touraine et al, 1975). Both had low proportions of T cells (measured by cytotoxicity with an anti-T serum) and raised B lymphocytes. One had low levels of thymus hormone activity in serum but near-normal proliferative responses to PHA, Con A and in mixed lymphocyte culture.

An increasing number of patients with defective cell-mediated immunity but normal or only slightly impaired antibody responses are being recognised. There is no adequate classification for this group and, with few exceptions (Rezza et al, 1974), the disorder has not been familial. Some have had low numbers of blood T lymphocytes and a primary defect in thymus function in a few is suggested by improvement in laboratory tests following thymus grafting. One such case (Businco et al, 1975) had low serum concentrations of thymic hormone activity. The presence of increased numbers of null cells which could be induced to make E rosettes or become susceptible to lysis by anti-T cell sera by incubation with thymus extracts or theophylline (Hayward and Graham, 1976) has also been observed and it may become possible to select patients for thymus graft treatment by this test.

Other conditions associated with defective cell-mediated immunity

Immunodeficiency with thrombocytopenia and eczema (Wiskott–Aldrich syndrome) is relatively well defined and the X-linked inheritance is compatible with a single gene defect. In most cases the proliferative response by blood lymphocytes to mitogens has been normal or only slightly low (Oppenheim, Blaese and Waldmann, 1970) but some have had low proportions of blood T lymphocytes. This apparent contradiction may be related in part to the tendency for the immunodeficiency to worsen with time. Up to half of patients have improved following injections of transfer factor (Spitler, Levin and Fudenberg, 1975) and this has coincided with increases in the percentage of blood E-rosette forming cells. Optimal responses to transfer factor have been claimed to occur in patients whose monocytes failed to bind IgG (Spitler et al, 1972) but lack of monocyte receptors for IgG in other patients is inconstant (Douglas and Goldberg, 1972).

Immunological findings in ataxia telangiectasia patients are variable: up to half have had very low serum levels of IgE and about a third are IgA deficient. Their blood B lymphocytes are generally present in normal numbers (Gajl-Peczalska, Lim and Good, 1975) and synthesise IgA in response to PWM stimulation (Wu et al, 1973) even if there is IgA deficiency. Evidence of defective cell-mediated immunity includes negative delayed hypersensitivity skin tests and, in some, reduced responses to PHA. Some patients have had normal numbers of blood E-rosette forming cells even though their PHA response was low (Yata and Goya, 1972); others have been reported as having reduced numbers of such cells.

Severe combined immunodeficiency

This is 'combined' because the effector limbs of both antibody and cell-mediated immunity are severely impaired. Transmission in the original cases was autosomal recessive and affected infants were very lymphopenic: this combination was interpreted as resulting from the failure of a common lymphoid stem cell to develop. The successful treatment of some affected infants with grafts of tissue-matched sibling bone marrow, which contained stem cells, was consistent with this view. However, other infants were described whose clinical course was as severe as the original cases but who were not lymphopenic and in whose families the transmission appeared to be X-linked. There was heterogeneity also in the morbid anatomical findings: many cases had gross hypoplasia of all lymphoid tissue, others had small thymuses with a few Hassal's corpuscles or lymphocytes.

Tests of lymphocyte subpopulations confirm the impression that the severe combined immunodeficiency syndrome includes a range of disorders with a common clinical expression, but they have not yet contributed greatly to classification or treatment. If there were complete failure of stem cell development a corresponding lack of T and B lymphocytes would be expected but this seems relatively uncommon. Seven of the last nine patients we have studied have had blood B lymphocytes in normal numbers per mm^3, in which case their proportion has been very high because there were few if any T cells. Detection of some B cell development is consistent with the presence of IgM in some of the longer surviving of these patients.

In the few cases in which the heavy chain class of B-cell immunoglobulin has been tested, all classes have been found: in two of these the sum of percentages of the individual classes exceeded 100, so some cells carried immunoglobulin of more than one heavy chain class. These may be immature B cells perhaps similar to cells found in fetuses which stain for multiple immunoglobulin classes but it is not known whether such cells resynthesise immunoglobulins of both classes following stripping or capping procedures. None of these infants had the autosomal recessive form of combined immunodeficiency associated with adenosine deaminase deficiency, in which the thymus has a few Hassal's corpuscles. The in vitro responses of one ADA-deficient patient's lymphocytes were improved when exogenous ADA was added to the cultures and following transfusion with a normal donor's erythrocytes, as a source of ADA, the patient's blood lymphocyte count rose and a thymus shadow appeared on x-ray (Polmar et al, 1975), so the ADA deficiency may be primary. If so, this will be the first defined form of combined immunodeficiency.

Rare patients have lacked blood lymphocytes with the surface characteristics of T or B lymphocytes or monocytes although cells with the morphology of lymphocytes were seen in blood films. Some of these cells may be potential T cells as demonstrated by induction of T antigens or E-rosette formation following incubation with thymus extracts.

Secondary immunodeficiency

Although this is very much commoner than primary immunodeficiency the effects on blood lymphocyte populations have been studied less. The commonest cause in the world must be malnutrition which, when severe, causes lymphopenia, lymphocyte depletion from lymph nodes, and involution of the thymus (Smyth et al, 1971; Schopfer and Douglas, 1976). The lymphopenia is probably due mainly to a reduction in numbers of T lymphocytes since it is predominantly T-dependent areas of lymphoid tissues which are depleted and the proportion of blood E-rosette forming cells is low (Ferguson et al, 1974). This is associated with a diminished proliferative response to PHA (Chandra, 1974). These effects are reversible with refeeding.

Malnutrition as a consequence of primary gut disease can cause similar reversible effects and we have seen low numbers of blood E-RFC with depressed PHA response in infants with severe diarrhoea following secondary disaccharidase deficiency or acrodermatitis enteropathica of folate-responsive sprue. However, such effects are not constant since normal lymphocyte responses in infantile intractable diarrhoea are also reported (Spirer et al, 1973). Variable results are also obtained in Crohn's disease as regards lymphocyte count, PHA response by blood lymphocytes and blood lymphocyte populations. In this disease lymphocytes may be lost into the intestine and this would be expected to deplete predominantly long-lived recirculating cells. Another possibility is that granulomas in lymphoid tissue interfere with lymphocyte recirculation, as has been observed in leprosy (Bullock, 1974).

Abnormal lymphatics in intestinal lymphagiecasia leak both protein (albumin and immunoglobulins) and lymphocytes into the intestinal lumen (Strober et al, 1967). Lymphopaenia is usual and in the few cases we have studied the loss affected T cells more than B cells and the PHA response by blood lymphocytes was low.

Sarcoidosis

Patients with sarcoidosis tended to have lower blood lymphocyte counts, lower numbers of blood E-rosette forming cells and raised SmIg positive cells (Ramachandar et al, 1975). There was no correlation with the clinical stage, tuberculin responsiveness or drug treatment. Hedfors (1975) also found reductions in E-RFC in sarcoidosis but no increase in EAC-RFC. However, the latter test may give a falsely low result if either circulating immune complexes or antilymphocyte antibodies are present so they do not necessarily conflict with those of Ramachandar et al (1975).

Hepatitis

Low numbers of E-RFC were observed in patients with acute or chronic hepatitis; however, they returned to normal in patients who recovered from the acute form of the disease (DeHoratius, Strickland and Williams, 1974).

Infections

Niklasson and Williams (1974) found a trend towards lower proportions of E-RFC in blood from a series of adults hospitalised with severe bacterial and viral infections. The fall was of about 10 per cent and was associated with increased SmIg$^+$ small lymphocytes (mostly IgG) and more unidentified, null, cells during the acute phase. In 4 of the 22 patients the rise in SmIg-positive cells was not associated with increases in percentage of EAC-rosette forming cells: perhaps the C3 receptors of the B cells of these four were already saturated with complement-fixing immune complexes. Reduced proportions of active rosettes were found by Wybran and Fudenberg (1973) during viral but not bacterial infections. In lepromatous leprosy both T- and B-cell levels may be depressed (Mendes, Kopersztych and Mota, 1974).

Non-lymphoid Malignancies

Both the effects of the disease and its treatment may contribute to the depressed delayed hypersensitivity skin responses (Israel, 1973) and reduced proliferation induced by PHA (Chretien et al, 1973) which are common in patients with advanced malignancy. Some patients with bronchial carcinoma and other solid malignancies have low numbers of blood E-RFC before treatment is commenced (Anthony et al, 1975; Potvin, Tarpley and Chretien, 1975). These observations have given rise to the somewhat speculative proposal that depressed (general) cell-mediated immunity may render individuals more susceptible to malignant disease. Although malignancy is common in patients with primary immuno-deficiencies, it is usually lymphoreticular in origin, except in ataxia telangiectasia. Cancer of almost all types occurs predominantly in the very young or old and workers in this field should make all efforts to include age-matched controls in their studies. This represents a serious omission in a number of published studies.

OTHER SECONDARY CHANGES IN BLOOD LYMPHOCYTE POPULATIONS

There are a few reports of positive correlations between depressed or absent delayed hypersensitivity skin tests or blood lymphocyte responses to PHA and low numbers of blood E-rosette forming cells in patients with secondary immunodeficiency associated with malignancy (Catalona et al, 1975) and its treatment by radiotherapy (Stjernsward et al, 1972). In patients taking steroids loss of cell-mediated responses is associated with reduction in numbers of blood E-RFC, possibly due to redistribution of cells (Fauci and Dale, 1975) while other drugs such as aspirin reduce PHA responsiveness without in-fluencing the proportions of T or B lymphocytes (Cront, Hepburn and Pitts, 1975). Patients receiving intensive immunosuppression after kidney grafting had reduced num-bers of blood E-RFC and low PHA responses. Before their immunosuppression was started they had normal numbers of blood E-RFC but low PHA response, which was attributed to inhibitory factors in uraemic plasma (Lopez et al, 1975). Low numbers of blood E-RFC with normal PHA response was found later, while on maintenance immunosuppression, and attributed to the inhibitory effect of antilymphocyte globulin on the formation of E rosettes.

Lymphoid Malignancies

In the past few years many laboratories have analysed leukaemic cells and lymphomas with T- and B-cell markers (reviewed by Preud'homme and Seligmann, 1974; Greaves,

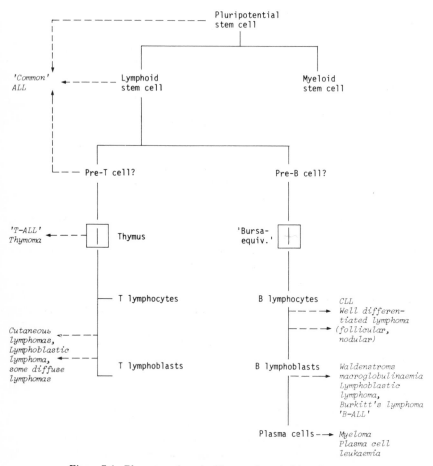

Figure 7.4 Phenotype 'map' of human lymphoid malignancies

1975; Edelson et al, 1975). These studies are aimed at an immunological categorisation of lymphoid neoplasms and they have provided reasonably consistent results as regards comparative cell surface phenotype; these are summarised in Figure 7.4. The exclusively T-cell phenotype of some of the cutaneous lymphomas (e.g. Sezary syndrome) is impressive (Edelson et al, 1975) as is the predominance of B cell features in CLL. Over 90 per cent of the latter studied have had μ and/or δ heavy chains on their CLL cells with either κ or λ light chains, but not both (Preud'homme and Seligmann, 1974). These observations, together with the idiotypic data (Fu, Winchester and Kunkel, 1975b) suggests that CLL, like most other human malignancies, has a monoclonal origin. IgG-positive CLL exists (Preud'homme et al, 1975) but is rare, corresponding approximately with the relatively low frequency of B lymphocytes with endogenously synthesised IgG in blood (see above). Surface phenotyping of CLL can occasionally be complicated by the IgG-binding activity of Fc receptors, or, more rarely, by cells with antibody activity against sheep red cells, making the cells E+ (Brouet and Prieur, 1974).

Table 7.9 Subgrouping of acute lymphoblastic leukaemias based on membrane marker analysis

Group	(%)[a]	E	HuTLA[b]	SmIg	HuBLAA[c]	ALL-A[d]	TTe[e]	MM[f]
'T-like ALL'	15–25	+	+	−	−	−	+	±
'B-like ALL'	1–3	−	−	+	+	−	−	−
'Common' ALL	60–80	−	−[g]	−	+	+	+	−
'Null' ALL	5–10	−	−	−	+ or −	−	+ or −	−

Data from references given below and Greaves, Janossy, Rapson, Hoffbrand and McCaffrey unpublished observations

[a] Proportion of patients (adults and children) diagnosed as ALL
[b] Anti-thymus serum (Brown et al, 1974; Greaves and Janossy, 1976)
[c] Anti-B lymphoid cell line p30 antigen (Schlossmann et al, 1976)
[d] Antisera to common ALL (Brown et al, 1975; Greaves, 1975)
[e] Terminal deoxynucleotidyl transferase enzyme (McCaffrey et al, 1974)
[f] Mediastinal thymic mass
[g] Kersey et al (1975) have reported that a proportion of E-, ALLs (i.e. probably 'common ALL') react with an antisera to human fetal thymus. This might indicate that some common ALL are derived from an immature T cell or T-cell precursor. However, the published data on this particular anti-HuTLA serum are insufficient to evaluate its specificity

Some CLL patients have a monoclonal protein in their serum which shares immunoglobulin heavy and light chain class and idiotype with the SmIg of the CLL cells. The association is commoner in another B-cell proliferative disorder, Waldenstrom's macroglobulinaemia, and it indicates that at least some of the cells derived from the abnormal clone were capable of differentiation into immunoglobulin-secreting cells. The lack of terminal differentiation in most cases of CLL may permit the cells to escape from normal feedback control.

Acute lymphoblastic leukaemia in both children and adults appear to consist of at least three distinct categories which morphologically are very similar but distinguishable by immunological (the membrane markers), histochemical and enzymatic criteria (Table 7.9). There is considerably less agreement on the divisions of lymphomas. It would appear, however, that the majority of the differentiated, follicular (or nodular) lymphomas are B lymphocyte-like counterparts of CLL (Salmon and Seligmann, 1974; Lukes and Collins, 1975). Some diffuse lymphomas and lymphoblastic lymphomas are T cell-like (Jaffe et al, 1975; Kaplan, Mastrangelo and Peterson, 1974). A proportion of poorly differentiated lymphomas and reticulum cell sarcomas may lack E-rosetting capacity and SmIg but may have C3 or Fc receptors.

Two key questions follow from this immunological phenotyping. Firstly, does a T-cell phenotype of a leukaemia or lymphoma necessarily mean that the 'target' cell in the disease is T lymphocyte? Whilst this could well be so it is probably impossible to prove and the alternative interpretation should always be borne in mind; namely that the disease process is initiated in a less-differentiated cell which retains at least a partial capacity to differentiate. Philadelphia chromosome-positive chronic myeloid leukaemia provides the obvious precedent—a stem cell defect reflected in excessive (monoclonal) production of granulocytes.

Secondly, does categorisation of lymphoid neoplasia based on membrane marker phenotypes have any practical value, which in effect means does typing of patient's cells in this way have prognostic significance? This remains to be seen. There are, however, indications that the T cell-like ALL group may have a worse prognosis than the common ALL group (Borella and Sen, 1973; Catovsky et al, 1974). It should be emphasised that T- and B-membrane markers may prove extremely useful in initial diagnosis in high count leukaemias or in lymphomas. They are, however, limited in so far as they, by definition, do not distinguish normal from malignant cells and therefore cannot be used to phenotype leukaemias in patients with few abnormal cells, or to assess patient response to therapy. Leukaemic-specific membrane markers may have much more value in this respect since the number of leukaemia cells can be accurately monitored during and after therapy (Greaves, 1975). Idiotypic immunoglobulin determinants on monoclonal B-cell malignancies are particularly interesting in this respect. Since these are effectively tumour-specific antigens they could be used to accurately monitor the numbers of malignant cells. Anti-idiotype antibody could also provide an extremely powerful specific therapeutic reagent (Stevenson and Stevenson, 1975).

CONCLUDING REMARKS

For many decades such simple clinical tests as the Schick and tuberculin tests have provided information on the integrity of the complex mechanisms which are involved in antibody and cell-mediated immunity. More recently it has become possible to distinguish directly between the lymphocyte populations which contribute to these responses but the tests involved are still crude compared with, for example, the sophistication with which antigen–antibody reactions can be described. Such lack of refinement makes the examination of cells difficult to standardise and so difficult to control: laboratories considering providing blood lymphocyte population analysis as a clinical service might bear in mind that this is expensive and sometimes difficult to interpret.

For the future, it is likely that blood lymphocyte population tests will contribute more to the diagnosis of severe immunodeficiency when we can distinguish between T (and perhaps B) cell subsets and quantitate suppressor cells in a well-defined in vitro system. There are therapeutic possibilities, too, if blood could be selectively enriched or depleted of defined populations. At a much more sophisticated level, our understanding of the different susceptibility of individuals to common diseases would be enormously enhanced if we could measure the clonal diversity of their lymphocytes.

Lymphocyte studies have depended heavily on the monoclonal lymphoproliferative disorders for evidence of specificity and it is in these disorders that knowledge of membrane properties (e.g. idiotypic antigens) might be used for a direct attack on the abnormal population.

REFERENCES

Abbas, A. K. & Unanue, E. R. (1975) Interrelationships of surface immunoglobulin and Fc receptors on mouse B lymphocytes. *Journal of Immunology*, **115**, 1665.
Anthony, H. M., Kirk, J. A., Madsen, K. E., Mason, M. K. & Templeman, G. H. (1975) E and EAC rosetting lymphocytes in patients with carcinoma of the bronchus. *Clinical and Experimental Immunology*, **20**, 41.
Arnaiz-Villena, A. & Festenstein, H. (1975) 4a (W4) and 4b (W6) human histocompatibility antigens are specifically associated with complement receptors. *Nature (London)*, **258**, 732.
Balch, C. M., Dagg, M. K., Lawton, A. R. & Cooper, M. D. (1975) *Federation Proceedings*, **34**, 994.
Barr, R. D. & Perry, S. (1976) Lysosomal acid hydrolases in human lymphocyte subpopulations. *British Journal of Haematology*, **32**, 565.
Beverley, P. B. (1976) Lymphocyte heterogeneity. In *T and B Lymphocytes in Immune Recognition*, ed. Loor F. and Roelants, G. E., New York: Wiley (in press).
Bianco, C., Patrick, R. & Nussenzweig, V. (1970) A population of lymphocytes bearing a membrane receptor for antigen–antibody complement complexes. *Journal of Experimental Medicine*, **132**, 702.
Bloom B, & David, J. (1976) *In Vitro Methods in Cell-mediated and Tumor Immunity*. New York: Academic Press (in press).
Borella, L. & Sen L. (1973) T cell surface markers on lymphoblasts from acute lymphocytic leukaemia. *Journal of Immunology*, **111**, 1275.
Brouet, J.-C., Preud'homme, J.-L. & Seligmann, M. (1975) The use of B and T membrane markers in the classification of human leukaemias, with special reference to acute lymphoblastic leukaemia. In *Blood Cells*, Vol. 1. Springer-Verlag.
Brouet, J.-C. & Prieur, A. M. (1974) Membrane markers on chronic lymphocytic leukaemia cells: A B cell leukaemia with rosettes due to antisheep erythrocyte antibody activity of the membrane bound IgM and a T cell leukaemia with surface Ig. *Clinical Immunology and Immunopathology*, **2**, 481.
Brown, G. & Greaves, M. F. (1974a) Cell surface markers for human T and B lymphocytes. *European Journal of Immunology*, **4**, 302.
Brown, G. & Greaves, M. F. (1974b) Enumeration of absolute numbers of T and B lymphocytes in human blood. *Scandinavian Journal of Immunology*, **3**, 161.
Bullock, W. E. (1974) Specificity of immunodeficiency in leprosy and other infections. In *Progress in Immunology, II*, **5**, 193.
Businco, L., Rezza, E., Giunchi, G. & Aiuti, F. (1975) Thymus transplantation. *Clinical and Experimental Immunology*, **21**, 32.
Catalona, W. J., Tarpley, J. L., Potvin, C. & Chretien, P. B. (1975) Correlations among cutaneous reactivity to BNCB, PHA induced lymphocyte blastogenesis and peripheral blood E rosettes. *Clinical and Experimental Immunology*, **19**, 327.
Catovsky, D., Goldman, J. M., Okos, A., Frisch, B. & Galton, D. A. G. (1974) T lymphoblastic leukaemia: a distinct variant of acute leukaemia. *British Medical Journal*, **2**, 643.
Chandra, R. K. (1974) Rosette forming T lymphocytes and cell mediated immunity in malnutrition. *British Medical Journal*, **iii**, 608.
Chess, L., MacDermott, R. P., Sondel, P. M. & Schlossman, S. F. (1974) Cells involved in human cellular hypersensitivity. In *Progress in Immunology II*, ed. Brent, L. & Holborow, J., Vol. 3, p. 125. Amsterdam: North Holland.
Chiao, J. W., Pantic, V. S. & Good, R. A. (1974) Human peripheral lymphocytes bearing both B-cell complement receptors and T cell characteristics for sheep erythrocytes detected by a mixed rosette method. *Clinical and Experimental Immunology*, **18**, 483.
Chretien, P. B., Crowder, W. L., Gertner, H. R., Sample, F. & Catalona, W. J. (1973) Correlation of pre-operative lymphocyte reactivity with the clinical course of cancer patients. *Surgery, Gynecology and Obstetrics*, **136**, 380.
Claman, H. N., Chaperon, E. A. & Triplett, R. F. (1966) Immunocompetence of transferred thymus-marrow cell combinations. *Journal of Immunology*, **97**, 828.
Cooper, M. D., Keightley, R. G. & Lawton, A. R. (1975) Defective T and B cells in primary immunodeficiencies. In *Membrane Receptors of Lymphocytes*, ed. Seligmann, M., Preud'homme, J. & Kourilsky, F. M. Amsterdam: North Holland.
Cooper, M. D. & Seligmann, M. (1976) B and T lymphocytes in immunodeficiency and of lymphoproliferate disease. In *B and T Cell Immune Recognition*, eds. Loor, F. & Roelants, G. E. Chichester: Wiley & Sons.
Cront, J. E., Hepburn, B. & Pitts, R. E. (1975) *New England Journal of Medicine*, **292**, 221.

Cunningham, B. A., Wang, J. L., Berggård, I. & Peterson, P. A. (1973) The complete amino acid sequence of β_2 microglobulin. *Biochemistry*, **12**, 4811.

Davies, A. J. S., Leuchars, E., Wallis, V., Marchant, R. & Elliot, E. V. (1967) The failure of thymus-derived cells to produce antibody. *Transplantation*, **5**, 222.

DeHoratius, R. J., Strickland, R. G. & Williams, R. C. (1974) T and B lymphocytes in acute and chronic hepatitis. *Clinical Immunology and Immunopathology*, **2**, 353.

Dickler, H. B. & Kunkel, H. G. (1972) Interaction of aggregated gamma-globulin with B lymphocytes. *Journal of Experimental Medicine*, **136**, 191.

DiGeorge, A. M. (1968) Congenital absence of the thymus and its immunologic consequences: concurrence with congenital hypoparathyroidism. In *Immunologic Deficiency Disease of Man*, ed. Bergsma, P. National Foundation.

Douglas, S. D. & Goldberg, L. S. (1972) Monocyte receptors for immunoglobulin and complement in immunologic deficiency disease. *Vox Sanguinis*, **23**, 214.

Douglas, S. D., Kamin, R. M. & Fudenberg, H. H. (1969) Human lymphocyte response to phytomitogens in vitro: normal, agammaglobulinaemic and paraproteinemic individuals. *Journal of Immunology*, **103**, 1185.

Dukor, P., Dietrich, F. M., Gisler, R. H., Schumann, G. & Bitter-Suermann, D. (1974) Possible targets of complement action in B cell triggering. In *Progress in Immunology, II*, ed. Brent, L. & Holborow, J., Vol. 3, p. 99. Amsterdam: North Holland.

Durandy, A., Wioland, M., Sabolobic, D. & Griscelli, C. (1975) Electrophoretic characteristics and membrane receptors of lymphocytes in primary immunodeficiency diseases. *Clinical Immunology and Immunopathology*, **4**, 440.

Dutton, R. W. & Mishell, R. I. (1967) Cell populations and cell proliferation in the in vitro response of normal mouse spleen to heterologous erythrocytes. *Journal of Experimental Medicine*, **126**, 443.

Edelson, R. I., Kirkpatrick, C. H., Shevach, E. M., Schein, P. S., Smith, R. N., Green, I. & Latzner, M. (1975) Preferential cutaneous infiltration of neoplastic thymus derived lymphocytes. *Annals of Internal Medicine*, **80**, 685.

Eisen, S. A., Wedner, H. J. & Parker, C. W. (1972) Isolation of pure human peripheral blood T-lymphocytes using nylon wool columns. *Immunology Communications*, **1**, 571.

Epstein, L. B. & Ammann, A. J. (1974) Evaluation of T lymphocyte effector function in immunodeficiency diseases: abnormality in mitogen-stimulated infection in patients with selective IgA deficiency. *Journal of Immunology*, **112**, 617.

Ezer, G. & Hayward, A. R. (1974) Inhibition of complement dependent lymphocyte rosette formation: a possible test for activated complement products. *European Journal of Immunology*, **4**, 148.

Fauci, A. S. & Dale, D. C. (1975) Alternate day prednisone therapy and human lymphocyte populations by surface markers. *Transplantation Reviews*, **16**, 114.

Feldman, M. & Pepys, M. B. (1974) Role of C3 on in vitro lymphocyte co-operation. *Nature (London)*, **249**, 159.

Ferguson, A. C., Lawlor, G. L., Neumann, C. G. et al (1974) Decresed rosette forming lymphocytes in malnutrition and intrauterine growth retardation. *Journal of Pediatrics*, **85**, 717.

Forni, L. & Pernis, B. (1975) Interactions between Fc receptors and membrane immunoglobulins. In *Membrane Receptors of Lymphocytes*, ed. Seligmann, M., Preud'homme, J.-L., & Kourilsky, F. M., p. 193. Amsterdam: North Holland.

Forsgren, A., Svedjelund, A & Wigzell, H (1976) Lymphocyte stimulation by protein A of *Staphylococcus aureus*. *European Journal of Immunology*, **6**, 207.

Frøland, S. S. & Natvig, J. B. (1973) Identification of three different human lymphocyte populations by surface markers. *Transplantation Reviews*, **16**, 114.

Frøland, S. S. & Natvig, J. G. (1972) Receptor Ig in the newborn. *Scandinavian Journal of Immunology*, **1**, 286.

Fu, S. M., Winchester, R. J. & Kunkel, H. G. (1975a) The occurrence of the HL-B alloantigens on the cells of unclassified acute lymphoblastic leukaemias. *Journal of Experimental Medicine*, **142**, 1334.

Fu, S. M., Winchester, R. J. & Kunkel, H. G. (1975b) Similar idiotypic specificity for the membrane IgD and IgM and human B lymphocytes. *Journal of Immunology*, **114**, 250.

Gajl-Peczalska, K., Lim, S. D. & Good, R. A. (1975) B lymphocytes in primary and secondary deficiencies of humoral immunity. In *Immunodeficiency in Man and Animals*, ed. Bergsma, D. et al. New York: Sinauer Association.

Geha, R., Rosen, R. S. & Merler, E. (1973) Identification and characterisation of subpopulations of lymphocytes in human peripheral blood after fractionation on discontinuous gradients of albumin. The cellular defect in linked agammaglobulinaemia. *Journal of Clinical Investigation*, **52**, 1726.

Gergely, P., Dzvonyar, J., Szegedi, G. et al (1974) T and B lymphocytes in pregnancy. *Klinische Wochenschrift*, **52**, 601.

Glick, B., Chang, T. S. & Jaap, R. G. (1956) The bursa of Fabricius and antibody production. *Poultry Science*, **35**, 224.

Goldblum, R. M., Lord, R. A., Cooper, M. D., Gathings, W. E. & Goldman, A. E. (1974) X-linked B lymphocyte deficiency. *Journal of Pediatrics*, **85**, 188.

Greaves, M. F. (1975) Clinical applications of cell surface markers. *Progress in Haematology*, **9**, 255.

Greaves, M. F. (1976) Virus receptors on lymphocytes. *Scandinavian Journal of Immunology*. Suppl. 5, 113.

Greaves, M. F. & Brown, G. (1973) A human B lymphocyte specific antigen. *Nature (London)*, **246**, 116.

Greaves, M. F. & Brown, G. (1974) Separation of human T and B lymphocytes. *Journal of Immunology*, **112**, 420.

Greaves, M. F., Brown, G. & Rickinson, A. (1975a) Epstein–Barr virus binding sites on lymphocyte subpopulations. *Clinical Immunology and Immunopathology*, **3**, 514.

Greaves, M. F., Falk, J. & Falk, R. (1975b) A surface antigen marker for human monocytes. *Scandinavian Journal of Immunology*, **4**, 80.

Greaves, M. F. & Janossy, G. (1976) Antisera to human T lymphocytes. In *In Vitro Methods in Cell-mediated and Tumor Immunity*, ed. Bloom, B. & David, J. New York: Academic Press.

Greaves, M. F., Raff, M. C. & Owen, J. J. T. (1973) *T and B Lymphocytes; their Origins, Properties and Roles in Immune Responses*. Amsterdam: Excepta Medica.

Hämmerling, G. J., Deak, B. D., Mauve, G., Hämmerling, U. & McDevitt, H. O. (1974) 'B' lymphocyte alloantigens controlled by the I region of the major histocompatibility complex in mice. *Immunogenetics*, **1**, 68.

Hayward, A. R. & Ezer, G. (1974) Development of lymphocyte populations in the human fetal thymus and spleen. *Clinical and Experimental Immunology*, **17**, 169.

Hayward, A. R. & Graham, L. (1976) Increased E rosette formation by fetal liver and spleen cells incubated with theophylline. *Clinical and Experimental Immunology*, **23**, 279.

Hayward, A. R. & Greaves, M. F. (1975a) Identification of cells with monocyte markers in panhypogammaglobulinaemia. *Scandinavian Journal of Immunology*, **4**, 75.

Hayward, A. R. & Greaves, M. F. (1975b) Central failure of B lymphocyte induction in panhypogammaglobulinaemia. *Clinical Immunology and Immunopathology*, **3**, 461.

Hedfors, E. (1975) Immunological aspects of sarcoidosis. *Scandinavian Journal of Respiratory Disease*, **56**, 1.

Ishii, Y., Koshiba, H., Keno, H., Maeyama, I., Takani, T., Ishibashi, F. & Kikuchi, K. (1975) *Journal of Immunology*, **11+**, 466.

Israel, L. (1973) Cell mediated immunity in lung cancer patients: data, problems and propositions. *Cancer Chemotherapy Reports Part 3*, **4**, 279.

Jaffe, E. S., Shevach, E. M., Sussman, E. H., Frank, M., Green, I. & Berard, C. W. (1975) Membrane receptor sites for the identification of lymphoreticular cells in benign and malignant conditions. *British Journal of Cancer* Suppl. 11, **31**, 107.

Jondal, M. & Klein, G. (1973) Surface markers on human B and T lymphocytes. II. Presence of Epstein–Barr virus receptors on B lymphocytes. *Journal of Experimental Medicine*, **138**, 1365.

Jondal, M., Klein, G., Oldstone, M. B. A., Bokish, V. & Yefenof, E. (1976) Surface markers of human B and T lymphocytes. VIII. The association between complement (C) and Epstein–Barr virus (EBV) receptors on human lymphoid cells. *Scandinavian Journal of Immunology* (in press).

Jondal, M., Wigzell, H. & Aiuti, F. (1973) Human lymphocyte subpopulations: classification according to surface markers and/or functional characteristics. *Transplantation Reviews*, **16**, 163.

Kaplan, J., Mastrangelo, R. & Peterson, W. D. (1974) Childhood lymphoblastic lymphoma, a cancer of thymus-derived lymphocytes. *Cancer Research*, **34**, 521.

Kersey, J., Nesbit, M., Hallgren, H., Sabad, A., Yunis, E. & Gajl-Peczalska, K. (1975) Evidence for origin of certain childhood acute lymphoblastic leukaemias and lymphomas in thymus-derived lymphocytes. *Cancer*, **36**, 1348.

Kreth, H. W. & Herzenberg, L. A. (1974) Fluorescence activated cell sorting of human T and B lymphocytes. I. Direct evidence that lymphocytes with a high density of membrane-bound immunoglobulin are precursors of plasmacytes. *Cell Immunology*, **12**, 396.

Kumagai, K., Abo, T., Sekizawa, T. & Sasaki, M. (1975) Studies of surface immunoglobulins on human B lymphocytes. 1. Dissociation of cell bound immunoglobulin with acid pH or at 36°. *Journal of Immunology*, **115**, 982.

Lawton, A. R., Self, K. S., Royal, S. A. & Cooper, M. D. (1972) Ontogeny of B lymphocytes in the human fetus. *Clinical Immunology and Immunopathology*, **1**, 104.

Lischner, H. W. & Huff, D. S. (1975) In *Immunodeficiency in Man and Animals. Birth Defects Original Article Series*, Vol. XI.

Litwin, S. D., Ochs, H. & Pollara, B. (1973) Surface immunoglobulins on blood lymphocytes of normal and immunodeficient persons studied by the mixed antiglobulin method. *Immunology*, **25**, 573.

Lopez, C., Simmons, R. L., Touraine, J. L., Park, B. H., Kiszkiss, D. F., Najarian, J. S. & Good, R. A. (1975) Discrepancy between PHA responsiveness and quantitative estimates of T cell numbers in human peripheral blood during chronic renal failure and immunosuppression after transplantation. *Clinical Immunology and Immunopathology*, **4**, 135.

Lukes, R. J. & Collins, R. D. (1975) New approaches to the classification of the lymphomata. *British Journal of Cancer*, Suppl. 11, **31**, 1.

McKenzie, I. F. & Snell, E. D. (1975) Ly-4.2: a cell membrane alloantigen of murine B lymphocytes. 1. Population studies. *Journal of Immunology*, **114**, 848.

Medawar, P. B. & Simpaon, E. (1975) *Nature (London)*, **258**, 106.

Mendes, N. F., Kopersztych, S. & Mota, N. G. S. (1974) T and B lymphocytes in patients with lepromatous leprosy. *Clinical and Experimental Immunology*, **16**, 23.

Miller, J. F. A. P. (1964) The effect of thymic ablation and replacement. In *The Thymus in Immunobiology*, ed. Good, R. A. & Gabrielson, A. E. New York: Harper and Row.

Miller, J. F. A. P. & Mitchell, G. F. (1968) Cell to cell interaction in the immune response, *Journal of Experimental Medicine*, **128**, 801.

Möller, G. (ed.) (1973) T and B lymphocytes in humans. *Transplantation Reviews*, **16**.

Möller, G. (ed.) (1975) Separation of T and B lymphocyte subpopulations. *Transplantation Reviews*, **25**.

Moretta, L., Ferrarini, M., Durante, M. L. & Mingari, M. C. (1975) Expression of a receptor for IgM by human T cells in vitro. *European Journal of Immunology*, **5**, 565.

Moscatelli, P., Bricarelli, F. D. & De Barbieri, A. (1973) Immunoglobulins on the surface of lymphocytes, their distribution in cord blood, newborns and infants affected with transient hypogammaglobulinaemia. *Helvetica paediatrica acta*, **28**, 553.

Mosier, D. E. & Johnson, B. M. (1975) Ontogeny of moise lymphocyte function. II. Development of the ability to produce antibody is modulated by T lymphocytes. *Journal of Experimental Medicine*, **141**, 216.

Müller-Hermelink, H. K. (1974) Characterisation of the B-cell and T-cell regions of human lymphatic tissue through enzyme histochemical demonstration of ATPase and S'-nucleotidase activities. *Virchows Archives, B, Cell Pathology*, **16**, 371.

Niklasson, P. M. & Williams, R. C. (1974) Studies of peripheral blood T and B lymphocytes in acute infections. *Information on Immunology*, **9**, 1.

Oppenheim, J. J., Blaese, R. M. & Waldmann, T. A. (1970) Defective lymphocyte transformation and delayed hypersensitivity in Wiskott Aldrich syndrome. *Journal of Immunology*, **104**, 835.

Owen, F. L. & Fanger, M. W. (1975) Studies on the human T lymphocyte population. III. Synthesis and release of lymphocyte receptor for sheep red blood cells by stimulated human T lymphoblasts. *Journal of Immunology*, **115**, 765.

Pepys, M., Sategna-Guidetti, C., Mirjah, D. D., Wansbrough-Jones, T. & Dash, A. C. (1976) Enumeration of immunoglobulin-bearing lymphocytes in whole peripheral blood. *Clincal and Experimental Immunology* (in press).

Piessens, W. F., Schur, P. H., Moloney, W C. & Churchill, W. H. (1973) Lymphocyte surface immunoglobulin. Distribution and frequency in lymphoproliferative diseases. *New England Journal of Medicine*, **288**, 176.

Plum, J. & Ringoir, S. (1975) A characterisation of human B and T lymphocytes by their lactate dehydrogenase isoenzyme pattern. *European Journal of Immunology*, **5**, 871.

Polliack, A. & de Harven, E. (1975) Surface features of normal and leukaemic lymphocytes as seen by scanning electron microscopy. *Clinical Immunology and Immunopathology*, **3**, 307.

Polmar, S. H., Wetzler, E., Stern, R. C. & Hirschorn, R. (1975) Restoration of in vitro lymphocyte responses with exogenous adenosine deaminase in a patient with severe combined immunodeficiency. *Lancet*, **ii**, 743.

Potvin, C., Tarpley, J. L. & Chretien, B. (1975) Thymus-derived lymphocytes in patients with solid malignancies. *Clinical Immunology and Immunopathology*, **3**, 476.

Preud'homme, J.-L., Brouet, J. C. & Seligmann, M. (1975) Lymphocyte membrane markers in human lymphoproliferative diseases. In *Membrane Receptors of Lymphocytes*, ed. Seligmann, M., Preud'homme, J.-L. & Kourilsky, F. M. Amsterdam: North Holland.

Preud'homme, J.-L. & Labaume, S. (1975) Immunofluorescent staining of human lymphocytes for the detection of surface immunoglobulins. *Annals of the New York Academy of Sciences*, **254**, 254.

Preud'homme, J.-L. & Seligmann, M. (1974) Surface immunoglobulins on human lymphoid cells. In *Progress in Clinical Immunology*, ed. Schwartz, R. S. Vol. 2, p. 121. New York: Grune and Stratton, Inc.

Raff, M. C. (1970) Two distinct populations of peripheral lymphocytes in mice distinguishable by immunofluorescence. *Immunology*, **19,** 637.

Raff, M. C. & Wortis, H. H. (1970) Thymus dependence of θ-bearing cells in the peripheral lymphoid tissues of mice. *Immunology*, **18,** 931.

Raff, M. C. (1971) Surface antigenic markers for distinguishing T and B lymphocytes in mice. *Transplantation Reviews*, **6,** 52.

Ramachandar, K., Douglas, S. D., Siltzbach, L. E. & Taub, R. N. (1975) Peripheral blood lymphocyte subpopulations in sarcoidosis. *Cell Immunology*, **16,** 422.

Reif, A. E. & Allen, J. M. V. (1964) The AKR thymic antigen and its distribution in leukaemias and nervous tissue. *Journal of Experimantal Medicine*, **120,** 413.

Rezza, E., Aiuti, F., Businco, L. & Castello, M. A. (1974) Familial lymphopenia with T lymphocytes defect. *Journal of Pediatrics*, **84,** 178.

Roitt, I. M., Greaves, M. F., Torrigiani, G., Brostoff, J. & Playfair, J. H. L. (1969) The cellular basis of immunological responses. *Lancet*, **ii,** 367.

Ross, G. D. & Polley, M. J. (1975) Specificity of human lymphocyte complement receptors. *Journal of Experimental Medicine*, **141,** 1163.

Ross, G. D., Rabellino, E. M., Polley, M. J. & Grey, H. M. (1973a) Combined studies of complement receptor and surface immunoglobulin bearing cells and sheep erythrocyte rosette forming cells in normal and leukemic human lymphocytes. *Journal of Clinical Investigation*, **52,** 377.

Ross, G. D., Polley, M. J., Rabellino, E. M. & Grey, H. M. (1973b) Two different complement receptors on B lymphocytes. One specific for C3b and one specific for C3b inactivator cleaved C3b. *Journal of Experimental Medicine*, **138,** 798.

Rowe, D. S., Hug, K., Forni, L. & Pernis, B. (1973) Immunoglobulin D as a lymphocyte receptor. *Journal of Experimental Medicine*, **138,** 965.

Sachs, D. & Dickler, H. (1975) The possible role of I region determined cell surface molecules in the regulation of immune responses. *Transplantation Reviews*, **22.**

Salmon, S. E. & Seligmann, M. (1974) B cell neoplasia in man. *Lancet*, **ii,** 1230.

Schiff, R. I., Buckley, R. B., Gilbertsen, R. B. & Metzgar, R. S. (1974) Membrane receptors and in vitro responsiveness of lymphocytes in human immunodeficiency. *Journal of Immunology*, **112,** 376.

Schopfer, K. & Douglas, S. D. (1976) In vitro studies of lymphocytes from children with Kwashiorkor. *Clinical Immunology and Immunopathology*, **5,** 21.

Schlossman, S. F., Chess, L., Humphreys, R. E. & Strominger, J. L. (1976) Distribution of Ia-like molecules on the surface of normal and leukaemic human cells. *Proceedings of the National Academy of Sciences* **73,** 1288.

Sidman, C. L. & Unanue, E. R. (1975) Development of B lymphocytes. I. Cell populations and a critical event during ontogeny. *Journal of Immunology*, **114,** 1730.

Siegal, F. P., Pernis, B. & Kunkel, H. G. (1971) Lymphoctytes in human immunodeficiency states: a study of membrane-associated immunoglobulins. *European Journal of Immunology*, **1,** 482.

Smith, M. D., Barratt, R. M., Hayward, A. R. & Soothill, J. F. (1975) The inhibition of complement dependent lymphocyte rosette formation by the sera of children with steroid sensitive nephrotic syndrome and other renal diseases. *Clinical and Experimental Immunology*, **21,** 236.

Smyth, P. M., Brerton-Stiles, G. G., Grace, H. J., Mafoyane, A., Schonland, M., Coovadia, H. M., Loening, W. E. K., Parent, M. A. & Vos, G. H. (1971) Thymolymphatic deficiency and depression of cell-mediated immunity in protein-calorie malnutrition. *Lancet*, **ii,** 939

Snell, G. D., Cherry, M., McKenzie, I. F. C. & Bailey, D. W. (1973) Ly-4, a new locus determining a lymphocyte surface alloantigen in mice. *Proceedings of the National Academy of Sciences*, **70,** 1108.

Spirer, Z., Tamir, I., Bogair, N. & Werbin, B. Z. (1973) Immunological functions in the intractible diarrhea syndrome of infancy. *Helvetica Pediatrica acta*, **28,** 301.

Spitler, L. E., Levin, A. S. & Fudenberg, H. H. (1975) Transfer factor II. Results of therapy. In *Immunodeficiency in Man and Animals*, ed Bergsma, D. et al. Sinauer Association, Sunderland, Mass, USA.

Spitler, L. E., Levin, A. S., Stites, D. P., Fudenberg, H. H., Pirofsky, B., August, C. S., Stiehm, E. R., Hitzig, W. H. & Gatti, R. A. (1972) The Wiskott Aldrich syndrome. *Journal of Clinical Investigation*, **51,** 3216.

Steel, C. M., Evans, J. & Smith, M. A. (1974) Physiological variation in circulating B cell: T cell ratio in Man. *Nature (London)*, **2, 7,** 387.

Stevenson, G. T. & Stevenson, F. K. (1975) Antibody to a molecularly-defined antigen confined to a tumour cell surface. *Nature*, **254,** 714.

Stites, D. P., Wybran, J., Carr, M. C. & Fudenberg, H. H. (1972) Development of cellular immune competence in man. In *Ontogeny of Acquired Immunity*. Ciba Foundation Symposium.

Stjernsward, J., Jondal, M., Vanky, F., Wigzell, H. & Sealy, R. (1972) Lymphopenia and change in distribution of human B and T lymphocytes in peripheral blood induced by irradiation for mammary carcinoma. *Lancet*, **i**, 1352.

Strelkauskas, A. J., Wilson, B. S., Dray, S. & Dodson, M. (1975) Inversion of levels of human T and B cells in early pregnancy. *Nature (London)*, **258**, 332.

Strober, W., Wochner, R. D., Carbone, P. P. & Waldmann, T. A. (1967) Intestinal lymphangiectasia: a protein losing enteropathy with hypogammaglobulinaemia, lymphocytopenia and impaired homograft rejection. *Journal of Clinical Investigation*, **46**, 1643.

Ting, A., Mickey, M. R. & Terasaki, P. I. (1976) B-lymphocyte alloantigens in Caucasians. *Journal of Experimental Medicine*, **143**, 981.

Touraine, J. L., Touraine, F., Dutruge, J., Gilly, J., Colon, S. & Gilly, R (1975) Immunodeficiency diseases. I. *Clinical and Experimental Immunology*, **21**, 39.

Van Boxel, J. A., Paul, W. E., Terry, W. D. & Green, I. (1972) IgD-bearing human lymphocytes. *Journal of Immunology*, **109**, 648.

Vitetta, E. S., Melcher, U., McWilliams, M., Lamm, M. E., Phillips, Q. & Uhr, J. W. (1975) Cell surface immunoglobulin XI. The appearance of an IgD-like molecule on murine lymphoid cells during ontogeny. *Journal of Experimental Medicine*, **141**, 206.

Vogler, L. B., Pearl, E. R., Gathings, W. E., Lawton, A. R. & Cooper, M. D. (1976) B-lymphocyte precursors in bone marrow in immunoglobulin deficiency diseases. *Lancet*, **ii**, 376.

Vossen, J. M. (1975) Membrane-associated immunoglobulin determinants on bone marrow and blood lymphocytes in the pediatric age group and on fetal tissues. *Annals of the New York Academy of Sciences*, **254**, 70.

Waldmann, T. A., Durm, U., Broder, S., Blackman, M., Blaese, R. M. & Strober, W. (1974) Role of suppressor T cells in pathogenesis of common variable hypogammaglobulinaemia. *Lancet*, **ii**, 609.

Warner, N. L. & Szenberg, A. (1964) Immunologic studies on hormonally bursectomized and surgically thymectomized chickens: dissociation of immunologic responsiveness. In *The Thymus in Immunobiology*, ed. Good, R. A. & Gabrielson, A. E. New York: Harper and Row.

WHO/IARC (1974) Identification, enumeration and isolation of B and T lymphocytes from human peripheral blood. *Scandinavian Journal of Immunology*, **3**, 521.

Winchester, R. J., Fu, S. M., Hoffman, T. & Kunkel, H. G. (1975a) IgG on lymphocyte surfaces; technical problems and the significance of a third cell population. *Journal of Immunology*, **114**, 1210.

Winchester, R. J., Fu, S. M., Wernet, P., Kunkel, H. G., Dupont, B. & Jersild, C. (1975b) Recognition by pregnancy serums of non-HLA alloantigens selectively expressed on B lymphocytes. *Journal of Experimental Medicine*, **141**, 924.

Wu, L. Y. F., Lawton, A. R. & Cooper, M. D. (1973) Differentiation capacity of cultured B lymphocytes from immunodeficient patients. *Journal of Clinical Investigation*, **52**, 3180.

Wybran, J. & Fudenberg, H. H. (1973) Thymus derived rosette forming cells in various human disease states: cancer, lymphoma, bacterial and viral infections. *Journal of Clinical Investigation*, **52**, 1026.

Yata, J. & Goya, N. (1972) Rosette formation with sheep erythrocytes. *Lancet*, **i**, 42.

Yoshida, T. O. & Andersson, B. (1972) Evidence for a receptor recognizing antigen complexed immunoglobulin on the surface of activated mouse thymus lymphocytes. *Scandinavian Journal of Immunology*, **1**, 401.

Yu, D. T. Y. (1975a) Human lymphocyte subpopulations: early and late rosettes. *Journal of Immunology*, **115**, 91.

Yu, D. T. U. (1975) Lymphocyte subpopulations. Human red blood cell rosette. *Clinical and Experimental Immunology*, **20**, 311.

Yu, D. T. Y., Peter, J. B., Paulus, H. E. & Nies, K. M. (1974) Human lymphocyte subpopulations. Study of T and B cells and their density distribution. *Clinical Immunology and Immunopathology*, **2**, 333.

8
ABNORMALITIES OF CIRCULATING PHAGOCYTE FUNCTION

Bengt Björkstén   Paul G. Quie

Phagocytic cells can be divided into two types: the circulating phagocytes, i.e. polymorphonuclear neutrophils, eosinophils, basophils and monocytes (Fig. 8.1); and fixed tissue phagocytes, i.e. Kupffer cells of the liver, microglial cells of the central nervous system and splenic and lymph node macrophages. The bone marrow is the source of tissue

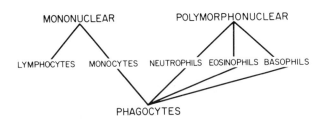

Figure 8.1   Nomenclature of circulating phagocytes

macrophages as well as circulating phagocytes. The cells which become macrophages are released into the circulation as immature monocytes and migrate to tissues where they mature to macrophages. The specialised nature of macrophages is a result of the peculiar environmental influence in the various organ systems where monocytes find their home (Van Furth, 1970).

Since the observations of Metchnikoff in 1891, it has been known that an intact phagocytic cellular response is essential for competent host bacterial defence. The function of the phagocytic system depends not only on an adequate number of cells and humoral factors but also on normal function of the phagocytic cells.

Clinically useful methods have been developed for studying different aspects of circulating phagocyte function; however, practical laboratory tests for evaluation of tissue macrophage function have not been devised. Discussion in this chapter will deal with abnormalities of circulating phagocytes, primarily neutrophil granulocytes and monocytes.

Circulating phagocytes show spontaneous amoeboid movements (random migration) and have the capacity for unidirectional movement towards attractant substances (chemotaxis). Factors attracting phagocytes are termed cytotaxins and include a number of products derived from serum and from microbial metabolism. They are primarily denatured

proteins and polypeptides. The motility of circulating phagocytes and pseudopod formation during phagocytosis are both thought to depend on actin and myosin, proteins which
involve the microtubule and microfilament system of the cells (Pollard and Weihing, 1974;
Stossel, 1975). Excellent comprehensive reviews of the chemotactic process have recently
been published (Gallin and Wolff, 1975; Wilkinson, 1974). A schematic representation of
responses of circulating phagocytes during the initial phases of inflammation is shown in
Figure 8.2.

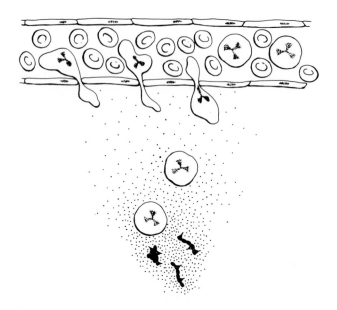

Figure 8.2   Early steps in the inflammatory response. Neutrophils adhere to the surface of capillaries
and venules, diapedese through spaces between endothelial cells and migrate toward an increased
concentration of cytotaxins. Cytotaxins are depicted by the small dots

Attachment of bacteria or other particles to the phagocytic membrane triggers formation of pseudopodia which surround the particle, fuse, and form a phagocytic vacuole
(Fig. 8.3A–D). Phagocytosis is more rapid if the particles have been opsonised, i.e. have
been coated with host factors which provide a ligand between microbe and phagocyte.
Opsonins include serum antibacterial antibodies and activated complement components,
notably C3b which may be activated by either the classical or the alternate (properdin)
pathway. Recent studies have shown that certain bacterial species, e.g. many strains of
E. coli, *S. pneumoniae*, *S. epidermidis*, *S. viridans* and *S. marcescens* efficiently activate
serum complement C3 to its opsonically active state C3b via the alternate pathway
(Björkstén et al, 1977; Fine, 1975; Forsgren and Quie, 1974; Simberkoff, Ricupero
and Rahal, 1976). Other bacterial species including *S. aureus*, *Pseudomonas aeruginosa*,
some strains of *E. coli* and some strains of *S. pneumoniae* are less capable of properdin
pathway activation (Björkstén et al, 1977; Fine, 1975; Forsgren and Quie, 1974).
Following ingestion, a series of distinct events occur including discharge of the granular
contents into the phagocytic vacuole, a burst of phagocyte metabolic activity, killing and
digestion of the ingested organisms (Fig. 8.3E–F). Circulating phagocytes have diverse

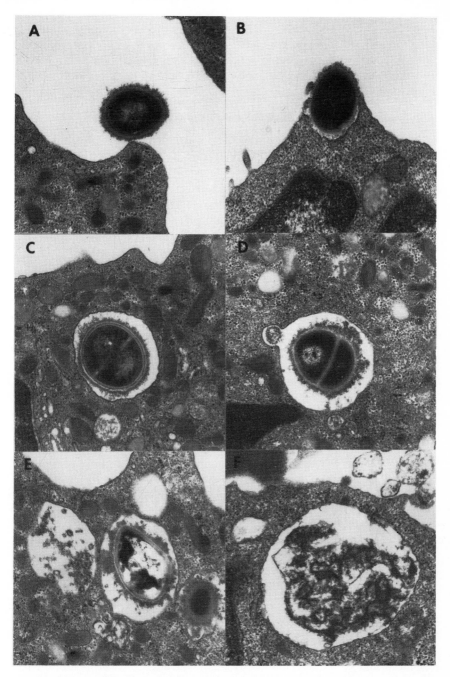

Figure 8.3 (× 21 150) Phagocytosis of *S. aureus* by a human neutrophil. A, Attachment of particle to cell membrane. B, Pseudopodia surround particle. C, Formation of a phagocytic vaculoe. D, Degranulation into phagocytic vacuoles. E and F, Lysis of the phagocytised bacterium. Electronmicrographs kindly supplied by Dr C. Carlyle Clawson, Department of Pediatrics, University of Minnesota. (Published with the permission of Polish Publishing C., Warsaw)

and complex antimicrobial systems including myeloperoxidase (MPO), lysozyme, lacto-ferrin, cationic proteins, acid and reactive oxygen radicals (superoxide, singlet oxygen, hydrogen peroxide and hydroxyl radicals). An excellent review of antimicrobial mechanisms in phagocytes has recently been published by Klebanoff(1975). For recent reviews on clinical conditions associated with phagocyte dysfunction, the reader is referred to *Lancet* (1974a) and Quie and Davis (1973).

Quantitative Disorders of Circulating Phagocytes

The most frequently encountered clinical problem of recurrent infections related to phagocyte dysfunction is neutropenia. This diagnosis can be made when there is persistent reduction in number of circulating neutrophils as well as in marginal and bone marrow pools of these cells. Greatly increased risk of bacterial or fungal infection occurs when there are less than 500 neutrophils per microlitre of blood. Abnormally low numbers of any of the other types of circulating phagocytes are not correlated with an increased risk of infection. In patients with neutropenia, infections are particularly common in the skin and in the respiratory tract as well as buccal and rectal mucosal ulceration.

Neutropenia may be a consequence of decreased production or increased destruction of neutrophils and may be primary or secondary to other conditions. Primary causes of decreased production of neutrophils include several hereditary conditions. Neutropenia caused by decreased production may be secondary to toxic effects of physical agents and drugs or to a number of diseases, e.g. leukaemia, neuroblastoma and infection. Increased destruction of neutrophils is seen in immune neutropenia and in hypersplenism. In some conditions, the number of circulating neutrophils may be low but marginal and bone marrow pools of these cells are normal, and there is a normal response to infection. Thus patients with this condition are not usually afflicted with recurrent infections. For a review of clinical conditions associated with neutropenia see Finch (1972) and Wintrobe et al (1974a).

METHODS OF INVESTIGATION

Peripheral blood leucocyte counts with evaluation of cell types by differential counts is a part of the routine laboratory evaluation of all patients suspected of infection. Many factors independent of infection, e.g. hunger, convulsion and strenuous physical activity (Finch, 1972; Wintrobe et al, 1974a) may rapidly change the body's distribution of leucocytes. Therefore data on peripheral leucocytes must be correlated with clinical and laboratory findings.

In cyclic neutrophilia, a variation in the number of peripheral leucocytes occurs in cycles of approximately three weeks (Wintrobe et al, 1974b). Repeated leucocyte counts are necessary for diagnosis of this rare condition. Counts should be done as early as possible when infections appear, and at regular intervals for several weeks.

Examination of a biopsy specimen of bone marrow from patients with neutropenia is frequently necessary to evaluate presence of neutrophil precursors.   .

Epinephrine and steroid tests offer fairly simple methods for evaluation of the relative sizes of the neutrophil marginating pool and the bone marrow reserve of mature granulocytes respectively (Dale et al, 1975; Deinard et al, 1974; Samuels, 1951; Storti, 1967). In the epinephrine test 0.4 ml 1:100 aqueous epinephrine per mm^2 is injected subcutaneously. Neutrophil counts are done on capillary blood specimens prior to and 15, 30, 45 and 60 min following administration of epinephrine. Normally, there is more than 45 per cent increase in circulating neutrophils after the injection. Steroids may be administered either as oral prednisolone (adult dose 10–80 mg) or intravenous hydrocortisone (50–100 mg). When the bone marrow reserves are adequate, there is a more than 50 per cent increase in peripheral blood neutrophil counts between 2 and 6 h after injection. Steroids have replaced the use of endotoxin for estimation of the bone marrow granulocyte pool.

Table 8.1 Clinical conditions with disorders of locomotion

A. Intrinsic (cellular) defects	
1. Isolated chemotactic defects—lazy leucocyte syndrome	Miller et al, 1971; Miller et al, 1973
2. Combined with eczema and high IgE	Dahl et al, 1976; Hill and Quie, 1974; Van Scoy et al, 1975
3. Combined with neutropenia and eosinophilia	Björkstén and Lundmark, 1976
4. Combined with defective cellular immunity	Clark et al, 1973; Snyderman et al, 1973
5. Chediak-Higashi syndrome	Clark and Kimball, 1971; Gallin, 1975; Root et al, 1972
6. Defective phagocytosis of killing	Boxer, Hedley-Whyte and Stossel, 1975b; Edelson et al, 1973; Miller, 1975; Steerman et al, 1971
7. Combined with rheumatoid arthritis and with cancer	Baum, 1975; Snyderman and Stahl, 1975
8. Effect of drugs	(see Table 8.2)
B. Extrinsic defects (abnormalities of humoral factors)	
1. Complement deficiency	Gallin, 1975
2. Presence of chemotaxis inhibitors:	
Hodgkin's disease	Ward and Berenberg, 1974
Liver cirrhosis	DeMeo and Andersen, 1972
Idiopathic	Smith et al, 1972; Soriano et al, 1973; Ward and Schlegel, 1969
3. Hyperosmolality	Bryant, Sutcliffe and McGee, 1972
C. Combined intrinsic and extrinsic or unclassified defects	
1. Newborn infants	Miller, 1971
2. Diabetes mellitus	Baum, 1975; Hill et al, 1974b; Miller and Baker, 1972
D. Increased chemotactic responsiveness	
Bacterial infections	Hill et al, 1974a

In patients with suspected increased destruction of neutrophils a search for neutrophil antibodies (Boxer et al, 1975a) and evaluation of splenic function may be of value. Other specialised methods for investigation of neutrophil production and turnover rates include bone marrow culture (Goldman and Sultan, 1975; McCulloch, 1975), use of DF ^{32}P-labelled neutrophils (Athens et al, 1959; Blume et al, 1968), and the measuring of serum muramidase levels (Blume et al, 1968; Fink and Finch, 1968). However, the value of these techniques in clinical practice has not been established.

Disorders of Locomotion

Defective granulocyte locomotion may result from intrinsic abnormalities of the phagocytes or from extrinsic factors. An outline of clinical conditions with abnormal neutrophil chemotaxis is shown in Table 8.1. In addition to patients with isolated defects of neutrophil locomotion (Miller et al, 1973; Miller, Oski and Harris, 1971), chemotactic defects combined with immunologic abnormalities in humoral immunity (Gallin, 1975; Steerman et al, 1971) and combined immune defects (Clark et al, 1973; Snyderman et al, 1973) have been reported in recent years. Reports include chemotactic defects of neutro-

Table 8.2   Pharmacologic agents which effect phagocyte function

Mode of action	Drug	References
Affecting cell membrane	Acetyl salicyclic acid	MacGregor et al, 1974
	Amphotericin B	Björkstén et al, 1976
	Chlorpromazine	Björkstén and Quie, 1976; Ruutu, 1972
	Concanavalin A	Berlin, 1972
	Corticosteroids	MacGregor et al, 1974; Mandell et al, 1970; Peters et al, 1972; Ward, 1966
	Ethanol	Brayton et al, 1970; MacGregor et al, 1974
	Levorphanol	Wurster et al, 1971
Affecting microfilaments	Cytochalasin B	Davis et al, 1971b; Zigmond and Hirsch, 1972
Affecting microtubules	Colchicine	Caner, 1965; Malawista and Bensch, 1967
	Vinblastine	Edelson and Fudenberg, 1973
Affecting postphagocytic metabolism	Ascorbic acid	MacGregor et al, 1974
	Phenylbutazone	Solberg, 1972b; Strauss et al, 1968
	Sulphonamides	Lehrer, 1971
Affecting intracellular levels of cyclic nucleotides:		
Increases cAMP (depression of chemotaxis)	Histamine, catecholamines prostaglandins E_1 and E_2	Hill et al, 1975; Rivkin et al, 1975
Increases cGMP (enhancement of chemotaxis)	Acetylcholine, phorbol myristate,	
	Prostaglandins $F_2\gamma$	Hill et al 1975
Unknown mechanisms		
Increases phagocytosis	Clofazimine	Brandt, 1971
Inhibits phagocytosis	Tetracycline	Forsgren, Schmeling and Quie, 1974
Inhibits chemotaxis	Gentamicin	Khan et al, 1975
Inhibits chemotaxis and phagocytosis	Chloroquine	Ward, 1966

phils in patients with recurrent staphylococcal infection, eczema, high levels of serum IgE and eosinophilia (Dahl, Greene and Quie, 1976; Hill and Quie, 1974; Van Scoy et al, 1975). Four siblings with defective chemotaxis, neutropenia, eosinophilia and combined immune deficiency were evaluated by one of us recently (Björkstén and Lundmark, 1976). This report and others (Miller et al, 1973; Van Scoy et al, 1975) document the familial nature of this disorder. These patients have many features in common which suggests that granulocyte dysfunction and cell-mediated immunity and humoral immunity may result from a common pathogenic denominator, i.e. defective monocyte-macrophage function, abnormal antigen processing or abnormal immunoregulation. The reader is referred to the recent report of Miller (1975) for a detailed review of chemotactic defects.

A number of drugs depress neutrophil chemotaxis (Table 8.2). Certain drugs, i.e. histamine, catecholamines and prostaglandins are believed to act by increasing intracellular levels of cAMP (Hill et al, 1975; Rivkin, Rosenblatt and Becker, 1975). The phagocyte membrane is affected by chlorpromazine (Björkstén and Quie, 1976), by amphotericin B (Björkstén, Ray and Quie, 1976) and possibly by corticosteroids (Ward, 1966). Cytochalasin B reversibly paralyses the contractile microfilament systems and has been shown to reversibly inhibit chemotaxis and phagocytosis (Davis, Estenson and Quie, 1971b; Zigmond and Hirsch, 1972). Disruption of microtubules may be associated with inhibition of chemotaxis by colchinine (Caner, 1965; Malawista and Bensch, 1967) and vinblastine (Edelson and Fudenberg, 1973). In a recent report zinc deficiency was suggested as a cause for defective chemotaxis (Huff et al, 1975).

Humoral chemotactic factors generated by the inflammatory response include components of the complement system. Activation of complement results in generation of chemotactically active serum factors; C3a, C5a, C567 (Gallin and Wolff, 1975; Müller-Eberhard, 1975; Wilkinson, 1974). The activation is carried out by both the classical and alternate pathways of complement activation. A deficiency of C3 or C5 alone usually does not inhibit chemotactic activity (Alper, Stossel and Rosen, 1975) since chemotactically active fragments can be elaborated by tissue proteases (Ward, 1972). However, deficiency of the early complement components may delay generation of chemotactic factors. Gallin reported recently that generation of chemotactic activity was delayed in C1r and C2 deficient sera. Furthermore, addition of the early complement components to deficient sera restored normal kinetics of chemotactic factor generation (Gallin, 1975). Purified preparations of human kallikrein and plasminogen activator have also been reported to be chemotactic for neutrophils and for monocytes (Gallin, 1975; Kaplan, Goetzl and Austen, 1973).

An inhibitor of chemotactic factors has been reported in several children with recurrent infections (Smith et al, 1972; Soriano et al, 1973; Ward and Schlegel, 1969), in patients with Hodgkin's disease (Ward and Berenberg, 1974), and with liver cirrhosis (DeMeo and Anderson, 1972). The circulating inhibitor in these patients appears to be an excess of a factor present in lesser amounts in normal serum. Monocytes from patients with Wiskott–Aldrich syndrome have decreased chemotactic responsiveness and plasma from the patients is inhibitory to normal monocytes (Altman, Snyderman and Blaese, 1974). In kwashiorkor, impaired kinetics of neutrophil chemotaxis has been reported in addition to other phagocyte abnormalities (Schopfer and Douglas, 1976).

It has been reported that neutrophil motility, adhesiveness and phagocytosis are inhibited by hyperosmolality (Bryant, Sutcliffe and McGee, 1972) and by hypo- or hyperglycaemia (Van Oss, 1971). These conditions may account for depressed phagocyte function in diabetes (Baum, 1975; Hill et al, 1974b; Miller and Baker, 1972). Neutrophils from patients with diabetes mellitus also have depressed chemotactic responsiveness when suspended in normal serum suggesting an intrinsic neutrophil defect. The nature of the defect in diabetic neutrophils remains unexplained, however, addition of insulin in vitro improves chemotactic responsiveness (Baum, 1975; Hill et al, 1974b).

METHODS FOR STUDYING DISORDERS OF LOCOMOTION

In 1962, Boyden introduced a new technique for the measurement of chemotaxis. He designed a chamber in which chemotactically active factors were separated from leucocyte suspensions by a micropore filter with 3 to 8 μm pore size so that cells required an active process of locomotion in order to squeeze through the filter. This technique is still the most widely used and accepted method for studying phagocyte locomotion. A cell suspension is placed in the upper part of the chamber and a solution of chemotactically active substance is placed in the lower chamber. During incubation, the chemotactic substance diffuses through the filter attracting cells which migrate through the filter towards the higher concentration of chemotactic attractant in the lower chamber. After incubation, filters are removed from the chemotactic chambers, fixed and stained with haematoxylin for cell counting.

Chemotaxis can be measured either by counting the number of cells which have reached the lower surface of the filter after a fixed time interval (DeMeo and Anderson, 1972; Hill, 1974a; Ward, 1966), or by measuring the distance cells have migrated in a given time (Wilkinson, 1974). Both methods give reproducible results in experienced hands and the correlation between them is usually very good. The proportion of the cell population responding to a chemotactic agent is measured by counting cells that have migrated through the filter at a certain time and the degree of response of a population of activated cells is determined by measuring the leading front of migrating cells. Fewer cells are needed for the leading front method, and the test is more rapid to perform, however, the percentage of cells responding to chemotactic stimulation cannot be determined by this method. For evaluation of increased chemotaxis the index method (counting the number of cells on the bottom of the filter) is preferred.

Gallin and co-workers (1973) have devised a radioassay of neutrophil chemotaxis in Boyden chambers employing ^{51}Cr-labelled cells. The upper and the lower parts of the cell chamber are separated by two micropore filters which after incubation are placed in individual γ-counter vials. Chemotaxis is expressed as the number of counts per minute (ct/min) in the lower filter with corrections made for variable incorporation of ^{51}Cr by the leucocytes. This method appears to be more sensitive over a wide range of cell responses than conventional filter methods. Also a larger number of samples can be processed in the laboratory.

A new method for evaluating chemotaxis and random migration in which phagocyte locomotion under agarose is assessed has recently been described (Cutler, 1974; Nelson, Quie and Simmons, 1975). Agarose plates are prepared and a series of three wells 2.4 mm in diameter spaced 2.5 mm apart are punched in the hardened agarose. The centre wells are filled with 10 μl of a leucocyte suspension (approximately 0.5×10^6 neutrophils). The outer wells are filled with the same volume of chemotactic factors and the inner wells with balanced salt solution without chemotactic factor. The dishes are incubated at 37°C in a humidified atmosphere during which period leucocytes migrate under the agarose layer. Migration is stopped and leucocytes are fixed by covering the plates with methanol and formaldehyde. The agarose gel is removed and the cells stained. The migration pattern is projected on a white background using a microprojector and the linear distance the cells have moved from the margin of the well toward the chemotactic factor in the outer well ('chemotaxis') and toward the control medium in the inner well ('spontaneous migration') is measured (Nelson et al, 1975). The advantages of measuring chemotaxis under agarose are (1) many tests can be performed with a single sample of cells, (2) filters which are notoriously variable are not used and (3) incubation time can be prolonged to 18 h for determining migration of eosinophils and monocytes. However it will be necessary to correlate this method with the more widely used filter method before its value for clinical studies is established.

In vivo migration of neutrophils may be evaluated by the skin window test described by Rebuck and Crowley in 1955. An area of about 1×1 cm on the volar surface of the forearm is abraded down to the corium with great care being taken to avoid puncture bleeding. Abrasion of the skin in a uniform fashion is necessary since the size and depth of the abrasion may significantly influence the number of exudate cells. The abraded area is covered by a clean coverslip which is removed at certain time intervals and stained to determine the number and type of cells adherent to the coverslip.

Quantitative estimations of the cellular response may be obtained using a small plastic chamber which can be emptied and filled without removal from the skin (Senn, 1972). Practical problems include chamber leakage and patient discomfort. Table 8.3 summarises the methods available for evaluating phagocytic cells locomotion.

Table 8.3 Methods for studying disorders of locomotion

A. Through filters
1. Chemotactic index
2. Leading front
3. ^{51}Cr method
B. Under agarose
C. In vivo (Rebuck technique)
1. Qualitative
2. Quantitative

Recently Mass et al (1975) suggested a virtually atraumatic technique to remove the stratum corneum of the skin with adhesive tape, leaving intact the underlying dermal layers including the skin capillaries. This method may prove very useful for evaluating the capacity of neutrophils to move across the endothelial and dermal barriers. However, the more traumatic 'abrasion methods' provide a combined assessment of in vivo neutrophil movement and of chemotactic factors in the patient's own tissue extracts.

A predominantly neutrophil response is normally observed in the 3 to 6 h coverslips, while monocytes dominate the 18 and 24 h exudates. Under normal conditions only few eosinophils are found, but the number may be much increased in allergic patients (Felarca and Lowell, 1969) and in patients with neutrophil or immunologic dysfunction (Björkstén and Lundmark, 1976).

The methods currently used for measuring chemotaxis are not well standardised and the results obtained when testing leucocytes from normal persons vary from day to day. Several controls must be assayed simultaneously and all test conditions should be performed in triplicate. Abnormal results obtained by either method should be repeated and preferably be confirmed using two separate methods.

Disorders of Phagocytosis, Microbial Killing and Metabolism

An immunologically specific response to surface antigens of microbes colonising the host is critical for phagocytosis of many microbial species. Therefore clinical conditions associated with impaired synthesis or abnormal loss of immunoglobulins are frequently associated with abnormal serum opsonic activity. Immunoglobulin disorders include genetic deficiencies of the immunoglobulin-producing system, i.e. agammaglobulinaemia as well as acquired abnormalities of synthesis or loss of immunoglobulins (Davis, 1973; Gotoff, 1973).

Phagocytosis of most microbial organisms is amplified by heat-labile opsonins derived from the complement system. Thus complement deficiencies as well as defective antibody synthesis may result in impaired phagocytosis and enhanced susceptibility to infection. Since a primary opsonic factor in the complement system is C3b, it is not surprising that patients with defective C3 have defective opsonic function and recurrent infections (Alper et al, 1970). Complement activation occurs via the alternate pathway in the absence of specific antibodies and normal function of this system may be especially important for opsonisation of organisms and phagocytosis in the early stages of infection, i.e. before specific antimicrobial antibodies have developed. Subnormal levels of components of the alternate pathway have been reported in newborn infants (Stossel, Alper and Rosen, 1973), in patients with sickle cells anaemia (Johnston, Newman and Struth, 1973) and in glomerulonephritis (McLean and Michael, 1973).

A number of pharmacologic agents inhibit neutrophil phagocytosis, e.g. chlorpromazine (Ruutu, 1972), levorphanol (Wurster et al, 1971), cytochalasin B (Malawista, Gee and Bensch, 1971). These drugs presumably impair membrane function or microfilament activity of the phagocytic cells. Inhibited neutrophil adhesiveness has been reported after in vivo exposure of leucocytes to ethanol, prednisone and acetyl salicylic acid (MacGregor, Spagnuolo and Lentneh, 1974). Thus corticosteroids impair several aspects of neutrophil function: motility (Ward, 1966), adhesiveness (MacGregor et al, 1974), and microbial killing (Mandell, Rubin and Hook, 1970). Phenylbutazone (Strauss, Paul and Sbarra, 1968) and sulphonamides (Lehrer and Cline, 1969) impair postphagocytic metabolic events in phagocytes. Enhancement of neutrophil phagocytosis in vitro and in vivo has been reported for clofazimine, a chemotherapeutic agent active against *M. leprae* (Brandt, 1971). A summary of pharmacologic agents which effect phagocyte function is shown in Table 8.2.

The discovery that neutrophils from patients with chronic granulomatous disease (CGD) are defective in bactericidal function established the concept that adequate phagocyte function as well as adequate numbers are necessary for antimicrobial defence (Holmes et al, 1966; Quie et al, 1967). The underlying mechanism for the defective killing of catalase producing microorganisms by CGD phagocytes is a deficiency of an oxidative metabolic response during phagocytosis (Root, 1975). As a result, reactive oxygen metabolites, i.e. superoxide, hydrogen peroxide, singlet oxygen or hydroxyl radicals are not formed and the microbicidal power of these cells is greatly diminished. Certain microorganisms without catalase produce oxygen radicals and these species are readily killed by CGD phagocytes.

Defective intracellular killing of microorganisms (both catalase positive and catalase negative) has been described in the Chediak–Higashi syndrome (Root, Rosenthal and Balestra, 1972) in complete absence of glucose-6-phosphate dehydrogenase (Cooper et al, 1972), in myeloperoxidase deficiency (Davis, Brunning and Quie, 1971a; Lehrer and Cline, 1969), and in patients with protein-calorie malnutrition (Schopfer and Douglas, 1976). In approximately 30 per cent of patients with acute leukaemia and in 15 per cent of patients with Down's syndrome (Gregory, 1972), defective phagocyte microbicidal activity has been described. Neutrophils from patients with severe acute infections (Solberg and Hellum, 1972) have a transient defect in bactericidal capacity which has been found to correlate with the presence of toxic neutrophils (McCall et al, 1971). A summary of clinical conditions with disorders of phagocytosis and killing is shown in Table 8.4.

METHODS FOR STUDYING INGESTION, KILLING AND OXIDATIVE METABOLISM

These are summarised in Table 8.5. Neutrophil adhesiveness can be studied by a recently described method employing nylon fibre columns (MacGregor et al, 1974). A

Table 8.4   Clinical conditions with disorders of phagocytosis and killing

A. Defective opsonisation	
1. Hypogammaglobulinaemia	*Lancet*, 1974a
2. Newborn infants	Forman and Stiehm, 1969
3. Complement deficiency	Miller and Baker, 1972
B. Other extrinsic defects	
1. Drugs—see Table 8.2	
2. Bacterial toxin	*Lancet*, 1974a
3. Hyperosmolarity	Bryant et al, 1972
C. Intrinsic disorders of killing	
1. Chronic granulomatous disease (CGD)	Quie et al, 1967
2. Chediak–Higashi syndrome	Root et al, 1972
3. Glucose-6-phosphate dehydrogenase (G-6-PD) deficiency	Cooper et al, 1972
4. Myeloperoxidase deficiency	Davis et al, 1971; Lehrer and Cline, 1969
5. Acute leukaemia	Gregory, 1972
6. Severe bacterial infection	McCall et al, 1971; Solberg and Hellum, 1972
7. Down's syndrome	Gregory, 1972
8. Protein-calorie malnutrition	Schopfer and Douglas, 1976

Table 8.5   Methods for studying disorders of phagocytosis and killing

A. Adhesion
   1. Granulocyte adherence to nylon fibre columns

B. Phagocytosis
   1. Counting of phagocytised particles under light microscope
   2. Colorimetric determination of phagocytised paraffin oil
   3. Phagocytosis of radiolabelled bacteria
   4. Quantitative immunoglobulin and complement determinations
   5. Determination of opsonic activity in normal and chelated serum

C. Phagocytosis and killing
   1. Bacterial and fungal killing assays

D. Metabolic response
   1. NBT test
   2. Chemiluminescence
   3. Oxygen consumption
   4. Hexose monophosphate shunt activity

E. Lysosomal enzyme quantitation

F. Myeloperoxidase determination

G. Electron microscopy

leucocyte suspension with a known number of neutrophils is passed through a nylon fibre column and the number of neutrophils adhering to the column during the passage is used as measure of adhesiveness. The method allows measurement of a single step in the phagocytic process; however, the full clinical importance of the method has not yet been established.

Methods for estimating phagocytosis include incubation of phagocytic cells with particles and counting the number of intraleucocytic particles in each phagocyte or the percentage of phagocytes which have ingested particles (Brandt, 1971; Ruutu, 1972). Magnification of phagocytic cells by electron microscopy can be useful in documenting intracellular location of particles. However, this technique is not practical for routine studies.

A major technical problem involving direct measurement of phagocytosis of bacteria by circulating phagocytes is efficient separation of cells containing particles from cell adherent particles. Controls necessary for each assay include bacteria and opsonins without phagocytes, phagocytes and bacteria without opsonin and stationary (non-rotating) tubes containing all reagents. When a method is established in a laboratory, it is necessary to demonstrate absence of particle migration at 4°, lack of apparent ingestion at zero time and demonstration of the maximum capacity for ingestion of the particles being studied.

In 1946, Maaløe devised a method to measure phagocytosis and intracellular killing of bacteria, based on differential centrifugation of bacteria and phagocytes and the counting of extracellular and intracellular bacteria. Most currently used methods for measuring phagocytosis and intracellular killing are modifications of the Maaløe technique. The rate of ingestion and killing can be separated by adding to the test mixtures phenylbutazone, which blocks intracellular killing (Solberg, 1972a), or lysostaphin (Tan, Watanakundkorn and Phair, 1971) or antibiotics (Alexander, Windhorst and Good, 1969; Solbert, 1972b) to kill extracellular bacteria. The bacterial killing test used in our laboratory involves incubation of neutrophils and bacteria at a ratio of about 1 : 1 (Quie et al, 1967). The suspension contains either 8 per cent fresh serum from a pool of normal donors to provide opsonin factors, or when opsonin activity is tested, dilutions of individual sera. The phagocytic mixtures are tumbled end-over-end at 37°C. A calibrated platinum loop is used to remove aliquots at 0, 30, 60 and 120 min and colony counts are done by incubating dilutions of the removed aliquots in nutrient agar. After 120 min incubation, the phagocytic mixtures are centrifuged, the supernatants are sampled to determine extracellular organisms which were not phagocytised, and the pellets are lysed in distilled water and surviving intracellular bacteria determined. Figure 8.4 illustrates essential steps in this procedure.

Recently Stossel et al (1972) have devised an assay for ingestion using paraffin oil particles containing oil red O. Leucocytes are incubated with particles and uningested particles are removed from the cells by differential centrifugation. The ingested paraffin oil is extracted from the cells and quantified spectrophotometrically. This method also allows separation of phagocytic vacuoles and analysis of vacuole contents.

A method for measuring phagocytosis using ^{3}H-thymidine labelled bacteria has been established in our laboratory (Verhoef et al, 1977). This method has been adapted from several reports describing phagocytosis of radiolabelled bacteria and is used for measuring phagocytosis of S. aureus, S. epidermidis, E. coli, Streptococcus and S. pneumoniae. The organisms are incubated in Mueller–Hinton broth containing 2 to 4 μCi of ^{3}H-thymidine per millilitre (6.7 Ci/mmol). After 18 h incubation (12–16 h for E. coli), S. aureus, S. epidermidis, E. coli and streptococcal cultures are harvested. When labelling S. pneumoniae, another 2 μCi/ml is added to the culture after 16 h and bacteria are harvested after another 3 h incubation. A labelling efficiency of approximately 1 c/600 to 1000 bacteria is achieved. This method has been used for evaluating kinetics of phagocytosis of different strains of bacteria within the same species; for detection of differences in opsonic activity in different sera and for determination of phagocytic capacity of neutrophils from patients with suspected phagocytic defects.

ANALYSIS OF SERUM OPSONINS

A detailed analysis of phagocytosis includes the differentiation of heat-labile and heat-stable opsonins, and quantitative measurements of both immunoglobulins and comple-

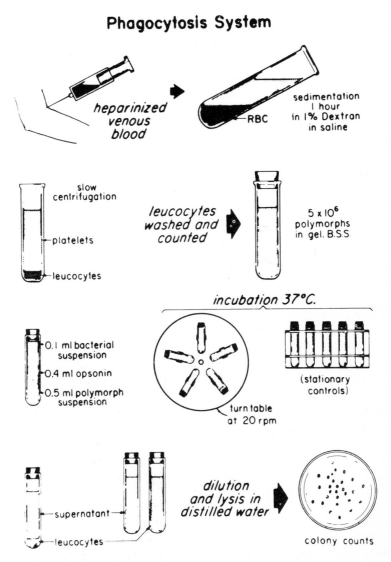

Phagocytosis System

Figure 8.4 Essential steps in the measurement of neutrophil bacterial killing by a modified Maaløe technique. This is the basic assay for measurement of bacteria killed which is used in the authors' laboratory

ment. Heat-labile magnesium-dependent opsonins include components of the classical and alternate pathways of complement activation; these can be differentiated by chelating serum with EGTA which binds calcium more avidly than magnesium. Since the classical pathway requires both Ca^{2+} and Mg^{2+}, while only the latter ion is needed for the alternate pathway, chelation of serum with 10 mM EGTA plus 10 mM Mg^{2+} provides a method for measuring alternate pathway activity (Forsgren and Quie, 1974). Although chelation of serum theoretically is simple, minor changes in the technique may lead to inhibition of both pathways and appropriate controls are necessary.

To evaluate serum opsonic capcity from patients suspected of defective phagocyte function, we use *S. aureus* 502A which only activates complement via the classical pathway, and a smooth, serum-resistant *E. coli* strain with the capacity to activate the alternate pathway. However, the assay is easily adapted to other microbial species. Since individual strains of different bacterial species, e.g. *E. coli* (Björkstén et al, 1977), *S. marcescens* (Simberkoff et al, 1976), *S. pneumoniae* (Fine, 1975) and possibly other species vary in opsonin requirements, using the strain causing the patient's infection may be particularly valuable.

NITROBLUE TETRAZOLIUM REDUCTION TEST

In 1968, Baehner and Nathan reported that neutrophils from patients with CGD lacked the ability to reduce nitroblue tetrazolium (NBT) into formazan in contrast to normal neutrophils and this NBT test was suggested as a diagnostic test for the disease. The same year Park, Fikrig and Smithwick (1968) introduced the NBT slide test which was recommended for differentiating between blood samples from patients with an untreated fungal or bacterial infection and from healthy persons or patients with viral infections or noninfectious disorders. The test was widely recommended for use in the differentiation of viral and bacterial infections; however, several more recent papers have seriously questioned the validity of the test for such purposes (*Lancet*, 1974b; Björkstén, 1974a; Steigbigel, Johnson and Remington, 1974).

When performing the NBT test, a strictly standardised technique is crucial, since many technical factors influence the test results (Björkstén, 1974a, b). The blood sample is mixed with an equal volume of 0.1 per cent NBT solution in sterile saline, incubated in a 37°C water bath for 25 min, and then smears of the mixtures are made on glass slides. The slides are fixed, counterstained and the neutrophils containing discrete intracellular deposits of nitroblue formazan are counted using a light microscope. Presently, the main indication for the NBT test would be as a simple screening test for chronic granulomatous disease. The test may also be of value in the differentiation between pyelonephritis and cystitis (Björkstén and DeChateau, 1975), in monitoring patients with an increased susceptibility to bacterial infections (Wollman et al, 1972), and in evaluating effectiveness of instituted antimicrobial therapy.

CHEMILUMINESCENCE

Chemiluminescence (CL) is the emission of light from chemical reactions. In neutrophils and monocytes increased CL occurs as a consequence of phagocytosis (Allen, Sternholm and Steele, 1972; Nelson et al, 1976). The precise source of CL obtained from the cells is not known, but it is believed to be due to highly unstable intermediate products of oxygen metabolism, either singlet oxygen per se or excited carbonyl groups derived from singlet oxygen-mediated oxidations (Allen et al, 1972). The amount of CL produced by the phagocytes depends on the degree and rate of phagocytosis, on a functioning oxidative cell metabolism, and on the nature of phagocytised particles. Phagocyte CL before and during phagocytosis can be accurately quantitated in a liquid scintillation counter which is adjusted for measuring CL. Under red illumination, a suspension of preopsonised particles (e.g. zymosan or different bacterial species) are transferred to dark-adapted counting vials. The background counts are recorded and then a leucocyte suspension is added to the test mixtures. CL is counted for 60 to 120 min and the results are graphed as counts per minute

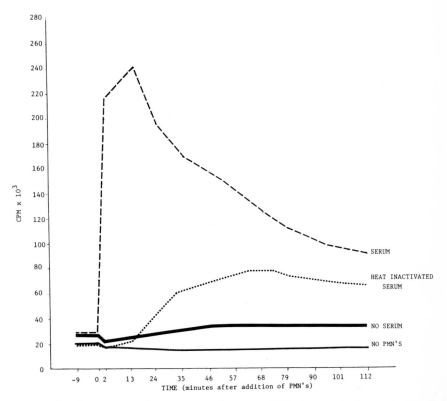

Figure 8.5   Chemiluminescence (in counts per minute, ct/min) by human phagocytes during phago-cytosis of zymosan particles in the presence of fresh serum, heat-inactivated serum or Hank's BSS. The figure shows a typical response

versus time on regular graph paper (Fig. 8.5). The method is simple to perform, rapid and has a high reproducibility (standard deviation is less than 5 per cent of mean) (Nelson et al, 1976).

Furthermore, since CL is a result of the end products of the oxidative metabolism, this, as a single technique, yields more information than measuring oxygen consumption, when evaluating patients with suspected defective phagocyte function. Chronic granulomatous disease leucocytes have a profoundly depressed CL and leucocytes from mothers of boys with X-linked CGD show a CL response intermediate between that of CGD patients and normal persons. Therefore, this is a useful method for diagnosis of a carrier state (un-published).

The CL response of phagocytes correlates with engulfment and therefore the method can be used to measure serum opsonic function (Grebner et al, 1977). The method can also be used to evaluate the influence of bacterial species with unusual virulence on the oxidative metabolism of host cells (unpublished).

PHAGOCYTIC OXIDATIVE ENZYMES

Quantitative measurement of phagocyte oxidative enzymes including myeloperoxidase, glucose-6-phosphate dehydrogenase, NADH and NAD-oxidase can be done; however, these assays are presently used only as research tools.

Several of the methods described in this chapter are not suitable for routine use in a small laboratory where the individual tests would be done only occasionally. Under such

Table 8.6   Clinical laboratory investigation of suspected phagocyte disorders

I. Suspected neutropenia
   A. Serial quantitative determinations of the different types of blood leucocytes
   B. Bone marrow examination
   C. Epinephrine and hydrocortisone tests

II. Suspected locomotion defect
   A. Leucocyte chemotactic activity
   B. Serum cytotaxins

III. Suspected phagocytosis and killing defect
   A. Nitroblue tetrazolium reduction test
   B. Maaløe bactericidal system using *S. aureus* and *E. coli*
   C. Chemiluminescence assay

circumstances, blood samples may be sent to a laboratory where tests for granulocyte function are done routinely. Blood samples may be transported at 4°C and storage for up to 12 h does not seriously impair phagocyte function if leucocyte clumping can be prevented (McCullogh, Weiblen and Quie, 1974). Serum samples for measuring opsonic activity should be sent frozen.

In Table 8.6 are listed methods which we routinely use in our laboratory for evaluation of patients with suspected phagocyte disorders. These methods are not necessarily the best ones in every respect; however, they are reasonably accurate and quite simple to perform.

As a first measure in the evaluation of phagocyte motility we study random migration and chemotaxis of leucocytes suspended in the patient's own plasma. If this is abnormal, chemotaxis of patient's phagocytes in control plasma and leucocytes from a healthy person in patient plasma is tested. The skin window method is used to study phagocyte locomotion in vivo. For most purposes the qualitative method using coverslips is the most suitable technique for evaluation of cell migration to an abraded area. The full cooperation of the patient is needed and he or she is preferably hospitalised when the test is done.

The first step to evaluate ingestion and killing by neutrophils or monocytes includes the use of the Maaøle system with two bacterial strains. This phagocytosis assay is less accurate than methods utilising radioactively labelled bacteria or oil droplets when precise evaluation of the kinetics of phagocytosis are required. The measurement of phagocyte chemiluminescence has replaced standard assays of oxygen uptake and hexose monophosphate shunt activity as the initial procedure for evaluation of phagocyte metabolic function.

Conclusion

The recognition of defective phagocyte function in patients is important since prompt and aggressive treatment is usually necessary when infections occur in these patients. Certain drugs may compromise phagocyte function which would require change of therapy. In addition some phagocyte disorders are familial in nature and precise definition of the defects are necessary for appropriate genetic counselling.

Careful laboratory investigation of abnormal cells from patients with phagocyte defects has led to entirely new concepts of mechanisms of cell function. For example, the relationship between oxidative metabolism and intracellular bacterial killing was not appreciated until phagocytic cells from patients with chronic granulomatous disease were shown to have both of these defects. Biochemical analysis of cellular and humoral factors from patients with disorders of phagocyte function will undoubtedly reveal other unrecognised mechanisms critical for host defence.

REFERENCES

Alexander, J. W., Windhorst, D. B. & Good, R. A. (1969) Improved tests for the evaluation of neutrophil function in human disease. *Journal of Laboratory and Clinical Medicine*, **72**, 136–148.

Allen, R. C., Stjernholm, R. L. & Steele, R. H. (1972) Evidence for the generation of an electronic excitation state(s) in human polymorphonuclear leukocytes and its participation in bactericidal activity. *Biochemistry Biophysics Research Communication*, **47**, 679–684.

Alper, C. A., Abramson, N., Johnston, R. B. Jr, Jandl, J. H. & Rosen, F. S. (1970) Increased susceptibility to infection associated with abnormalities of complement-mediated function and of the third component (C3). *New England Journal of Medicine*, **282**, 349–354.

Alper, C. A., Stossel, T. P. & Rosen, F. S. (1975) Genetic defects affecting complement and host resistance to infection. In *The Phagocytic Cell in Host Resistance*, ed. Bellanti, J. A. & Dayton, D. H., National Institute of Child Health, pp. 127–138. New York: Raven.

Altman, L. C., Snyderman, R. & Blaese, R. M. (1974) Abnormalities of chemotactic lymphokine synthesis and mononuclear leukocyte chemotaxis in Wiskott–Aldrich syndrome. *Journal of Clinical Investigation*, **54**, 486–493.

Athens, J. W., Mauer, A. M., Ashenbrucher, H., Cartwright, G. E. & Wintrobe, M. M. (1959) Leukokinetic studies. I. A method for labeling leukocytes with diisopropylfluorophosphate (DFP[32]). *Blood*, **14**, 303–333.

Baehner, R. L. & Nathan, D. G. (1968) Quantitative nitroblue tetrazolium test in chronic granulomatous disease. *New England Journal of Medicine*, **278**, 971–976.

Baum, J. (1975) Chemotaxis in human disease. In *The Phagocytic cell in Host Resistance*, ed. Bellanti, J. A. & Dayton, D. H., National Institute of Child Health, pp. 283–293. New York: Raven.

Berlin, R. D. (1972) Effect of concanavalin A on phagocytosis. *Nature (New Biology)*, **235**, 44–45.

Björkstén, B. (1974a) The influence of technical factors on the NBT test. *Scandinavian Journal of Haematology*, **12**, 46–50.

Björkstén, B. (1974b) The nitroblue tetrazolium (NBT) test. A methodological and clinical study. *Umeå University Medical Dissertation*, **15**.

Björkstén, B. & DeChateau, P. (1975) Use of the nitroblue tetrazolium (NBT) test in the differentiation between pyelonephritis and cystitis. *Acta paediatrica scandinavia*, **64**, 182–186.

Björkstén, B. & Lundmark, K. M. (1976) Recurrent bacterial infections in four siblings with neutropenia, eosinophilia, hyperimmunoglobulinemia A and defective neutrophil chemotaxis. *Journal of Infectious Disease*, **133**, 63–71.

Björkstén, B. & Quie, P. G. (1976) Effect of phenothiazines and related compounds on chemotaxis by human polymorphonuclear leukocytes. *Infection and Immunity*, **14**, 948–950.

Björkstén, B., Bortolussi, R., Quie, P. G. & Gothefors, L. (1977) Interaction of *E. coli* strains with serum and neutrophils. Variability in response and lack of relationship to K1 antigen. *Journal of Pediatrics*, **89**, 892–897.

Björkstén, B., Ray, C. S. & Quie, P. G. (1976) Inhibition of human neutrophil chemotaxis and chemiluminescence by amphotericin B. *Infection and Immunity*, **14**, 129–134.

Blume, R. S., Bennett, J. M., Yankee, R. A. & Wolff, S. M. (1968) Defective granulocyte regulation in the Chediak–Higashi syndrome. *New England Journal of Medicine*, **279**, 1009–1015.

Boyden, S. (1962) The chemotactic effect of mixtures of antibody and antigen on polymorphonuclear leukocytes. *Journal of Experimental Medicine*, **115**, 453–466.

Boxer, L. A., Greenberg, M. S., Boxer, G. J. & Stossel, T. P. (1975a) Autoimmune neutropenia. *New England Journal of Medicine*, **293**, 748–753.

Boxer, L. A., Hedley-Whyte, E. T. & Stossel, T. P. (1975b) Neutrophil actin dysfunction and abnormal neutrophil behavior. *New England Journal of Medicine*, **291**, 1093–1098.

Brandt, L. (1971) Enhancing effect of clofazimine (B663) on the phagocytosis of neutrophilic leukocytes *in vitro*. *Scandinavian Journal of Haematology*, **8**, 265–269.

Brayton, R. G., Stokes, P. E., Schwartz, M. S. & Louria, D. B. (1970) Effect of alcohol and various diseases on leukocyte mobilization, phagocytosis and intracellular bacterial killing. *New England Journal of Medicine*, **282**, 123–128.

Bryant, R. E., Sutcliffe, M. C. & McGee, Z. A. (1972) Effect of osmolalities comparable to those of the renal medulla on function of human polymorphonuclear leukocytes. *Journal of Infectious Diseases*, **126**, 1–10.

Caner, J. E. Z. (1965) Colchicine inhibition of chemotaxis. *Arthritis and Rheumatology*, **8**, 757–760.

Clark, R. A. & Kimball, H. R. (1971) Defective granulocyte chemotaxis in the Chediak–Higashi syndrome. *Journal of Clinical Investigation*, **50**, 2645–2652.

Clark, R. A., Root, R. K., Kimball, H. R. & Kirkpatrick, C. H. (1973) Defective neutrophil chemotaxis and cellular immunity in a child with recurrent infections. *Annals of Internal Medicine*, **78**, 515–519.

Cooper, M. R., DeChatelet, L. R., McCall, C. E., LaVia, M. F., Spurr, C. L. & Baehner, R. L. (1972) Complete deficiency of leukocyte glucose-6-phosphate dehydrogenase with defective bacterial activity. *Journal of Clinical Investigation*, **51**, 769–778.

Cutler, J. E. (1974) A simple *in vitro* method for studies on chemotaxis. *Proceedings of the Society for Experimental Biology and Medicine*, **147**, 471–474.

Dahl, M. V., Greene, W. H. & Quie, P. G. (1976) Infection, dermatitis, elevated IgE and impaired neutrophil chemotaxis. *Archives of Dermatology*, **112**, 1387–1390.

Dale, D. C., Fauci, A. S., Guerry, D. & Wolff, S. M. (1975) Comparison of agents producing a neutrophilic leukocytosis in man. *Journal of Clinical Investigation*, **56**, 808–813.

Davis, A. T., Brunning, R. O. & Quie, P. G. (1971a) Polymorphonuclear myeloperoxidase deficiency in a patient with myelomonocytic leukemia. *New England Journal of Medicine*, **285**, 789–790.

Davis, A. T., Estenson, R. D. & Quie, P. G. (1971b) Cytochalasin B. III. Inhibition of human polymorphonuclear leukocyte phagocytosis. *Proceedings of the Society for Experimental Biology and Medicine*, **137**, 161–164.

Davis, S. D. (1973) Antibody deficiency disorders. In *Immunologic Disorders in Infants and Children*, ed. Stiehm, E. R. & Fulginiti, V. A., pp. 184–198. Philadelphia: W. B. Saunders.

Deinard, A. S., Fortuny, I. E., Theologides, A., Anderson, G. L., Boen, J. & Kennedy, B. J. (1974) Studies on the neutropenia of cancer chemotherapy. *Cancer*, **33**, 1210–1218.

DeMeo, A. N. & Andersen, B. R. (1972) Defective chemotaxis associated with a serum inhibitor in cirrhotic patients. *New England Journal of Medicine*, **286**, 735–740.

Edelson, P. J. and Fudenberg, H. F. (1973) Effect of vinblastine on the chemotactic responsiveness of normal neutrophils. *Infection and Immunity*, **8**, 127–129.

Edelson, P. J., Stites, D. P., Gold, S. & Fudenberg, H. F. (1973) Disorders of neutrophil function. Defects in the early stages of the phagocytic process. *Clinical and Experimental Immunology*, **13**, 21–28.

Felarca, A. B. & Lowell, F. C. (1969) Local effects of cortisol in the time course of eosinophilotaxis with the use of an improved technique. *Journal of Allergy*, **43**, 114–118.

Finch, S. C. (1972) Granulocytopenia. In *Hematology*, ed. Williams, W. J., Beutler, E., Erslev, A. J. & Rundles, R. W., pp. 628–654. New York: McGraw-Hill.

Fine, D. P. (1975) Pneumococcal type-associated variability in alternate complement pathway activation. *Infection and Immunity*, **12**, 772–778.

Fink, M. E. & Finch, S. C. (1968) Serum muramidase and granulocyte turnover. *Proceedings of the Society for Experimental Biology and Medicine*, **127**, 365–367.

Forman, M. L., & Stiehm, E. R. (1969) Impaired opsonic activity but normal phagocytosis in low birthweight infants. *New England Journal of Medicine*, **281**, 926–931.

Forsgren, A. & Quie, P. G. (1974) Influence of the alternate complement pathway on opsonization of several bacterial species. *Infection and Immunity*, **10**, 402–404.

Forsgren, A., Schmeling, D. & Quie, P. G. (1974) Effect of tetracycline on the phagocytic function of human leukocytes. *Journal of Infectious Diseases*, **130**, 412–415.

Gallin, J. I. (1975) Abnormal chemotaxis: cellular and humoral components. In *The Phagocytic Cell in Host Resistance*, ed. Bellanti, J. A. & Dayton, D. H., National Institute of Child Health, pp. 227–243. New York: Raven.

Gallin, J. I., Clark, R. A. & Kimball, H. R. (1973) Granulocyte chemotaxis: an improved in vitro assay employing ⁵¹Cr-labeled granulocytes *Journal of Immunology*, **111**, 233–240.

Gallin, J. I. & Wolff, S. M. (1975) Leukocyte chemotaxis: physiological considerations and abnormalities. *Clinics in Haematology*, **4**, 567–607.

Goldman, J. M. & Sultan, C. (1975) Clinical applications of bone-marrow culture. *Lancet*, **ii**, 696–699.

Gotoff, S. (1973) Acquired and transient immunodeficiency disorders. In *Immunologic Disorders in Infants and Children*, ed. Stiehm, E. R. & Fulginati, V. A., pp. 303–330. Philadelphia: W. B. Saunders.

Grebner, J., Mills, E. L., Holmes, B. H. & Quie, P. G. (1977) Comparison of phagocytic and chemiluminescence response of human polymorphonuclear neutrophils. *Journal of Laboratory and Clinical Medicine*, **89**, 153–159.

Gregory, L. (1972) Leukocyte function in Down's syndrome and acute leukemia. *Lancet*, **i**, 1359–1361.

Hill, H. R., Estenson, R. D., Quie, P. G., Hogan, N. A. & Goldberg, N. D. (1975) Modulation of human neutrophilic chemotactic response by cyclic 3′5′-guanosine monophosphate and cyclic 3′5′-adenosine monophosphate. *Metabolism*, **24**, 447–456.

Hill, H. R., Gerrard, J. M., Hogan, N. A. & Quie, P. G. (1974a) Hyperactivity of neutrophil leukotactic response during active bacterial infection. *Journal of Clinical Investigation*, **53**, 996–1002.

Hill, H. R., Sauls, H. A., Dettloff, J. L. & Quie, P. G. (1974b) Impaired leukotactic responsiveness in patients with juvenile diabetes mellitus. *Clinical Immunology and Immunopathology*, **2**, 395–403.

Hill, H. R. & Quie, P. G. (1974) Raised serum IgE levels and defective neutrophil chemotaxis in three childten with eczema and recurrent bacterial infections. *Lancet*, **i**, 183–187.

Holmes, B., Quie, P. G., Windhorst, D. B. & Good, R. A. (1966) Fatal granulomatous disease of childhood: an inborn error of phagocyte function. *Lancet*, **i**, 1225–1228.

Huff, J. C., Weston, W. L., Nelder, K. H. & Hambidge, K. M. (1975) Defective monocyte chemotaxis and zinc deficiency in acrodermatitis entheropathica. *Clinical Research*, **23**, 229A.

Johnston, R. B., Jr, Newman, S. L. & Struth, A. G. (1973) An abnormality of the alternate pathway of complement activation in sickle-cell disease. *New England Journal of Medicine*, **288**, 803–808.

Kaplan, A. P., Goetzl, E. J. & Austen, K. F. (1973) The fibrinolytic pathway of human plasma. II. The generation of chemotactic activity by activation of plasminogen proactivator. *Journal of Clinical Investigation*, **52**, 2591–2595.

Khan, A. J., Evans, H. E., Glass, L. & Khan, P. (1975) Defective in vitro neutrophil chemotaxis induced by gentamicin. *15th Interscience Conference on Antimicrobial Agents and Chemotherapy*, Washington, DC, Abstract 65.

Klebanoff, S. J. (1975) Antimicrobial mechanisms in neutrophilic polymorphonuclear leukocytes. *Seminars in Hematology*, **12**, 117–142.

Lancet (1974a) Disorders of neutrophil function. *Lancet*, **i**, 438–440.

Lancet, (1974b) Another look at the N.B.T. test. *Lancet*, **i**, 664–665.

Lehrer, R. I. (1971) Inhibition by sulphonamides of the candidiacidal activity of human neutrophils. *Journal of Clinical Investigation*, **50**, 2498–2505.

Lehrer, R. I. & Cline, M. J. (1969) Leukocyte myeloperoxidase deficiency and disseminated candidiasis: the role of myeloperoxidase in resistance to *Candida* infection. *Journal of Clinical Investigation*, **48**, 1478–1488.

Maaløe, O. (1946) *On the Relation Between alexin and Opsonin*, 186 pp. Copenhagen: Munksgaards.

MacGregor, R. R., Spagnuolo, P. J. & Lentneh, A. Z. (1974) Inhibition of granulocyte adherence by ethanol, prednisone and aspirin measured with an assay system. *New England Journal of Medicine*, **291**, 642–646.

Malawista, S. E. & Bensch, K. G. (1976) Human polymorphonuclear leukocytes: demonstration of microtubules and effect of colchicine. *Science*, **156**, 521–522.

Malawista, S. E., Gee, J. B. L. & Bensch, K. G. (1971) Cytochalasin B reversibly inhibits phagocytosis: functional, metabolic and ultrastructural effects in human blood and rabbit alveolar macrophages. *Yale Journal of Biology and Medicine*, **44**, 286–300.

Mandell, G. L., Rubin, W. & Hook, E. W. (1970) The effect of an NADH oxidase inhibitor (hydrocortisone) on polymorphonuclear leukocyte bactericidal activity. *Journal of Clinical Investigation*, **49**, 1381–1388.

Mass, M. F., Dean, P. B., Weston, W. L. & Humbert, J. R. (1975) Leukocyte migration in vivo: a new method study. *Journal of Laboratory and Clinical Medicine*, **86**, 1040–1046.

McCall, C. E., Caves, J., Cooper, R. & DeChatelet, L. (1971) Functional characteristics of human toxic neutrophils. *Journal of Infectious Diseases*, **124**, 68–75.

McCulloch, E. A. (1975) Granulopoiesis in cultures of human haemopoietic cells. *Clinics in Haematology*, **4**, 509–533.

McCullough, J., Weiblen, B. & Quie, P. G. (1974) Chemotactic activity of human granulocytes preserved in various anticoagulants. *Journal of Laboratory and Clinical Medicine*, **84**, 902–906.

McLean, R. H. & Michael, A. F. (1973) Properdin and C3 proactivator: alternative pathway components in human glomerulonephritis. *Journal of Clinical Investigation*, **52**, 634–644.

Metchnikoff, E. (1968) *Lectures on the Comparative Pathology of Inflammation*. Delivered at the Pasteur Institute in 1891. (Translated by Starling, F. A. & Starling, E. H.) New York: Dover Publications.

Miller, M. E. (1971) Chemotactic function in the human neonate: humoral and cellular aspects. *Pediatric Research*, **5**, 487–492.

Miller, M. E. (1975) Pathology of chemotaxis and random mobility. *Seminars in Hematology*, **12**, 59–82.

Miller, M. E. & Baker, L. (1972) Leukocyte function in juvenile diabetes mellitus. Humoral and cellular aspects. *Journal of Pediatrics*, **81**, 979–982.

Miller, M. E. & Nilson, U. R. (1970) A familial deficiency of the phagocytosis-enhancing activity of serum related to a dysfunction of the fifth component of complement (C5). *New England Journal of Medicine*, **282**, 354–358.

Miller, M. E., Norman, M. E., Koblenzer, P. J. & Schonauer, T. (1973) A new familial defect of neutrophil movement. *Journal of Laboratory and Clinical Medicine*, **82**, 1–8.

Miller, M. E., Oski, F. A. & Harris, M. B. (1971) Lazy leukocyte syndrome: a new disorder of neutrophil function. *Lancet*, **i**, 665–669.

Müller-Eberhard, H. J. (1975) Complement and phagocytes. In *The Phagocytic Cell in Host Resistance*, ed. Bellanti, J. A. & Dayton, D. H., National Institute of Child Health, pp. 87–97. New York: Raven.

Nelson, R. D., Mills, E. L., Simmons, R. L. & Quie, P. G. (1976) The chemiluminescence response of phagocytizing human monocytes (in press).

Nelson, R. D., Quie, P. G. & Simmons, R. L. (1975) Chemotaxis under agarose: a new and simple method for measuring chemotaxis and spontaneous migration of human polymorphonuclear leukocytes and monocytes. *Journal of Immunology*, **115**, 1650–1656.

Park, B. H., Fikrig, S. M. & Smithwick, E. M. (1968) Infections and nitroblue tetrazolium reduction by neutrophils. A new diagnostic aid. *Lancet*, **ii**, 532–534.

Peters, W. P., Holland, J. F., Hansjoeg, S., Rhomberg, W. & Banerjee, T. (1972) Corticosteroid administration and localized leukocyte mobilization in man. *New England Journal of Medicine*, **286**, 342–345.

Pollard, T. D. & Weihing, R. A. (1974) Actin and myosin and cell movement. *CRC Critical Review in Biochemistry*, **2**, 1–65.

Quie, P. G. & Davis, A. T. (1973) Phagocytic and granulocytic disorders. In *Immunologic Disorders in Infants and Children*, ed. Stiehm, E. R. & Fulginiti, V. A. ,pp. 273–288. Philadelphia: W. B. Saunders.

Quie, P. G., White, J. G., Holmes, B. & Good, R. A. (1967) In vitro bactericidal capacity of human polymorphonuclear leukocytes: diminished activity in chronic granulomatous disease of childhood. *Journal of Clinical Investigation*, **46**, 668–679.

Rebuck, J. W. & Crowley, J. H. (1955) A method of studying leukocytic function in vivo. *Annals of New York Academy of Science*, **59**, 757–805.

Rivkin, I., Rosenblatt, J. & Becker, E. L. (1974) The role of cyclic AMP in the chemotactic responsiveness and spontaneous motility of rabbit peritoneal neutrophils. The inhibition of neutrophil movement and the elevation of cyclic AMP levels by catecholamines, prostaglandins, theophylline and cholera toxin. *Journal of Immunology*, **115**, 1126–1134.

Root, R. K. (1975) Comparison of other defects of granulocyte oxidative killing mechanisms with chronic granulomatous disease. In *The Phagocytic Cell in Host Resistance*, ed. Bellanti, J. A. & Dayton, D. H., National Institute of Child Health, pp. 201–219. New York: Raven.

Root, R. K., Rosenthal, A. S. & Balestra, D. J. (1972) Abnormal bactericidal, metabolic and lysosomal functions of Chediak–Higashi syndrome leukocytes. *Journal of Clinical Investigation*, **51**, 649–665.

Ruutu, T. (1972) Effect of phenothiazines and related compounds on phagocytosis and bacterial killing by human neutrophilic leukocytes. *Annales medicine experimentalis et biologiae Fenniae*, **50**, 24–36.

Samuels, A. J. (1951) Primary and secondary leukocyte changes following the intramuscular injection of epinephrine hydrochloride. *Journal of Clinical Investigation*, **30**, 941–947.

Schopfer, K & Douglas, S. D. (1976) Neutrophil function in children with kwashiorkor. *Journal of Laboratory and Clinical Medicine*, **88**, 450–461.

Senn, H. J. (1972) Infectabwehr bei Hämoblasten: Funktionelle Studien über Leukozytenmobilisation beim gesunden und kranken Menschen. *Experimentelle Medizin Pathologie und Klinik*, **36**, Berlin: Springer.

Simberkoff, M. S., Ricupero, I. & Rahal, J. R., Jr (1976) Host resistance to *Serratia marcescens* infection: serum bactericidal activity and phagocytosis by normal blood leukocytes. *Journal of Laboratory and Clinical Medicine*, **87**, 206–217.

Smith, C. W., Hellers, J. C., Dupree, E., Goldman, A. S. & Lord, R. A. (1972) A serum inhibitor of leukotaxis in a child with recurrent infections. *Journal of Laboratory and Clinical Medicine*, **79**, 878–885.

Snyderman, R., Altman, L. C., Frankel, A. & Blaese, R. M. (1973) Defective mononuclear leukocyte chemotaxis: a previously unrecognized immune dysfunction. Studies in a patient with chronic mucocutaneous candidiasis. *Annals of Internal Medicine*, **78**, 509–513.

Snyderman, R. & Stahl, C. (1975) Defective immune effector function in patients with neoplastic and immune deficiency diseases. In *The Phagocytic Cell in Host Resistance*, ed. Bellanti, J. A. & Dayton, D. H., National Institute of Child Health, pp. 267–281. New York: Raven.

Solberg, C. O. (1972a) Protection of phagocytized bacteria against antibodies. *Acta medica scandinavica*, **191**, 383–387.

Solberg, C. O. (1972b) Enhanced susceptibility to infection. A new method for the evaluation of neutrophil granulocyte functions. *Acta pathologica et microbiologica scandinavica*, Section B, **80**, 10–18.

Solberg, C. O. & Hellum, K. B. (1972) Neutrophil granulocyte function in bacterial infections. *Lancet*, **ii**, 727–730.

Soriano, R. B., South, M. A., Goldman, A. S. & Smith, C. W. (1973) Defect of neutrophil motility in a child with recurrent bacterial infections and disseminated cytomegalovirus infection. *Journal of Pediatrics*, **83**, 951–958.

Steerman, R. L., Snyderman, R., Leiken, S. L. & Colten, H. R. (1971) Intrinsic defect of the polymorphonuclear leukocyte resulting in impaired chemotaxis and phagocytosis. *Clinical Experimental Immunology*, **9**, 939–946.

Steigbigel, R. T., Johnson, P. K. & Remington, J. S. (1974) The nitroblue tetrazolium reduction versus conventional hematology in the diagnosis of bacterial infection. *New England Journal of Medicine*, **290**, 235–238.

Storti, E., Lusbarghi, E., Grignaffini, G. F. & Sgandurra, A. (1967) Biological and clinical significance of the adrenalin test in haematology. *Haematologia*, **1**, 27–34.

Stossel, T. P. (1975) Phagocytosis: recognition and Ingestion. *Seminars in Hematology*, **12**, 83–116.

Stossel, T. P., Alper, C. A. & Rosen, F. S. (1973) Opsonic activity in the newborn: role of properdin. *Pediatrics*, **52**, 134–137.

Stossel, T. P., Mason, R. J., Hartwig, J. & Vaughan, M. (1972) Quantitative studies of phagocytosis by polymorphonuclear leukocytes: use of emulsions to measure the initial rate of phagocytosis. *Journal of Clinical Investigation*, **51**, 615–624.

Strauss, R. R., Paul, B. B. & Sbarra, A. J. (1968) Effect of phenylbutazone on phagocytosis and intracellular killing by guinea-pig polymorphonuclear leukocytes. *Journal of Bacteriology*, **96**, 1982–1990.

Tan, J. S., Watanakundkorn, C. & Phair, J. P. (1971) A modified assay of neutrophil function: use of lysostaphin to differentiate defective phagocytosis from impaired killing. *Journal of Laboratory and Clinical Medicine*, **78**, 316.

Van Furth, R. (1970) Origin and kinetics of monocytes and macrophages. *Seminars in Hematology*, **7**, 125–141.

Van Oss, C. J. (1971) Influence of glucose levels on the in vitro phagocytosis of bacteria by human neutrophils. *Infection and Immunity*, **4**, 54–59.

Van Scoy, R. E., Hill, H. R., Ritts, R. E., Jr & Quie, P. G. (1975) Familial neutrophil chemotaxis defect, recurrent bacterial infections, mucocutaneous candidiasis, and hyperimmunoglobulinemia E. *Annals of Internal Medicine*, **82**, 766–771.

Verhoef, J., Peterson, P. K., Sabath, L. D. & Quie, P. G. (1977) Phagocytosis and intracellular survival of staphylococci. An assay using ³H-thymidine labeled bacteria and human polymorphonuclear leukocytes. *Journal of Immunological Methods* (in press).

Ward, P. A. (1966) The chemosuppression of chemotaxis. *Journal of Experimental Medicine*, **124**, 209–226.

Ward, P. A. (1972) Complement-derived chemotactic factors and their interactions with neutrophilic granulocytes. In *Biological Activities of Complement*, ed. Ingram, D. G., pp. 108–116. Basel: S. Karger.

Ward, P. A. & Berenberg, J. L. (1974) Defective regulation of inflammatory mediators in Hodgkin's disease. Supernormal levels of chemotacticfactor inactivator. *New England Journal of Medicine*, **290**, 76–80.

Ward, P. A. & Schlegel, R. J. (1969) Impaired leukotactic responsiveness in a child with recurrent infections. *Lancet*, **ii,** 344–347.

Wilkinson, P. C. (1974) *Chemotaxis and Inflammation*, 214 pp. Edinburgh and London: Churchill Livingstone.

Wintrobe, M. M., Lee, G. R., Boggs, D. R., Bithell, T. C., Athens, J. W. & Foerster, J. (1974a) Variations of leukocytes in disease. In *Clinical Hematology*, 5th edn, pp. 1266–1312. Philadelphia: Lea and Febiger.

Wintrobe, M. M., Lee, G. R., Boggs, D. R., Bithell, T. C., Athens, J. W. & Foerster, J. (1974b) Quantitative, morphologic and functional disorders of the granulocyte and monocyte-macrophage system. In *Clinical Hematology*, 5th edn, pp. 1313–1355. Philadelphia: Lea and Febiger.

Wollman, M. R., David, D. S., Brennan, B. L., Lewy, J. E., Stenzel, K. H., Rubin, A. L. & Miller, D. R. (1972) The nitroblue tetrazolium test. Usefulness in detecting bacterial infections in uraemic and immunosuppressed renal transplant patients. *Lancet*, **ii,** 289–293.

Wurster, N., Elsbach, P., Simon, E. J., Pettis, P. & Lebow, S. (1971) The effects of the morphine analogue levorphanol on leucocytes. Metabolic effects at rest and during phagocytosis. *Journal of Clinical Investigation*, **50,** 1091–1099.

Zigmond, S. H. & Hirsch, J. G. (1972) Effects of cytochalasin B on polymorphonuclear leukocyte locomotion, phagocytosis and glycolysis. *Experimental Cell Research*, **73,** 383–393.

9
THE CLINICAL USE OF ANTILYMPHOCYTE GLOBULIN

A. D. Barnes

Over the past 25 years disorders of the immune system have been implicated in an increasing number of clinical situations. In some circumstances there appears to be a damaging over-activity, and in therapy measures designed to dampen the response have been used. In other circumstances disease is associated with a lack of immune responsiveness, and therapy is aimed at stimulating the immune system in a variety of ways. One of the major limitations of the currently available measures that alter the immune response is their lack of specificity. Other drawbacks are the inability to assess the potency of such measures, and their inability to abolish immunological memory. The latter aspect of the immune response and indeed many other of its functions are controlled by the various subpopulations of lymphoid cells. It is not surprising, therefore, that antisera directed against lymphocytes have been used as a therapeutic tool in clinical practice in circumstances where a dampening down of immune responsiveness is indicated. This chapter reviews the clinical experience with antilymphocyte serum (or, in practice, the globulin fraction of such serum, ALG) and draws conclusions as to its future role.

EARLY EXPERIMENTS WITH ALG

The earliest description of a material which was akin to ALG was by Metchnikoff (1899). During the subsequent 50 years there were scattered reports which showed that the sera from animals injected with spleen, lymph node, thymus, tonsil, kidney, liver, heart or blood from other species were cytoxic in vitro to lymphoid cells of the donor species. When these sera were injected in vivo they had a variable effect. Some caused lymphopenia, often transient, some lymphoid hypoplasia, some were acutely toxic and others had no apparent effects.

It was not until Waksman and his colleagues (1961) showed that an ALG suppressed delayed hypersensitivity responses in rats that its clinical use was really considered. It was in the field of organ transplantation that the main clinical interest lay. Woodruff and Anderson (1963) produced a potent ALG which prolonged the survival of skin allografts and suppressed delayed hypersensitivity reactions. Since then there have been studies of the in vivo and in vitro effects of sera raised against almost every combination of cell type and in a very large number of species combinations. This review will be confined to those animal studies which are directly relevant to the clincal use of ALG or are important in understanding its mode of action.

Patients for whom treatment with ALG may be considered vary from those who are clearly mounting an immune response which is damaging to them (e.g. the allografted patient) to those whose primary disease process is thought to be immunologically mediated (e.g. multiple sclerosis) although the precise mechanisms are obscure. Some of the 'diseases' are acute and others are chronic or episodic. Although it is easy to document the start of an immunological reaction against an allograft it is impossible to determine the start of naturally occurring immunologically mediated disease. In the latter it is not until some tissue destruction has taken place that the 'disease' becomes clinically apparent. The symptoms and signs may be the result of progressive immunological damage or to scarring or healing of the first attack. The latter is unlikely to be influenced by ALG but may be influenced by steroids.

THE PRODUCTION OF ALG FOR CLINICAL USE

One of the greatest difficulties facing anyone working with ALG in the laboratory or clinic is to obtain a standard preparation. The potency of the preparation depends on whether the animal producing the serum makes appropriate antibodies to the right antigens on the heterologous lymphocytes which are used to raise the antilymphocyte serum. There are many different antigens on a lymphoid cell, some carry organ specificity, some allo-specificity and some xeno-specificity. There is evidence (Rogers, 1975) that the different antigenic specificities are on separate molecules in the cell surface membrane.

In order to obtain larger quantities of uniform serum it has become customary to pool the serum from a batch of immunised animals. Unfortunately this can pose problems if an animal produces a 'toxic' antibody which thus contaminates a large pool of serum. A nephritogenic agent was produced in the pool prepared for the first Canadian Medical Research Council trial of ALG in renal transplantation. Pooling sera also has the effect of diluting highly active sera with ones that are less active or have no activity at all. On the other hand pooling is the only practical way of producing a standardised product for large scale clinical use (Fig. 9.1).

Production of Antigen

Many types of cell have been used as sources of antigens to produce human ALG, but nowadays only antisera raised to cultured human lymphoblasts or to thymocytes are in general use.

Antispleen cell sera

These were easy to produce and were used extensively in renal transplantation by Starzl and his colleagues (1967). However these preparations often have high antierythrocyte and antiplatelet activity which is undesirable as absorption is necessary. In animal models antispleen sera have a lower and more variable immunosuppressive activity than other sera.

Antiperipheral blood (buffy coat) sera

This is a more readily available source of antigen than spleen as the buffy coat can be removed from blood in the preparation of frozen red cells and plasma protein preparations by the blood banks. The problem is that it is difficult to obtain a bulk antigenic preparation sufficiently free from erythrocytes and platelets to enable a serum to be produced that is low in anti-red cell and platelet activity.

Antithoracic duct cell sera

A very pure preparation of lymphocytes free from erythrocytes is obtained by cannulation of the thoracic duct. This procedure has been performed as an immunosuppressive measure in patients awaiting renal transplantation, but only produces relatively small quantities of lymphocytes at any one time. Such an antigen is, therefore, unsuitable for

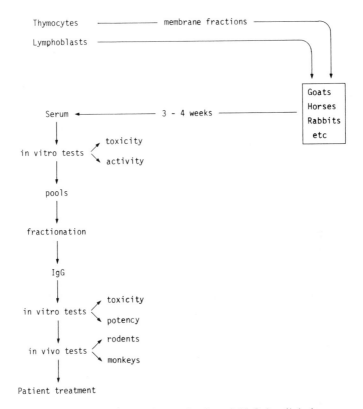

Figure 9.1   Flow chart for the production of ALG for clinical use

the large-scale production of ALG. The same applies to lymph node cell lymphocytes as a source of antigen for the preparation of ALG.

Antithymocyte sera

Human thymuses can be obtained from children undergoing open heart surgery where the gland is often subtotally removed for technical surgical reasons without harm to the patient. These provide a very pure preparation of lymphoid cells. The sera raised against thymocytes in most animal models are particularly potent and reliable immunosuppressive agents. They have low titres of erythrocyte and platelet antibodies and often do not require absorption. There are problems in the commercial production of such reagents but they can be used as the standard against which to compare other products. If thymic, splenic or lymph node stroma is induced in the immunising injection, antibodies fixing to the renal glomerular basement membrane may be produced, and may lead to subsequent renal damage in the grafted recipient.

Anticultured lymphoblast sera

There are now many virus-transformed human lymphoblast lines which are capable of being grown in bulk tissue culture. In this way many kilograms of lymphoid cells can be obtained free from erythrocytes, platelets and organ stroma. Moreover, the cell production can be geared to the immunisation protocol, without having to depend on the availability of clinical specimens at variable intervals (Sell et al, 1973). The use of this antigen does depend on the assumption that cultured transformed cells retain the surface antigens relevant to the induction of immunosuppressant antibodies.

FORM OF THE ANTIGEN

At the time when only clinical sources of antigen for ALG production were available these were obtained irregularly making immunisation schedules difficult to standardise. Therefore methods of storing antigen were investigated. Bulk storage of living cells in liquid nitrogen was feasible but very expensive. However, a cell membrane preparation which could be extracted from lymphoid tissue retained antigenic activity. Antisera raised against such a membrane preparation compared very well with those made against fresh whole cells so that any immunisation schedule was possible and the dose of antigen (number of cells) given at any one time could be varied at will.

The use of adjuvant

In most immunisation schedules the use of adjuvant allows the dose of antigen to be reduced, but adjuvants widen the spectrum of antibodies produced. In clinical ALG production adjuvants were used especially when the antigen sources were limited. However, if a larger dose of antigen without adjuvant was used less unwanted and potentially toxic antibodies were produced and the resultant sera required little or no absorption. Levey and Medawar (1966) produced in rabbits a good antimouse ALG by repeated intravenous injections of mouse lymphocytes. Barnes et al (1972) have confirmed this in rabbits with repeated intravenous injections of human thymocytes and in fact have shown, as have Binns et al (1971), that for man multiple subcutaneous, intramuscular and intraperitoneal administration with adjuvant produces a good ALG in several species.

Short or prolonged immunising schedules

There is no general agreement concerning a good in vitro test which correlates with the in vivo immunosuppressive activity of ALG. It is clear that sera which have no in vitro lymphocytotoxic activity will not be immunosuppressive, but conversely sera with very high cytotoxic titres may be inactive immunosuppressive agents in vivo. There are now many studies to show that the best immunosuppressive activity is obtained in the fourth week from the start of immunisation. If immunisation is continued for longer than four weeks, or is repeated after an interval, the cytotoxic titre will be higher but the immunosuppressive potency, as measured by skin graft survival, will be shorter. It is, therefore, uneconomical to take serum for more than three to four weeks after the peak of activity has been reached. New animals should then be used.

The species to immunise

Many species have been used for human ALG production and the decision as to which to use depends on availability, size, ease of handling, animal sensitisation in the population and potency of the sera obtained. Horses were used first as there was much experience in using horse antisera in man. It has been found, however, that horse ALG is probably not as active as some other types and horse sensitisation is common in the population. Rabbits probably produce the most potent ALG for human use, but are more expensive as only a small volume of serum can be obtained from each animal, and therefore production costs are high. Goats, pigs, sheep, cows and dogs can all be used to produce a good ALG. In my experience pig and cow ALGs are reliable and easy to produce; also prior sensitivity in the population is rare. It is important to have available products from more than one species so that should a patient be sensitised to one species another can be used.

Serum Processing

Test bleeds from individual animals, or small pools of animals in the case of rabbits, are tested for potential activity and toxicity. Sera with absent or very low cytotoxic activity, very high haemolytic or antiplatelet activity, and glomerular basement membrane fixation (Taylor, 1970) are excluded.

Sera are then processed in pools to produce the IgG fraction. The most frequent techniques use ammonium sulphate and DEAE Sephadex bulk fractionation or forced flow electrophoresis (Moberg et al, 1970). This usually yields a product which is 95 per cent IgG. The processing is performed in a sterile laboratory to reduce the possibility of producing pyrogens.

ALG is tested in vitro for cytotoxic, haemolytic, antiplatelet and antiglomerular basement membrane activity. Other in vitro tests are also performed which may correlate with in vivo immunosuppressive activity. These include rosette inhibition, mixed agglutination titres, lymphocyte opsonisation and many others. No single test or tests can be recommended as absolutely reliable and the choice is very much the personal preference of the investigator (Southworth et al, 1970; Greaves et al, 1969; Long et al, 1969). In vivo tests usually include acute toxicity studies in mice and rats, pyrogen tests in rabbits and skin allograft survival tests in monkeys (Balner, Eyzvoogel and Cleton, 1968).

The most commonly used in vivo method for testing human ALG for immunosuppressive activity is by its effect on the survival of skin allografts in monkeys. A 'good' product doubles or trebles skin allograft survival. However, in a series of experiments on the use of ALG alone to prolong renal allografts in monkeys, it was found that graft survival was not prolonged beyond controls, although the same ALG at the same dosage had doubled skin graft survival in other groups of the same species (Barnes et al, unpublished observations).

The product is then tested for sterility and packed in suitable storage volumes for clinical use. Most investigators store ALG at $-20°C$. Others prefer to store it at $5°C$ and to limit the storage time. There is conflicting evidence over the stability of ALG on long-term storage at any temperature (Courtney et al, 1975). ALG has been freeze-dried and reconstituted for clinical use. Freezing and freeze-drying can lead in some products to aggregation of the γ-globulin molecules, which is made worse by shaking during thawing or reconstitution. The microaggregates may be responsible for anaphylactic reactions when ALG is administered intravenously. Aggregates can be removed by ultracentrifugation immediately prior to clinical administration but this makes for great difficulties in clinical practice. Aggregate formation is a characteristic of ALG or IgG rather than ALS or whole serum. Thawing and refreezing also encourage aggregation. Aggregates probably increase the immunogenicity of ALG and hence restrict the time over which it may be administered without being subjected to immune elimination.

Route of Administration

Subcutaneous

This was the most commonly used route. It is safer when the ALG has a tendency to aggregate but it is painful, especially if a large volume (e.g. 20 ml) of ALG is given. Some products in some patients give very little local reaction whereas in other patients they produce large areas of brawny oedema, which can be extremely painful, and which leaves the skin over the sites looking as if it had been badly sunburned.

Intramuscular

This tends to have similar results to the subcutaneous route, but in our experience is even more painful.

Intravenous

This route has many advantages over the subcutaneous one and is being used more widely but there are problems with some products. If ALG is administered too rapidly (more than 4 mg/kg/h) there may be a hypotensive episode due to bradykinin release from the destroyed circulating lymphocytes (Bradley et al, 1971).

ALG can be administered by this route in at least three ways:

(i) by routine intravenous drip diluted in 250 to 500 ml normal saline,
(ii) as a concentrated solution via a syringe pump, and
(iii) by hand injection through a syringe.

After injection of the concentrated solution into a peripheral vein, the vein should be flushed with normal saline to reduce the incidence of venous thrombosis. Many clinicians prefer to inject ALG into a large vein via an indwelling central venous catheter. This may act as a portal for entry of organisms and lead to septicaemia, which is a major hazard in immunosuppressed patients. In patients undergoing renal transplantation, thrombosis of a vein is a serious complication, since, should the transplant fail, it reduces the superficial veins available for life-saving dialysis. ALG should never be injected into a dialysis arteriovenous fistula or shunt as this will almost invariably induce clotting.

In the present state of ALG preparations, they should always be administered by medical practitioners who know how to do so, and also know what complications to expect. This responsibility should not be delegated to nurses, although they may be called upon to monitor the pulse, temperature and blood pressure at least half-hourly during each administration and for 4 h thereafter.

THE CLINICAL USE OF ALG

Renal Transplantation

It is particularly in this field that one would expect a benefit to be seen from the ability of ALG to suppress completely the T-cell mediated cellular rejection of the transplanted kidney. Despite the use of ALG in cadaveric renal transplantation for a decade variations in the product and lack of controls reported in the trials make an assessment of its true value impossible even today (1976).

The longest experience reported in the literature is that of Starzl and his colleagues (1967), but neither in this nor any of their subsequent reports have there been adequate controls of transplanted patients who did not receive ALG. The control groups were retrospective, being those patients treated before the introduction of this reagent. The earlier sequential groups suggested a benefit but this could be explained by the authors achieving better results because of greater experience in the overall management of the transplanted patient. The ALG used in these patients was derived from horse antihuman spleen cell antiserum and it was given as a series of intramuscular injections for approximately four months and in addition to standard prednisone and azathioprine therapy. Five years later Starzl and his colleagues (1972) reviewed their experience of ALG after another 160 renal transplant patients had been treated. The benefits seen in the earlier series were less clear-cut and they conclude that whereas prednisone is indispensible for human renal allotransplantation the role of ALG is uncertain.

Shiel and his colleagues (1972, 1973) reported a sequential series of patients treated with prednisone and azathioprine alone, and with horse ALG or goat ALG. They claimed an unacceptable level of complications with horse ALG but a 12 per cent improvement in graft success with goat ALG. This is now given routinely in a dose of 10 mg/kg daily for five days following renal transplantation and these authors claim results with cadaveric transplantation which are better than the world experience. The ALG used in this trial was derived from antithymocyte serum and was made in small batches which had rather variable in vitro characteristics. No correlation with in vivo immunosuppressive results appeared in these reports. None was recorded by Shiel et al and the ALG used by Starzl's group showed no immunosuppressive effect on skin allografts in monkeys.

Simmons and his colleagues (1972a) reported their experience of 169 uncontrolled patients undergoing renal transplantation, and receiving horse ALG raised against cultured lymphoblasts. They claim that ALG was beneficial particularly in high risk elderly or diabetic patients receiving cadaveric grafts, in whom they were able to lower doses of prednisone. This claim is supported by the suggestion that patients who received the higher dose of ALG had the best graft survival. However this is not a fair assessment as the ALG dose was dictated by the patient's tolerance of it. Mannick and his colleagues (1972) using rabbit antithymocyte serum claimed that they obtained most benefit in patients who had been previously sensitised against transplantation antigens. At a symposium in Bad Soden in Germany in 1972 (Bad Soden Symposium, 1972) surgeons from America and Europe reported their experiences in the field of clinical renal transplantation and none of these communications indicated any definite benefit in using ALG. At a second symposium in London in 1975 a similar group of clinicians were likewise unable to be convinced of the benefit of ALG as an addition to the immunosuppressive regime. Some clinicians regarded their product as having minimal toxicity and some benefit, whereas others considered that the recipients of ALG might be more susceptible to overwhelming infections and be more likely to die from these with functioning transplants (Michel et al, 1975; Bach et al, 1973; Barnes, Samson and Hall, 1976). At a recent meeting of transplant surgeons there was a further series of reports of the use of ALG in renal transplantation (Transplantation Society Conference, 1977). These reports highlighted the marked variation in benefit between batches of supposedly standard preparations. A true assessment of the beneficial claims must await full publication of the studies. Much of the benefit claimed rests on the poor results of patients who did not receive ALG.

The dosage of ALG given in the various clinical series has varied considerably. Some of the doses have been scaled up on a mg/kg basis from rodent or monkey experiments. A summary of some of the schedules that have been used is given in Table 9.1, but this is not complete. Varying proportions of the patients have had the course of treatment curtailed because of the side-effects of ALG, in particular pain and allergic reactions.

Table 9.1 Examples of the variations in ALG dosage schedule given to patients following renal transplantation

Author	Species	Route	mg/kg	Duration
Starzl et al (1967)	Horse	i.m.	4–5	Four months
Mannick et al (1972)	Rabbit	s.c.	1.5	Five injections alternate days
Simmons et al (1972a, b)	Horse	i.v.	10	Daily 14 days
		i.v.	25	Daily 14 days
Shiel et al (1972, 1973)	Horse	i.m.	0.75	One week to three months
	Goat	i.v.	3–6	One week to three months
		i.v.	10	Daily five days
Barnes et al (1976)	Cow	i.v. or s.c.	7–14	Daily 10 days
	Pig	i.v. or s.c.	7–14	Daily 10 days
	Rabbit	i.v. or s.c.	7–14	Daily 10 days
Kountz[a]	Horse	i.v.	10	Daily 14 days

[a] Reported in Transplantation Society Conference 6 (1977)

Skin Transplantation

Although this form of transplantation forms the basis of almost all experimental work on this subject it might be asked whether there was any evidence of the beneficial effect of ALG on skin grafts in man. Monaco and his colleagues (1967) and Simmons and his colleagues (1972b) have shown that ALG prolongs the survival of skin allografts in man in relation to the dosage administered, 20 mg/kg being more effective than 4 mg/kg by a factor of 50 per cent. Although it might appear attractive to use ALG to prolong the survival of skin allografts in patients with burns too extensive to be treated by autografts alone there are few convincing reports of its success. In these circumstances because of the risks of infection corticosteroids might be contraindicated (Diethelm et al, 1972, 1974).

Liver Transplantation

There are only two centres in the world with a large experience of liver transplantation. Putnam et al (1976) claim that ALG is essential for the success of such grafts. Calne (1976) claims similar grafting success and never uses ALG. It should be remembered that allograft rejection is less vigorous in liver grafts than in kidney or heart grafts.

Heart Transplantation

At the world's most active heart transplant centre in Stanford, California, it is claimed that ALG is an essential component of the post-transplant immunosuppressant regime (Caves et al, 1973). There are no controls for this claim. Not only is a long course of ALG started at the time of transplantation but the dose is increased at the time of a clinical rejection episode. A similar regime has been used in renal transplantation but there is no evidence that ALG alone can reverse an acute rejection episode in renal transplantation. At present it must be accepted that heart and kidney transplants may differ in this respect.

Bone Marrow Transplantation

Bone marrow transplantation is immunologically very much more complex than renal transplantation (see Chap. 10). A prospective recipient will almost certainly have received, prior to the decision to transplant, multiple infusions of whole blood, leucocytes or platelets, usually from many donors. This usually results in sensitisation of the recipient against one or more of the histocompatibility antigens, and may lead to a more vigorous host versus graft (HVG) rejection. Moreover, the cells of a prospective bone marrow donor have the capability of reacting against the histocompatibility antigens of the recipient, and can give rise to a graft versus host (GVH) reaction. The marrow donor may have been presensitised by pregnancy or transfusion so that a more violent GVH reaction may occur. Attempts are made to reduce to a minimum these two-way reactions in marrow allografting by using mixed lymphocyte reactions to exclude highly reactive donors but such tests are imperfect.

It was logical therefore to use ALG in an attempt to reduce the GVH and HVG reaction in clinical bone marrow transplantation. ALG may be given to the donor, the donor cells may be exposed to ALG in tissue culture and ALG may be given to the recipient. Donor pretreatment is not usually regarded as ethical. There is no evidence to date to support the usefulness of the in vitro culture of bone marrow with ALG. However, Storb (1976) has found that after a marrow allotransplant in patients with aplastic anaemia, receiving cyclophosphamide and procarbizine treatment, ALG can effectively control acute episodes of GVH reaction. It is of interest that ALG therapy is effective in these patients, many of whom have had multiple sensitising blood transfusions. This may be the first demonstration in man that ALG can abolish immunological memory.

Theoretically it should be possible to process bone marrow transplants in vitro using sera specifically reactive against certain cell types. For example, in a patient with red cell aplasia it should be possible to exclude from the graft all but the precursors of the erythrocyte series; so far this approach has not been possible clinically. There are many differences between the reactions of rodents and of primates in experimental bone marrow transplantation, and many practical problems remain to be solved in this field.

CLINICAL USES OF ALG OTHER THAN FOR ORGAN TRANSPLANTATION

Compared with the allografting of tissues the rationale for the clinical use of ALG in non-transplant situations is less clear. Over the years a wide variety of diseases have been thought to be due to a hyperactive or an inappropriately active immune system. These are the so-called autoimmune diseases. However, the evidence that an immune reaction is the prime cause of the disease is usually weak; in none is it as clear-cut as in the allograft reaction. The current orthodox therapy for many of these diseases is prednisone with or without the addition of azathioprine or cyclophosphamide. In many cases this therapy is ineffective and in some the dosage required is toxic.

This had led a few clinicians to use ALG in these conditions usually when the conventional therapy has failed. However, there are problems in assessing its value. For most of these uncommon diseases the clinical course is variable, the criteria for diagnosis are inexact and subject to variable interpretation, and in most cases no exact animal model exists. Therefore controlled clinical trials are not available and many of the reports are anecdotal or concern a small series of uncontrolled patients.

Multiple Sclerosis

The aetiology of multiple sclerosis is unknown in man but there are several models of experimental encephalomeylitis in rats, guinea-pigs and mice. Waksman and his colleagues (1961) showed that ALG could have a beneficial effect on allergic encephalomyelitis in rats. Field (1969) showed a similar benefit in guinea-pigs. ALG could prevent the development of the disease but was not of value therapeutically once the disease was clinically established. Rook and Webb (1970) showed that the course of a virus-induced encephalomyelitis in mice could be altered beneficially by ALG. The benefit appeared to be due to an effect on cell-mediated immunity rather than to a reduction of specific antibody production.

It was not surprising, therefore, that ALG should be used therapeutically in multiple sclerosis. The studies of Pirofsky and his colleagues (1972) are typical of several uncontrolled clinical accounts. They suggest that clinical benefit may sometimes be observed. However, multiple sclerosis is a very difficult disease to assess because there are frequent changes in activity occurring spontaneously. Pirofsky claims two fair therapeutic responses and three failures in five patients treated.

Ring and his colleagues (1974) again in an uncontrolled series claim that they have prevented further deterioration of multiple sclerosis patients by adding ALG to other immunosuppressive regimes. They claim that patients who have had symptoms for less than 10 years are more likely to respond, since after this time the cerebral changes are more likely to be degenerative rather than inflammatory. The course of therapy they advocate is at least three weeks of intravenous therapy at more than 10 mg/kg ALG daily. Antithoracic duct serum was more effective than antilymphoblast serum.

Several uncontrolled trials are in progress at present. In one, under the aegis of the United Kingdom MRC, routine immunological assessment is carried out in parallel with the clinical assessment. Knight et al (1976) have shown that there is good evidence of immunosuppression in these patients as measured by in vitro tests, but a long-term clinical assessment is not yet available.

One problem with long-term use of ALG is the development of antibodies to the heterologous γ-globulin in the recipient which leads to rapid immune elimination. Tolerance to ALG can be achieved either by using large doses of ALG for short periods or by a desensitising procedure with normal globulin of the appropriate species (Taub et al, 1969).

Myasthenia Gravis

One of the most effective forms of treatment for myasthenia gravis is thymectomy. Some patients respond well only to relapse at a later date. Pirofsky and his colleagues (1972) report four excellent and four fair results with two failures in a group of 10 patients.

At this centre five patients have been treated each with a 10-day course of ALG (Barnes, 1976). All the patients had had a thymectomy with a good response some years (3–20 years) previously, although they had all relapsed, and were experiencing very troublesome side-effects from their medication. ALG appeared to be beneficial in four patients, allowing the cholinergic drugs to be reduced. In one patient a response to a course of ALG was obtained on two separate occasions one year apart. As in multiple sclerosis, the assessment of a response in patients with myasthenia gravis is very difficult. A controlled clinical trial is needed but this is difficult to arrange because of the rarity of the disease in its severe form, unresponsive to conventional therapy. Such evidence as there is suggests that ALG is most likely to be beneficial in treating a relapse after a successful thymectomy, possibly because it causes the elimination of T-cells that are colonising other lymphoid organs following the thymectomy.

Systemic Lupus Erythematosus, Polyarteritis Nodosa and Other Disorders

While evidence of benefit from ALG in the neurological field is scarce, evidence in other fields is even scarcer. Most of the reports are of a few isolated patients with a wide range of presenting symptoms who have had a wide variety of preceding or concurrent treatments. These have often included prednisone and azathioprine or cyclophosphamide. The course of the patient has varied from the dramatic improvement to no improvement and death.

We have given a 10-day course of ALG to each of five patients with acute severe renal impairment requiring dialysis, in whom the clinical and biopsy evidence indicated a diagnosis of polyarteritis nodosa. Three of the five had a clinical response and one has normal renal function more than four years later. These patients did not receive any other immunosuppressive therapy. A further patient presented with asthma which was treated with corticosteroids with partial benefit. He then had a massive patchy bowel infarction which histologically was due to polyarteritis. He then received ALG and an increase in prednisone. He died some four months later from intraperitoneal infection and small bowel fistulation but there were no further asthmatic attacks and at autopsy there was no evidence of polyarteritis. This suggests that ALG may have been beneficial in this case. The use of ALG in such cases is encouraging, because in the experience of most clinicians their prognosis is very poor. However, many more patients will need to be treated before a role for ALG can be defined.

A few patients with chronic hepatitis, rheumatoid arthritis, amyotrophic lateral sclerosis, diffuse encephalomyelitis, hypertrophic neuritis, Guillain Barré syndrome, scleroderma, Hammond–Rich syndrome, eosinophilic enteritis and lymphosarcoma have been treated with no benefit.

A few patients with autoimmune haemolytic anaemia, with or without an underlying lymphoma, have been treated with benefit. This follows the report by Denman and his colleagues (1967) that ALG suppresses the Coombs-positive anaemia in NZB mice. In none of the lymphoma patients was there any evidence of the exacerbation of the lymphoma under ALG treatment (Pirofsky et al, 1972).

From a theoretical standpoint, ALG should be used early in the acute stages of an 'autoimmune' disease as it is less likely to have an effect on the late disease, which is the result of scarring following the earlier damage. From the results so far reported many patients appear to have been treated late, after there had been no response to conventional treatment, usually corticosteroids. Nowadays it could be argued that a course of ALG is safer than a course of high dosage prednisone and should be used as an initial treatment. There are, of course, still hazards from ALG and the risks should be carefully considered before starting treatment.

ALG AND NEOPLASIA

Following the initial report of Penn and his colleagues (1969) that there was an increased incidence of tumours in transplanted patients receiving ALG many attempts have been made to find a connection between ALG therapy and an increased incidence of neoplasms. Reducing the number of T-cells might interfere with immune surveillance; also it has been shown that ALG can facilitate the induction of experimental tumours in animals (Balner and Dersjant, 1969; Zipp and Kountz, 1971). On the other hand several studies have failed to show an increase in spontaneous tumour formation after acute or chronic ALG therapy in patients. The only increases in malignancy in transplanted patients which are statistically significant are those of reticulum cell sarcoma (350 times normal) and lymphoma (35 times normal). There is no evidence that ALG administration increases this risk. However, at least one reticulum cell sarcoma has developed at the site of ALG injection. Any reports of tumours following renal transplantation should be regarded critically since tumours are not uncommon in a dialysis population. For example, at this centre recently a patient who had been maintained on regular haemodialysis for six years, was unexpectedly found to have a thyroid carcinoma while undergoing an operation for removal of the parathyroid glands. This could well have not come to light until after renal transplantation and possible ALG therapy. Last year three other patients on long-term dialysis presented with neoplasms from a population of about 100 on dialysis. In a series of 350 cadaveric renal transplants in our hospital over eight years, of whom 65 received ALG, only one patient developed neoplasia, and that patient had not received ALG.

In fact, ALG has been used in therapy in a small group of patients with lymphatic leukaemia or lymphomata who were resistant to more orthodox treatment. It is claimed that ALG can control the haemolytic process which sometimes occurs in these conditions (Pirofsky et al, 1972). It may be in the future that ALG could be of value in combination with drug therapy in lymphoid malignancies.

COMPLICATIONS OF ALG THERAPY

ALG may lead to therapeutic problems because of contained impurities, allergic reactions to the heterologous proteins and excessive immunosuppression.

Most of the unwanted antibodies and pyrogens can be excluded from material used clinically by scrupulous attention to detail during production of the ALG. Only rarely should a product with dangerous haemolytic, thrombocytolytic or antiglomerular basement membrane (nephritogenic) activity pass the laboratory screening. With a biological product it is always to be expected that variations may occur which fail to be detected in vitro or in laboratory animals but are of importance clinically. One variation that is commonly seen is that of the pain induced on subcutaneous or intramuscular injection. There is an element of patient pain threshold variation but some ALG preparations give more pain than others. The same applies to the frequency of thrombophlebitis after intravenous administration into peripheral veins.

The administration of any heterologous protein can cause an allergic response in the recipient, either as a result of presensitisation or later in the course of ALG administration from antibody production. Urticaria is common and is not usually of importance clinically. It does not require ALG therapy to be discontinued and can be controlled by antihistamines. Serum sickness occurs occasionally some days after starting therapy. This is due to antigen–antibody complex production and dictates cessation of ALG therapy. Rarely acute anaphylaxis occurs which can be fatal. Hydrocortisone and adrenaline should be available for emergency use at all times when ALG is being given and the staff should be aware of the earliest symptoms and signs of anaphylaxis.

ALG enhances the growth of viruses in many experimental animals (Edelmann and Wheelock, 1968; Hirsch and Murphy, 1968; Gaugas and Rees, 1968). Unfortunately there is no conclusive evidence in clinical practice. Some authors, including ourselves, have observed a higher incidence of deaths from infection following cadaveric renal transplantation with ALG than in controls whereas other series find no difference. As about 50 per cent of the deaths following renal transplantation are due to or are accompanied by infection an effect of ALG is difficult to determine.

INDUCTION OF TOLERANCE TO ALG

ALG is at least as immunogenic, if not more so, than the normal immunoglobulin from the same species. The antibodies produced markedly reduce the half-life of ALG by causing immune elimination. This renders a dose of ALG ineffective. Knight (1976) has attempted to render the recipient tolerant of the heterologous protein by giving intravenously a large (tolerogenic) dose of normal IgG. This enabled a protracted course of ALG to be given without antibody formation against the ALG. This technique is not appropriate to the administration of ALG in the near emergency situation of cadaveric renal transplantation, but such an approach may be of value in other circumstances.

THE FUTURE OF ALG THERAPY

Less has been published on ALG recently than two or three years ago. This is because ALG went through a honeymoon when many types were used by numerous clinicians in a wide variety of conditions often with no controls. We are now in a consolidation period where some clinicians have become disenchanted with ALG while others are involved in clinical trials or new treatment schedules for ALG. The manufacturers are attempting to provide more standardised products at a reasonable price, free from unwanted immune reactions, which would replace the clinicians' home-made concoctions. Currently a recommended course of commercially available ALG costs £500 to £1500 ($1000 to $3000) so that it is very important to define its clinical role. Much work needs to be done using ALG with forms of immunosuppression other than non-specific ones like prednisone and azathioprine. There are indications that ALG can be used to increase the potency of the specific forms of immunosuppression involving the use of specific antigen or enhancing sera when a cocktail of these materials is used. It is to be expected that satisfactory results will be dependent on the correct dosage and timing of the individual treatment regimes. Despite the lull I do not think we have heard the last of ALG as a clinical tool but I believe that we will not use it in its present manner for much longer.

REFERENCES

Bach, M. C., Sahyoun, A., Adler, J. L., Schlesinger, R. M., Breman, J., Madras, P., P'eny, F. & Monaco, A. P. (1973) High incidence of fungal infections in renal transplantation patients treated with antilymphocyte and conventional immunosuppression. *Transplantation Proceedings*, **5,** 549–553.

Bad Soden Symposium on ALG (1972) *Behringwerke Research Communications*, **51.** Behringwerke AG, Marburg.

Balner, H., Eyzvoogel, V. P. & Cleton, F. J. (1968) Testing of anti-human lymphocyte sera in chimpanzees and lower primates. *Lancet*, **i,** 19–22.

Balner, H. & Dersjant, H. (1969) Increased onocogenic effect of methylcholanthrine after treatment with antilymphocyte serum. *Nature*, **224,** 376–378.

Barnes, A. D., Hawker, R. J., Cowdell, E. I., Dickerson, C., Dukes, H., Griffin, H., Crozier, B., Fejfar, J., Robinson, B. H. B. & Blainey, J. D. (1972) The production of immunosuppressive antisera. *Proceedings of EDTA*, **9,** 364–370.

Barnes, A. D. (1976) The use of antithymocyte globulin in myasthenia gravis. *Postgraduate Medical Journal*, **52,** 112.

Barnes, A. D., Sansom, J. R. & Hall, C. L. (1976) A randomized prospective clinical trial of antilymphocyte globulin in 100 cadaveric renal transplants. *Postgraduate Medical Journal*, **52,** 75–76.

Binns, R. M., Simpson, E., Nehlsen, S. L. & Ruskiewicz, M., (1971) A method of producing immunosuppressive antilymphocyte serum in pigs and ruminants. *Transplantation Proceedings*, **3,** 784–788.

Bradley, J., Cuschieri, A., Mason, K. & Moran, B. (1971) Kinin liberation during therapy with anti-lymphocyte globulin. *Lancet*, **ii,** 578–581.

Calne, R. Y. (1976) *Postgraduate Medical Journal*, **52,** 108 (in discussion).

Caves, P. K., Stinson, E. B., Griepp, R. B., Rider, A. K., Dong, E. & Shumway, N. E. (1973) Results of 54 cardiac transplants. *Surgery*, **74,** 307–314.

Courtney, J. S., Thomas, D., Mosedale, B., Damjonovic, V. & Phillips, A. W. (1975) Studies in the stability of the antilymphocyte globulins. *Transplantation*, **19,** 394–399.

Davis, R. C., Nabreth, D. C., Olssen, C. A., Idelson, B. A., Schmitt, G. W., Cho, S. I. & Mannick, J. A. (1974) Use of rabbit ATG in cadaveric kidney transplantation. *Transplantation Proceedings*, **6,** 67–70.

Denman, A. M., Denman, E. J. & Holborrow, E. J. (1967) Suppression of Coombs positive haemolytic anaemia in N.Z.B. mice by antilymphocyte globulin. *Lancet*, **i,** 1084–1086.

Diethelm, A. G., Dimick, A., Shaw, J. F., Baker, H. & Wilson, S. P. (1972) Management of the severely burned child utilising skin allografts modified by equine antithymocyte globulin. *Behringwerke, Research Communications*, **51.**

Diethelm, A. G., Dimick, A., Shaw, J. F., Baker, H. & Phillips, S. J. (1974) Treatment of the severely burned child with skin transplantation modified by immunosuppressive therapy. *Annals of Surgery*, **180,** 814.

Edelman, R. & Wheelock, E. F. (1968) Enhancement of replication of vesicular stomatitis virus in human lymphocyte cultures treated with heterologous antilymphocyte serum. *Lancet*, **i,** 771–773.

Field, E. J. (1969) Antilymphocyte serum in experimental allergic encephalomyelitis. *British Medical Journal*, **2,** 758–760.

Gaugus, J. M. & Rees, R. J. W. (1968) Enhancing effect of antilymphocyte serum on mycobacterial infections in mice. *Nature*, **219,** 408–409.

Greaves, M. F., Tursi, A., Playfair, J. H. L., Torrigiani, G., Zamir, R. & Roitt, I. M. (1969) Immunosuppressive potency and in vitro activity of antilymphocyte globulin. *Lancet*, **i,** 68.

Hirsch, M. S. & Murphy, F. A. (1968) Effects of antilymphoid sera on viral infections. *Lancet*, **2,** 37–40.

Knight, S. C., Abbosh, J. & Lance, E. M. (1976) The effect of intensive immunosuppression on the *in vitro* activity of lymphocytes from multiple sclerosis patients. *Postgraduate Medical Journal*, **52,** 131–134.

Levey, R. H. & Medawar, P. B. (1966) The production of antilymphocyte serum in rabbits. *Annals of the New York Academy of Sciences*, **129,** 164.

Long, D. A., Edwards, D. C., Phillips, A. W. & Woiwod, A. J. (1969) Large scale production of antilymphocyte antibody. *Proceedings of the Royal Society of Edinburgh*, **70,** 346–354.

Mannick, J. A., Nabreth, D. C., Olsson, C. A. & Davis, R. C. (1972) Early low dose rabbit ALG therapy in cadaveric renal transplantation. *Transplantation Proceedings*, **4,** 497–499.

Metchnikoff, E. (1899) Études sur la résorption des cellules. *Annales de l'institut Pasteur*, **13,** 737.

Michel, R. P., Guttman, R. D., Knaack, J., Klassen, J., Bendoim, J. G. & Morehouse, D. D. (1975) Antilymphocyte globulin in renal transplantation. *Archives of Surgery*, **110,** 90–93.

Moberg, A. W., Gewurz, H., Jetzer, T., Simmons, R. L. & Najarian, J. S. (1970) Forced flow electrophoretic purification of antihuman antilymphoblast globulin. *Surgery*, **65**, 862–869.

Monaco, A. P., Wood, M. L. & Russell, P. S. (1967) Some effects of purified heterologous antihuman lymphocyte serum in man. *Transplantation*, **5**, 1106.

Penn, I., Hammond, W., Brettsneider, L. & Starzl, T. E. (1969) Malignant lymphomas in transplantation patients. *Transplantation Proceedings*, **1**, 106.

Pirofsky, B., Ramirez-Moghadam, J. C., Bardana, E. J. & Reid, H. (1972) Medical uses of antithymocyte antisera therapy. *Behringwerke Research Communications*, **51**, 183.

Putnam, C. W., Beart, R. W., Bell, R. H. & Starzl, T. E. (1976) Hepatic transplantation in 1975. *Postgraduate Medical Journal*, **52**, 104–108.

Ring, J., Lob, G., Angstwurm, H., Brass, B., Bockmund, H., Seifert, J., Coulin, K., Frick, E., Martin, J. & Brendel, W. (1974) Intensive immunosuppression in the treatment of multiple sclerosis. *Lancet*, **ii**, 1093–1096.

Rogers, K. (1975) Personal communication.

Rook, G. A. W. & Webb, H. E. (1970) Antilymphocyte serum and tissue culture used to investigate role of cell-mediated response in viral encephalitis in mice. *British Medical Journal*, **2**, 210–212.

Sell, K., Woody, J., Smith, J., Darrow, C. & Kayhoe, D. (1973) Evaluation of human cultured lymphoblasts as a source of antigen for production of immunosuppressive antilymphocyte sera. *Transplantation Proceedings*, **5**, 541–547.

Shiel, A. G. R., Mears, D., Kelly, G. E., Stewart, J. H., Johnson, J. R., Tiller, D., Gallery, E. D. M. & Duggan, G. (1972) A controlled trial of antilymphocyte globulin therapy (ALG) in man. *Transplantation Proceedings*, **4**, 501–505.

Shiel, A. G. R., Kelly, G. E., Mears, D., May J., Johnson, J. R., Ibels, L. S. & Stewart, J. H. (1973) Antilymphocyte globulin in patients with renal allografts from cadaveric donors. Late results of a controlled trial. *Lancet*, **i**, 227–228.

Simmons, R. L., Condie, R. & Najarian, J. S., (1972a) Antilymphoblast globulin for renal allograft prolongation. *Transplantation Proceedings*, **4**, 487–490.

Simmons, R. L., Moberg, A. W., Condie, R. & Najarian, J. S. (1972b) Prolongation of skin allografts in man using antilymphoblast globulin. *Behringwerke Research Communications*, **51**, 149–153.

Southworth, J. G., Ohanion, S. H., Plate, J. M. & Amos, D. B. (1970) Heterologous antihuman and antimouse sera prepared in horse, goat, rabbit and cow. *Federation Proceedings*, **79**, 101–102.

Starzl, T. E., Marchioro, T. L., Porter, K. A., Iwasaki, Y. & Cirelli, G. J. (1967) The use of heterologous antilymphoid agents in canine renal and liver homotransplantation and in human renal homotransplantation. *Surgery, Gynecology and Obstetrics*, **124**, 301–318.

Starzl, T. E., Groth, C. G., Kashiwagi, N., Putnam, G. W., Corman, J. L., Halgrimson, C. G. & Penn, I. (1972) Clinical experience with horse antihuman ALG. *Transplantation Proceedings*, **4**, 491–495.

Storb, R., Weiden, P. L. & Thomas, E. D. (1976) The use of anti-thymocyte serum in clinical and experimental marrow transplantation. *Postgraduate Medical Journal*, **52**, 96–101.

Taub, R. N., Kochwa, S., Brown, S. M., Rubin, R. D. & Dameshek, W. (1969) Antigen-induced immunological tolerance in man to equine antihuman thymocyte gamma-globulin. *Lancet*, **2**, 521–523.

Taylor, H. E. (1970) The occurrence of glomerular basement membrane reactive antibodies in antihuman antithymocyte globulin. *Transplantation Proceedings*, **2**, 413–416.

Transplantation Society Conference 6, New York, August 1976. To be published in *Transplantation Proceedings* (1977).

Waksman, B. H., Arboruys, S. & Arnason, B. J. (1961) The use of specific 'lymphocyte antisera' to inhibit hypersensitive reactions of the delayed type. *Journal of Experimental Medicine*, **114**, 997.

Woodruff, M. F. A. & Anderson, N. (1963) The effect of lymphocyte depletion by thoracic duct fistula and administration of anti-lymphocytic serum on the survival of skin homografts in rats. *Nature*, **200**, 702.

Zipp, P. & Kountz, S. L. (1971) Analysis of the immunosuppressive and oncogenic effects of heterologous antilymphocyte serum. *American Journal of Surgery*, **122**, 204–208.

10
REPLACEMENT THERAPY IN IMMUNODEFICIENCY

Rebecca H. Buckley

From the wealth of information now accumulated in the world's literature about the various immunodeficiency diseases and the therapies presently available for them, two important points emerge relevant to the subject of this article. The first is that well-defined immunodeficiency, the only true indication for replacement therapy, is rare (Medical Research Council, 1971) and the second is that currently available forms of therapy for such defects leave much to be desired. The latter is particularly true with respect to prevention of infections of the respiratory and gastrointestinal systems in patients with these disorders, primarily because of the lack of any effective way of replacing secretory IgA antibodies at mucous membrane surfaces except by complete immunologic reconstitution through transplantation of immunocompetent tissue. An even greater problem exists for those patients with deficits in thymus-dependent (T) or cell-mediated immune (CMI) function, however, where immunocompetent tissue grafts again provide the only hope for significant or long-term correction. Unfortunately, due to the biological laws governing transplantation immunology the latter therapy is available to only a select few with particular forms of immunodeficiency (Buckley, 1973).

TREATMENT OF HUMORAL IMMUNODEFICIENCY

In those conditions characterised by deficiencies in specific humoral immunity, there is undoubtedly benefit from the systemic replacement of IgG antibodies through administration of whole plasma or immunoglobulin concentrates. The successes noted following humoral replacement therapy for the first such host defect found to predispose to severe recurrent infections (Bruton, 1952) led for a time, however, to rather widespread and indiscriminate use of gammaglobulin injections in patients with recurrent respiratory infections who were not documented to be immunodeficient (Miller, 1969). Further misuse of this form of therapy has been fostered by physicians' use of improper diagnostic tests and inappropriate normative laboratory values in evaluating pediatric-age patients with suspected host deficits. This has led to frequent erroneous diagnoses of humoral immunodeficiency and often to years of unnecessary gammaglobulin injections in children. The only presently acceptable indication for use of humoral replacement therapy for prevention of recurrent infections is the clear demonstration of a host deficit in this limb of the immune system.

Professor Buckley is the recipient of Allergic Diseases Academic Award No. A170830-03.

Indications and Contraindications

Passive antibody therapy is indicated in all immunodeficiency states where severe impairment in antibody formation is demonstrated (Fudenberg et al, 1971; Cooper et al, 1973). These include especially those primary immunodeficiency diseases characterised by low or undetectable quantities of all five serum immunoglobulins, e.g. the 'a-' or 'hypo-' gammaglobulinaemias. In addition, humoral replacement therapy is indicated for patients with X-linked immunodeficiency with hyper-IgM and even for normogamma-globulinaemic immunodeficient patients who are shown to have marked impairment in their abilities to produce specific antibodies following immunisation. Deficits in humoral immunity in which replacement therapy with gammaglobulin or plasma is not indicated, however, include transient hypogammaglobulinaemia of infancy and selective IgA deficiency. In the former situation, these infants usually have the capacity to make specific antibodies normally following immunisation, despite low concentrations of all or some of the immunoglobulins during the first 15 to 18 months of life. Administration of passive antibody could suppress this ability and do more harm than good. In the case of selective IgA deficiency the lack of appropriate replacement therapy is unfortunate, since it is in all probability the most common of the well-defined immunodeficiency disorders and a high percentage of individuals with this defect are subject to chronic and recurrent respiratory infection (Buckley, 1975a). Patients with selective IgA deficiency usually have the ability to produce antibodies of the other immunoglobulin classes normally, however. Indeed a significant proportion of such individuals produce antibodies to IgA (Vyas, Levin and Fudenberg, 1970), and these have been implicated as the cause of anaphylactic transfusion reactions in some of these patients (Vyas, Perkins and Fudenberg, 1968; Schmidt, Taswell and Gleich, 1969). For this reason, humoral replacement therapy is contraindicated in this form of immunodeficiency. Moreover, even if products containing IgA could be given safely to patients with selective IgA deficiency, they still could not effect replacement of that immunoglobulin at mucous membrane surfaces, as mentioned above. This is due to the fact that secretory IgA in normal individuals derives from paragut and pararespiratory lymphoid tissue and is not transported from the intravascular compartment to external secretions, as originally thought. Indeed, even after intravenous infusions of large volumes of IgA-containing plasma into one agammaglobulinaemic patient, an increase in IgA could not be detected in his external secretions, and radiolabelled IgA infused into normal subjects could not be demonstrated in saliva or breast milk (Stiehm, Vaerman and Fudenberg, 1966).

Types of Therapy

Replacement therapy for correction of deficits in humoral immunity consists of the administration of either immune serum globulin (ISG) or normal plasma at regular intervals throughout the life of the patient. The commercially available ISG can be given only by the intramuscular route, but experimental intravenous forms of ISG are presently under investigation.

Immune serum globulin (ISG) for intramuscular use
This material is ordinarily prepared from outdated blood bank plasma or from placentas by the alcohol–salt fractionation method of Cohn et al (1950) and is supplied commercially

in solutions containing 14.5 to 16.5 g/100 ml of IgG (Heiner and Evans, 1967). Although these prepartions consist principally of IgG, they have also been shown to contain varying quantities of IgA, IgM, IgD, albumin, β1C, transferrin and placenta-specific proteins. The content of these latter proteins depends primarily upon whether the material is derived from plasma or placental sources but also upon technical variations in their preparation (Heiner and Evans, 1967). Gammaglobulin derived from placentas usually contains more IgA, IgM and IgD than does that prepared from plasma (Heiner and Evans, 1967), but the quantities of these proteins present even in the placentally derived preparations (less than 5 per cent of the total protein for any one of the immunoglobulins A, M or D) are probably inconsequential from a clinical standpoint in view of the very short half-lives of these immunoglobulins (Waldmann and Strober, 1969). The one exception to this statement is that patients with selective IgA deficiency may have life-threatening anaphylactic reactions to the small amount of IgA present in ISG preparations (Vyas et al, 1968). Gammaglobulin prepared by the alcohol–salt fractionation method has been found to be remarkably stable, showing little change in concentration of gamma-migrating protein or clinical effectiveness when stored at 4°C for as long as four years (MacKay, Vallet and Cambridge, 1973). Such preparations have been shown to aggregate and fragment, however, as well as to demonstrate anticomplementary activity to varying degrees upon storage. These changes occur more often in preparations from which ethanol is not completely removed by dialysis and in those contaminated to a greater degree by endogenous plasmin (MacKay et al, 1973). This anticomplementary activity is due to the formation of aggregates which have the ability to activate the complement system (Christian, 1960); it is to this property that clinical reactions to gammaglobulin injections have often been attributed (Richerson and Seebohm, 1966). The half-life of IgG in such preparations has been shown to vary from 17.5 to 22.1 days, with a mean of 19.8 days in normal subjects (Janeway et al, 1968). It is likely to be even longer in agammaglobulinaemic patients, since the mean half-life of IgG given in plasma or isolated from it by ion-exchange cheomatography was shown to be 32 days in five such patients studied by Stiehm et al (1966). The half-life is also likely to be affected by the clinical state of the patient, since other studies also showed a shortened survival for IgG in these patients during episodes of infection (Stiehm et al, 1966).

The recommended dose of ISG for the treatment of primary humoral immunodeficiency is 0.1 g/kg month (0.6 to 0.7 ml/kg month) after a loading dose of two to three times that amount. These doses, of necessity, require the administration of large volumes by the intramuscular route resulting in great discomfort to the recipient. It is generally considered inadvisable to give more than 20 to 30 ml at a time, or 40 ml per month, and no more than 5 ml per injection site because of this and other reasons discussed below. Many physicians who treat older patients with severe humoral deficiency recommend giving 10 ml/week of ISG to avoid giving too large a dose at any one time. The preferred injection sites are the buttocks, but the anterior thighs and deltoids may also be used. It is well to point out that the dose recommended above has been arrived at empirically from arbitrary clinical trials (Medical Research Council, 1971; Janeway et al, 1967) but that in practice it has seemed to be nearly as effective as twice that amount (Medical Research Council, 1971). Since half the above recommended dose was ineffective in one large study (Medical Research Council, 1971), and since there is considerable variability in immunoglobulin and antibody content from lot to lot of the commercially available preparations, further investigation of optimal dosage is needed. Furthermore, there would appear to be a need for establishing routine objective parameters for use in following the efficacy of therapy in such patients in addition to the subjective evaluations of clinical effectiveness.

ADVERSE REACTIONS TO ISG

As mentioned above, there are several theoretically possible adverse effects from the administration of homologous antibody globulins. In addition, there are well-documented adverse reactions to ISG because of problems unique to its fractionation and administration. The repeated large volumes administered intramuscularly to patients with immunodeficiency not only cause a great deal of pain but are a source of considerable psychological difficulty in some children with these defects. Adverse local reactions which have been encountered include sterile abscesses, fibrosis and sciatic or other nerve injuries. Infrequent but sometimes serious systemic reactions were also reported by the British Medical Research Council Working Party on Hypogammaglobulinaemia to have affected 32 out of 175 (18 per cent) patients treated over an 11 year period with ISG, and one death occurred (Medical Research Council, 1971). It became necessary to discontinue therapy in five of these patients, in part because of such reactions. As noted above, systemic reactions in agammaglobulinaemic patients are believed to be due to entry of aggregated immunoglobulin molecules into the intravascular compartment during administration of the large intramuscular volumes. This is thought to result in activation of the complement system and generation of anaphylotoxin and other vasoactive substances (Richerson and Seebohm, 1966). In one agammaglobulinaemic patient, however, the reaction was thought to be due to an antibody to aggregated gammaglobulin in the recipient's serum which could be demonstrated by agar gel diffusion (Ellis and Henney, 1969). Systemic reactions to ISG injections have also been noted in patients with selective IgA deficiency who have antibodies to IgA (Vyas et al, 1968). Symptoms of such reactions may appear from seconds to minutes to several hours after the injections and include flushing and facial swelling, dyspnoea, cyanosis, anxiety, nausea, vomiting, malaise, hypotension and even loss of consciousness. The treatment should be the immediate administration of epinephrine and antihistamines.

In the Medical Research Council Working Party on Hypogammaglobulinaemia study (1971) it was noted that agammaglobulinaemic boys with affected male relatives were significantly spared from systemic reactions and that the frequency of such reactions did not appear to correlate with the degree of anticomplementary activity of the batches of gammaglobulin employed. Indeed, the distribution of reactions among the 40 different batches used was random. These observations led members of the Working Party to suggest that the mechanism of the reaction may be related to the underlying disease of the recipient. It was also noted that such reactions could start at any stage of treatment and that the incidence did not change with length of therapy, arguing against a mechanism involving some form of immunisation. In any case, until more is known about the nature of such reactions, patients with a history of such reactions should be given a small test dose of ISG from a different supplier before such therapy is resumed. The test dose should be given in an extremity so that a tourniquet may be applied in the event of any sign of an adverse reaction. Skin testing with ISG preparations was found to be of no help in guiding the course of future therapy in such patients (Medical Research Council, 1971; Barunden et al, 1962).

Intravenous gammaglobulin preparations

These ISG preparations have all been treated in some way to render them aggregate-free and to eliminate anticomplementary activity. While several have undergone testing or are being tested in carefully supervised clinical trials, they are not available commercially since none has been licensed for general use in the United States. There are several advantages to the administration of ISG by the intravenous route: (1) much larger doses can be given than would be possible by the intramuscular route, (2) the action is more rapid, (3) there is no loss due to local proteolysis and (4) the therapy is far less painful. Unfortunately, reactions to intravenous infusions of unmodified ISG are more frequent and more severe in patients who stand to benefit most from them—e.g. patients with antibody deficiency—than in normals, for reasons which are poorly understood (Barunden et al, 1962). The symptoms and signs of such reactions are similar to those occurring with intramuscular ISG injections but may also include chills, fever, pallor and fatigue beginning 1 to 2 h after the infusion.

There has been considerable interest for over a decade now in the development of ISG preparations which would be safe for intravenous use, and several approaches have been tried (Barunden et al, 1962). These include: (1) physical removal of high molecular weight aggregates by ultracentrifugation or gel filtration, (2) treatment of the preparations with proteolytic enzymes, (3) treatment with certain chemicals which affect specific sites on the gammaglobulin molecule or with sulph-hydryl bond reducing agents and (4) incubation of these preparations at a low pH for varying periods of time. Successful removal of aggregates by ultracentrifugation requires an extremely high centrifugal force and does not appear to be practical for the large-scale production of ISG for intravenous use.

Treatment of such preparations with proteolytic enzymes such as trypsin, pepsin, or plasmin eliminates anticomplementary activity quite effectively and renders them safe for intravenous use (Janeway et al, 1968; Jager, 1967; Simons, Schumacher and Fowler, 1968). Unfortunately, however, immunoglobulin molecules which have been subjected to enzymatic treatment fragment into low molecular weight subunits which are more rapidly cleared from the circulation than the intact molecule, thereby compromising the duration of the passive immunity rendered. Plasmin-treated gammaglobulin preparations appear to be far superior to those treated with other proteolytic enzymes, since a considerable proportion of the plasmin-treated material retains a sedimentation coefficient of 6.5S and a half-life of 18 days, both just slightly less than those of intact IgG (Janeway et al, 1968).

Most promising, however, are preparations which have been rendered free of anticomplementary activity by treatment with sulph-hydryl bond reducing agents followed by alkylation with iodoacetamide. The immunoglobulins in these preparations reportedly retain the sedimentation characteristics and antibody potency of those in the untreated material and no low molecular weight fragments are generated. Apparently the IgG molecules remain held together by non-covalent bonds; it is not clear why anticomplementary activity is lost by this treatment. Some of these preparations are currently undergoing initial clinical trials, and the doses being given are roughly those recommended for the intramuscular preparations.

Plasma infusions

There are several obvious advantages to the use of plasma infusions in the therapy of severe humoral immunodeficiencies: (1) antibodies of all five immunoglobulin classes can be provided in significant quantities, (2) such intravenous infusions are far less painful than intramuscular ISG injections and thus have greater patient acceptability, (3) adverse reactions are few and (4) higher serum immunoglobulin concentrations can be effected than with intramuscular ISG injections. In addition, the donor can be immunised to provide higher titres of some antibodies than can be achieved with pooled gammaglobulin. The disadvantages include: (1) the potential danger of transmitting homologous serum hepatitis, (2) the risk of graft-versus-host (GVH) disease in infants with severe combined immunodeficiency disease from residual immunocompetent cells contained in most plasma preparations and (3) the inconvenience or impracticality of performing plasmaphaereses on a regular basis in some clinical settings. The risk of homologous hepatitis can be greatly reduced by careful donor selection, using guidelines described below. The danger of GVH can be avoided either by carefully removing all cellular elements, by irradiating the plasma sufficiently to destroy the GVH potential of the immunocompetent cells, or both. Finally, enlisting the aid of regional blood banks in conducting donor plasmaphaereses helps to reduce the impracticality of this form of therapy.

We first became impressed with the potential usefulness of plasma infusions for therapy of immunodeficiency while using them as a sustaining measure in infants with severe combined immunodeficiency who were awaiting transplantation (Buckley, 1972). For use in those patients, we either removed all cellular elements from the plasmas by high-speed centrifugation or irradiated them with 3000 rad prior to their administration. GVH did not occur in any of the patients as a consequence of infusion of plasma so treated, and we found that we achieved nearly adult levels of each of the three major immunoglobulins and normal antibody titres to a number of antigens.

Following our experience in those patients, we became interested in the use of plasma therapy in patients whose defects involved mainly the humoral limb of the immunologic system. Stimulating this interest was the fact that several patients with infantile X-linked agammaglobulinaemia whom we were following required chronic antibiotic therapy, in addition to injections of gammaglobulin at doses of 100 mg/kg every three weeks, in order to remain free of overt lower respiratory infection. A review of the literature on the use of plasma therapy in immunodeficiency revealed that it had been employed on only a very limited basis, the experience of Stiehm et al, (1966) being the most extensive.

Because of the potential advantages of this form of replacement, however, we began six and a half years ago to evaluate periodic plasma infusions in the treatment of immuno-deficiency and have used them to treat fifteen patients with severe humoral immunodefi-ciency followed at this institution during this period. The group includes four patients with infantile X-linked agammaglobulinaemia, nine with common variable immuno-deficiency or B-lymphocyte agammaglobulinaemia and two with X-linked immuno-deficiency with hyper-IgM. All plasma donors have been carefully screened for a histoy of hepatitis and by testing their sera for hepatitis B-antigen by counterelectrophoresis and, more recently, radioimmunoassay. In most cases a 'buddy' system is used whereby the same donor, usually a parent, is used repeatedly. This minimises the hepatitis risk since once a donor is established as being safe the danger of his transmitting hepatitis in the future is negligible. For two patients, their husbands serve as donors and for one, a brother. One patient has no relatives suitable for periodic plasma donations and he is currently receiving plasma from a group of professional blood donors whose blood has been used repeatedly for other recipients in whom there has been no subsequent development of homologous hepatitis. In most instances, the donors are of the same ABO and Rh blood types as the recipient but, in two cases, there are minor mismatches, e.g. the donor plasmas contain antibodies in low titre against recipient red cell antigens. In these cases, appropriate soluble blood group substances are added to the plasmas to neutralise the antibodies prior to infusion into the patients.

The dose of plasma employed varies according to the donor's serum IgG concentration but is usually selected to provide the recipient with 100 mg/kg IgG every three weeks and, in most cases, is approximately 10 ml/kg. As with ISG therapy, the dose for the first treat-

Table 10.1 Comparison of serum immunoglobulin concentrations in patients with deficits in humoral immunity three weeks after plasma infusions or gammaglobulin injections

Patient	Treatment status		IgG (mg/100 ml)	IgA (mg/100 ml)	IgM (mg/100 ml)
1		Pre-plasma	125	0	0
	3 weeks	Post-plasma[a]	256	9	4
2		Pre-plasma	50	0	0
	3 weeks	Post-plasma[a]	262	9	4
3		Pre-plasma	56	13	11
	3 weeks	Post-plasma[b]	249	18	15
4		Pre-plasma	205	5	6
	3 weeks	Post-plasma[c]	231	7	5
5		Pre-γ-globulin	125	0	0
	3 weeks	Post-γ-globulin	148	0	0
6		Pre-γ-globulin	65	0	15
	3 weeks	Post-γ-globulin	155	0	9
7		Pre-γ-globulin	47	0	9
	3 weeks	Post-γ-globulin	103	0	9
8		Pre-γ-globulin	130	0	0
	3 weeks	Post-γ-globulin	170	0	0
9		Pre-γ-globulin	25	0	11
	3 weeks	Post-γ-globulin	145	0	18
10		Pre-γ-globulin	60	0	0
	3 weeks	Post-γ-globulin	102	0	0

[a] Average values from 23 three-week posttreatment sera
[b] Average values from five three-week posttreatment sera
[c] Average values from two three-week posttreatment sera
Reproduced from Buckley, R. H. (1972) *American Journal of Diseases of Children*, **124**, 376–381. American Medical Association Specialty Journals, Chicago

ment is usually twice that amount. The results of serum immunoglobulin measurements three weeks after plasma infusions in the first four patients begun on this form of therapy are presented in Table 10.1 and compared with results of similar measurements in six other agammaglobulinaemic patients three weeks after they had received 0.6 ml/kg of ISG intramuscularly (Buckley, 1972).

Serum IgG concentrations averaged 113 mg/100 ml higher in the plasma-treated group than in the gammaglobulin treated group and low but higher than baseline concentrations of IgA and IgM could be detected after three weeks in the plasma-treated but not in the ISG-treated patients. In addition, as shown in Table 10.2, only one gammaglobulin-treated patient had detectable anti-B antibodies, none had antibodies to A cells or diphtheria toxoid, and all had low to absent antitetanus antibody titres. All plasma-treated patients, on the other hand, had normal antibody titres to tetanus toxoid and low titres to diphtheria toxoid. One type O recipient of type O plasma had near normal isohaemagglutinin titres. One possible reason for the lower antibody titres in the gammaglobulin-treated group is the fact that samples of three different commercial sources of ISG showed marked variability in their content of antitetanus antibody and each had very low titres of anti-diphtheria antibody (Table 10.2). Another possible cause of both the lower immuno-globulin concentrations and lower antibody titres in the ISG-treated patients three weeks posttreatment is that denaturation of gammaglobulin takes place during the alcohol-salt fractionation procedure and more rapid catabolism of this preparation occurs due to proteolysis by local tissue enzymes in the intramuscular injection sites.

Table 10.2   Comparison of antibody titres[a] in immunodeficiency patients three weeks after treatment with plasma or gammaglobulin

Patient	Treatment status		Blood type	Anti-A	Anti-B	Tetanus	Diphtheria
1[b]		Donor	A+	0	256	5×10^5	81
		Pre-plasma	O+	0	0	243	0
	3 weeks	Post-plasma	—	0	0[c]	2×10^4	81
2[b]		Donor	A+	0	256	5×10^5	81
		Pre-plasma	AB+	0	0	0	0
	3 weeks	Post-plasma	—	0	0	2×10^4	27
3[d]		Donor	O+	256	256	12.9×10^7	0
		Pre-plasma	O+	0	0	0	0
	3 weeks	Post-plasma	—	16	4	4.3×10^7	0
Commercial		Co.A	—	0	0	1.6×10^6	81
globulin		Co.B	—	0	0	6×10^4	9
		Co.C	—	0	0	3.5×10^9	243
4[b]	3 weeks	Post-γ-globulin	—	0	0	243	0
5[b]	3 weeks	Post-γ-globulin	—	0	0	81	0
6[b]	3 weeks	Post-γ-globulin	—	0	0	243	0
7[b]	3 weeks	Post-γ-globulin	—	0	4	0	0
8[b]	3 weeks	Post-γ-globulin	—	0	0	243	0

[a] Expressed as reciprocal of highest dilution giving positive reaction
[b] Infantile X-linked agammaglobulinaemia
[c] A and B blood group substances added to donor plasma before infusions
[d] Acquired hypogammaglobulinaemia, details reported elsewhere
Reproduced from Buckley, R. H. (1972) *American Journal of Diseases of Children*, **124**, 376–381. American Medical Association Specialty Journals, Chicago

The results of our experience with plasma therapy in the other 11 patients are in keeping with those described above for the first four, except that we find we are unable to maintain serum immunoglobulin concentrations of that magnitude in our larger teenage and adult patients because of difficulty in obtaining the volumes of plasma required to achieve the dosage given above. In addition, we have observed evidence for more rapid catabolism of the infused immunoglobulins in two patients who experienced acute episodes of infec-tion. In general, however, the clinical statuses of all of these patients have improved con-siderably since plasma therapy was initiated. Only one has experienced a serious infection, and this was meningitis due to an enterovirus. All patients formerly requiring chronic antibiotic therapy in addition to ISG have been able to discontinue it and the frequency of required courses of antibiotics has been reduced in all.

ADVERSE REACTIONS TO PLASMA
In contrast to our initial experience in which we observed no adverse effects from plasma therapy in any of the patients during the first two and a half years of our evaluation, we have subsequently encountered adverse reactions in four patients, one of whom is not

included in the above group of 15 since therapy could not be started because of the adverse effect. In keeping with the observation by the British Medical Council Working Party on Hypogammaglobulinaemia (1971) that boys with affected lateral male relatives were significantly spared from adverse reactions to ISG, we have seen no reactions in any of our patients with infantile X-linked agammaglobulinaemia.

Each of the four patients in whom we have observed untoward reactions had normal percentages of peripheral blood B-lymphocytes bearing surface immunoglobulins of the IgM and IgD classes and were diagnosed as having B-lymphocyte agammaglobulinaemia. In one patient, the reaction occurred only when he received plasma from his mother and not when he received it from his brothers. The reaction began approximately 1 h after the infusion was started, after he had received one full unit of plasma, and was characterised by chills, fever, and a drop in his peripheral blood leucocyte count. The mother's plasma was later found to contain cytotoxic antibodies to HLA antigens present on the patient's leucocytes. In a second patient with B-lymphocyte agammaglobulinaemia, who was unusual in that he had an elevated serum IgE concentration (800 i.u./ml), a reaction of generalised urticaria and angioedema was noted when he received plasma from his father but did not occur when he received plasma from a paternal uncle. In the third patient with B-lymphocyte agammaglobulinaemia, a reaction characterised by chills but no fever or chest oppression began 1 to 2 h after onset of the infusion on two occasions, followed by prolonged lethargy. The aetiologies of the reactions in the latter two patients remain undefined. There were no signs of haemolytic transfusion reactions, direct Coombs' tests were negative, and $\beta 1C$ levels did not change. In the case of the third patient, he had received plasma from the same donor on other occasions with no untoward effects. He is now receiving plasma from a pool of professional donors matched for the same blood type without adverse effects.

The fourth patient's reaction was very different from the aforementioned. This occurred in a girl who had a serum IgG concentration of 280 mg/100 ml, no detectable IgA by single radial diffusion, an IgM concentration of 14 mg/100 ml, and impaired antibody formation to a number of antigens. Since she had normal percentages of immunoglobulin-bearing B-lymphocytes, her findings were considered to be most consistent with a diagnosis of B-lymphocyte (or common variable) hypogammaglobulinaemia. She has no history of ever having received blood transfusions or ISG. Within seconds after beginning a compatible paternal plasma infusion, the patient experienced a sensation of tightness of the skin of her face, intense dyspnoea, moderate cyanosis, vomiting, defecation, mild hypertension and subsequent somnolence. The plasma was discontinued immediately; only a total of 15 ml was given. There were no changes in her vital signs other than the transient blood pressure rise, and she did not require treatment with emergency medications. All signs of the reaction subsided within 1 h except for the somnolence, which lasted several hours. There was no evidence of a haemolytic transfusion reaction and a direct Coombs' test shortly after the reaction was negative. Her serum $\beta 1C$ concentration in a sample collected 15 min following the reaction was slightly higher than that in a sample obtained immediately before the infusion was begun.

Subsequent analysis of the patient's pretreatment serum in the laboratory of Dr H. H. Fudenberg revealed that it contained a titre of 1:640 of anti-IgA antibodies, as detected by the chromic chloride passive haemagglutination method. Moreover, the antibodies reacted with all of several different IgA myeloma protein coats, indicating that they did not have allospecificity. The reaction experienced by this patient is similar to the anaphylactic transfusion reactions reported in patients with selective IgA deficiency who had anti-IgA antibodies (Vyas et al, 1968; Schmidt et al, 1969). The unusual feature of this patient, however, is that although she had no detectable serum IgA she did not have normal or elevated concentrations of IgG and IgM, as is usually seen in patients with selective IgA deficiency. This experience indicates that anti-IgA antibodies may exist in patients other than those with typical selective IgA deficiency. We feel that it is imperative that this possibility be investigated prior to beginning replacement therapy in other patients with absent serum IgA who have significant quantities of immunoglobulins of the other two major classes, even though the concentrations may be abnormally low.

Risks in Subjects with Normal Immunocompetence

While undoubtedly many persons with normal humoral immunity have received injections of immune serum globulin (ISG, gammaglobulin) without apparent adverse effects, several reports of putative allergic reactions following such injections have been made, and there are a number of theoretical dangers to this usually unnecessary practice. Plasma infusions and ISG injections have been shown to commonly induce antibodies to immunoglobulin alloantigens genetically different from those of the recipient (Allen and Kunkel, 1966; Stiehm and Fudenberg, 1965). In experimental animals, antiallotype antibodies have been found to suppress antibody formation in fetuses having immunoglobulins of the particular allotype (Herzenberg et al, 1967). From these observations, it has been postulated that maternal antibodies to human fetal immunoglobulin allotypes could have a role in the production of transient immunodeficiency disease of infancy; no firm evidence for this has been forthcoming, however.

Heiner has reported that ISG preparations derived from placentas also contain non-immunoglobulin proteins that appear to represent placenta-specific antigens (Heiner and Evans, 1967). Heterologous antisera prepared against placental ISG produced arcs on immunoelectrophoresis against placentally derived ISG that were not seen with anti-whole human serum antisera. These arcs were still produced after absorption of the anti-placental ISG antisera with normal human serum but not after absorption with minced placental tissues. It is not known whether administration of such preparations to female children or to women in the child-bearing age has resulted in any of the theoretically possible adverse consequences of immunisation against placental antigens.

Finally, in addition to the above considerations, it is also possible that passive antibody in the form of gammaglobulin injections or plasma infusions given normal individuals may suppress endogenous antibody formation to antigens they have not previously encountered. There is ample evidence for this phenomenon in experimental studies in animals, and it was on this rationale that the administration of anti-Rh (D) gammaglobulin preparations to Rh (D) negative women at delivery was begun to prevent formation of antibodies to fetal red cell Rh (D) antigens. While the success of the latter form of passive immunotherapy is unquestioned, the extent to which antibodies to other antigens have been suppressed by such therapy has not been examined in man.

TREATMENT OF CELLULAR IMMUNODEFICIENCY

The only certain effective replacement therapy for cellular immunodeficiency at present is the successful transplantation of a suitable immunocompetent tissue. Clearly, bone marrow remains the tissue of choice for such transplants whenever histocompatible donors are available. Most patients will not, however, be fortunate enough to have compatible potential donors, so alternative forms of therapy must be sought in order to avoid the uniformly fatal outcome in these patients if left untreated or if treated with incompatible bone marrow. Unfortunately, no other therapy has approached the measure of success achieved by bone marrow transplantation in patients with severe cellular immunodeficiency, although some alternatives appear to show promise. Humoral replacement therapy has been of limited value in the treatment of patients with defects in cellular immunity, but it is certainly indicated in those patients who have combined humoral and cellular immunodeficiencies.

Indications and Contraindications

A histocompatible immunocompetent tissue transplant has the theoretical possibility of succeeding in any immunodeficient patient who is completely lacking in thymus-dependent immunity. In actual practice, the only immunodeficient patients for whom this is a clear therapeutic indication at present are those with either severe combined immunodeficiency disease, the DiGeorge syndrome or the Nezelof syndrome. In other types of immunodeficiency, there is usually sufficient graft rejection capacity that even histocompatible marrow or other tissues are rejected unless the recipient is preconditioned with high doses of irradiation or immunosuppressive drugs. The only bone marrow transplants in immunodeficient patients without impaired CMI, were in three boys who had congenital X-linked agammaglobulinaemia (Buckley, 1973). These were all unsuccessful, in that the grafts either failed to take or survived only transiently, despite pretreatment of one such patient with large doses of cyclophosphamide. No changes occurred in the immunologic capacities of these patients, and graft-versus-host (GVH) reactions were not observed.

Other types of immune deficits which have been treated with bone marrow cells include: The Wiskott–Aldrich syndrome (two patients), chronic mucocutaneous moniliasis (two patients), and ataxia-telangiectasia (one patient) (Buckley, 1971). In these conditions, T-cell immunity is impaired but not absent, hence it is likely that allogeneic marrow grafts even from HLA compatible donors would eventually be rejected. Indeed, successul engraftment with long-term chimerism was achieved in only one such patient, a boy with Wiskott–Aldrich syndrome who was pretreated with lethal doses of cyclophosphamide (Bach et al, 1968). In view of our present limited understanding of the basic abnormalities in most types of immunodeficiency and the extreme hazards attendant to immunosuppressing an already immunocompromised host, this is generally considered inadvisable.

Transplants of mature immunocompetent tissues are contraindicated in patients with profound deficits in CMI when no histocompatible donors are available. This is due to the fact that grafts of such tissues present certain unique problems not seen in other types of organ and tissue transplantation. In this situation, not only can an immunocompetent host reject the graft, but the grafted immunocompetent cells can reject the host, invariably producing a fatal reaction (graft-versus-host disease) in histoincompatible transplants when the host is not capable of rejecting the graft. Moreover, it appears to be the only form of transplantation where strict mixed leucocyte culture (MLC) compatibility between donor and recipient is required for success. As will be discussed below, however, histoincompatible immunocompetent cells from fetal tissues such as thymus and liver appear to be exceptions to this rule, i.e. despite major histocompatibility differences between the fetal donor and a severely immunocompromised recipient, engraftment can occur without subsequent fatal GVH disease (Buckley et al, 1976).

Once the diagnosis of a severe cellular immune deficient has been established, a search for a compatible donor should begin immediately, since life-threatening infection and clinical deterioration may soon develop. Except in rare instances of genetic recombination, histocompatible donors will be found only among the patient's siblings. These siblings are identified by tissue typing and mixed lymphocyte culture studies of the patient's immediate family.

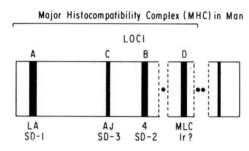

Figure 10.1   Schematic diagram of the genetic structure of the region of human chromosome number 6 determining the structure of the major transplantation antigens of man (the HLA complex). The most recent letter designation of these loci (agreed upon at the 1975 Histocompatibility Testing Workshop) is given on the top of the chromosomal diagram, and synonyms that have appeared in earlier literature are placed below each of the gene symbols.

The genetic control of determinants responsible for the characteristics of the major histocompatibility system in man is determined by genes located on a single pair of chromosomes (Thorsby, 1974). A schematic of the human autosome bearing the major histocompatibility region is shown in Figure 10.1. The region comprises at least three HLA loci, designated as A, B and C, the gene products of which are detected serologically in lymphocyte cytotoxicity tests, and a fourth locus, designated as D, the gene products of which can be detected usually only in MLC studies. The important concept to keep in mind is that all of these loci are closely linked and there is a low cross-over frequency. Hence, with a given family, all of the loci of this region are usually transmitted to offspring en bloc so that compatibility for one usually means compatibility for all.

This means, as shown in Figure 10.2, that for each sibling there is a one in four chance that he or she will be both HLA and MLR identical to the patient. In the schematic in Figure 10.2, the letters a, b, c and d are arbitrary symbols designating the four parental autosomes which carry fixed combinations of alleles controlled by the four major histocompatibility loci. This fixed combination is called a haplotype. There are two pairs of identical siblings among the offspring in this family, two with the haplotypes ac and two with haplotypes bc. Obviously, parents will usually differ from each of their offspring by one haplotype. Except in some consanguinous marriages where this is not the case and in one example of modification of a maternal immune response (Buckley et al, 1971b), all parent to offspring transplants in severe combined immunodeficiency have therefore resulted in fatal graft-versus-host disease in the infants.

In rare instances, recombination has occurred within the major histocompatibility region so that the inheritance of one or more of the serologically defined HLA (A, B, or

C locus) antigens does not follow that of the MLR or D locus antigens (Yunis and Amos, 1971). In such instances, siblings may be HLA non-identical but MLR identical or vice versa. Two patients with severe combined immunodeficiency have been treated success-fully with bone marrow from MLR identical but HLA non-identical relatives and fatal graft-versus-host disease did not occur (Vossen et al, 1973; DuPont et al, 1973). In contrast, marrow from an HLA identical, MLR non-identical unrelated donor produced fatal

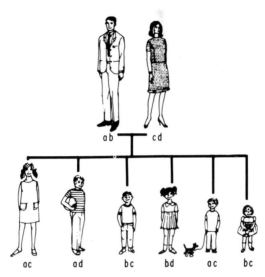

Figure 10.2   Schematic representation of the inheritance of the HLA system. The letters a, b, c, and d are arbitrary symbols for the four parental chromosomes bearing the HLA region. The four closely linked genes in this region on each chromosome are usually transmitted to the offspring en bloc, and the fixed combination of a, b, c, and d loci antigens is referred to as a haplotype. There are two pairs of HLA identical siblings among the offspring in this family, two with the haplotypes ac and two with bc. (Reproduced from Amos, D. B. (1971) In *Diseases of the Kidney* 2nd edn, ed. Strauss, M. B. & Welt, L. G. Boston: Little, Brown and Company, with permission)

graft-versus-host disease in another such infant, indicating the critical importance of MLR compatibility in bone marrow transplantation (DuPont et al, 1974). Current efforts in several centres are directed toward means of identifying MLR compatible unrelated individuals. As unlikely as success may seem in this endeavour, the genetic linkage dis-equilibrium which exists between the B and D loci puts this within the realm of possibility. Indeed, two such donors have been found recently for infants with severe combined immu-nodeficiency who had no compatible sibling donors by screening tor MLR compatibility with a large panel of unrelated individuals having the same B locus antigens as the patient (DuPont et al, 1974; Horowitz et al, 1975).

Types of Therapy

The types of therapy that have been tried in patients with cellular immunodeficiency include immunocompetent tissue grafts and administration of either transfer factor or thymosin.

Immunocompetent tissue grafts

Three types of immunocompetent tissues have been used in such attempts: bone marrow, fetal thymus and fetal liver.

BONE MARROW TRANSPLANTATION

It is now nine years since the first successful bone marrow transplant was performed to correct severe combined immunodeficiency disease (Gatti et al, 1968). Since that time, the immunologic capacities of over 35 immunodeficient patients have been reconstituted by transplants of histocompatible marrow (number estimated from reports collected at the Second Workshop of the International Cooperative Group for Bone Marrow Transplantation in Severe Combined Immunodeficiency, 1975). In addition, it has been estimated that an approximately equal number of unsuccessful attempts have been made to achieve immunologic reconstitution by bone marrow transplantation in immunodeficient infants and children.

In all instances where success was achieved, the donor and recipient were shown to be histocompatible in mixed leucocyte culture but not necessarily for the serologically defined HLA antigens (Gatti et al, 1968; Buckley et al, 1971a; DuPont et al, 1973). The donor in the majority of cases was a histocompatible sibling, but in a few instances was another relative who, because of consanguinity or recombinational events within the major histocompatibility complex, was compatible with the patient at the MLR locus (Gatti et al, 1968; DuPont et al, 1973; Vossen et al, 1973). All incompatible marrow grafts given infants with severe combined immunodeficiency disease either led to fatal GVH or were unsuccessful because the infant died of complications of the primary disease without evidence of adequate immunologic reconstitution (Buckley et al, 1971a; Buckley, 1973.)

Since no other therapy has approached the measure of success achieved by bone marrow transplantation, it is clear that it remains the treatment of choice for infants with severe combined immunodeficiency who have histocompatible potential donors. As death almost invariably occurs during infancy in that condition, definitive treatment offers the only hope of survival. Patients with thymic hypoplasia (the DiGeorge syndrome) or the Nezelof syndrome have not been treated with bone marrow cells (see Fetal Thymus Transplantation below), but this approach should be as effective in these patients as in severe combined immunodeficiency if fetal thymus transplantation is unsuccessful or not feasible.

The objective of marrow transplantation is to replace defective or absent cells of the recipient with functionally normal donor immunocompetent cells capable of reproducing themselves. Among the various cells present in bone marrow is a self-replicating cell that can give rise to either erythrocytes or granulocytes (Wu et al, 1967), and probably also to megakaryocytes and immunocompetent T and B cells (Wu et al, 1968), although the evidence for the latter is inconclusive. Many have been of the opinion that it is the attributes of this pluripotential stem cell (Nowell et al, 1970) that account for marrow's ability to correct both haematopoietic cell failure and deficits in adaptive immunity. It is equally likely, however, that immunologic reconstitution may occur on the basis of adoptive transfer of cells in bone marrow that have already begun differentiation pathways to become mature T and B cells while in the donor.

Information derived from successful cases of bone marrow transplantation in severe combined immunodeficiency to date not only does not allow conclusions as to which mechanism of correction is operative but also does not establish the nature of the primary defect or defects in such infants. In one instance of successful reconstitution by bone marrow, fetal thymus was also given (de Koning et al, 1969); in others, peripheral blood lymphocytes or unfractionated marrow (which possibly contained peripheral blood lymphocytes influenced by donor thymus) were given which could have effected adoptive transfer of immunity. Successful reconstitution of immunologic capacity has been achieved by bone marrow transplantation in both male and female patients with severe combined immunodeficiency disease including those with and without adenosine deaminase deficiency. Thus all presently recognised varieties of this defect are correctable by this procedure.

If a histocompatible donor is found for an infant with severe combined immunodeficiency, transplantation of bone marrow should be performed as rapidly as possible. For reasons to be mentioned later, this should be done after first having made certain that treatment for any existing *Pneumocystis carinii* pneumonia is well under way. The technique of bone marrow grafting is the simplest of all transplantation procedures, offers little risk to the donor, and involves removal of a tissue that is readily regenerated. It has been found that multiple small volume aspirations (0.1–0.3 ml) yield the greatest number of nucleated marrow cells with the least amount of contamination by peripheral blood lymphocytes, which have greater graft-versus-host potential. This is usually accomplished while the donor is under general anaesthesia (Thomas and Storb, 1970). The aspirates are drawn into sterile heparinised syringes and ejected into tissue culture medium by passage through needles of increasingly smaller size or through sterile metal mesh screens to remove bony spicules. The marrow cells are then administered to the patient usually by the intravenous route, or by the intraperitoneal route. The optimal number of cells needed for successful immunologic reconstitution is not yet established but cell numbers required have ranged from 9 to 50 million nucleated marrow cells per kilogram body weight of recipient (DuPont et al, 1974). Factors determining cell needs are not yet known but it is possible that infants with ADA deficiency, infants receiving unrelated MLR compatible marrow, or those receiving cells by the intraperitoneal route may require higher numbers of cells (DuPont et al, 1974).

Following the administration of the bone marrow cells, success can be documented by observing for either direct (confirmed by the presence in the recipient of one or more donor markers) or indirect (appearance of a donor immune function) evidence of engraftment. Three types of markers have been found helpful in identifying donor characteristics in marrow recipients: karyotypic markers, red and white cell antigenic markers, and serum allotypic markers. If donor and recipient are of opposite sex, karyotypic markers are most useful and can be detected sooner (after two weeks) than antigenic markers, since detection of the latter is difficult until donor cells have replicated sufficiently for the antigens to be detected (usually after about one month). Serum immunoglobulin allotypic markers are useful in documenting chimerism of immunocompetent cells. Any of these markers, if present, provide direct evidence of engraftment.

If they are not available or cannot be detected, indirect evidence of engraftment must be relied upon. Improved immunologic function in patients with severe combined immunodeficiency is strong indirect evidence of engraftment. In those infants whose immunological defect has been corrected by histocompatible allogeneic bone marrow transplantation, there has been considerable variability in the times of appearance of various donor immune functions (Table 10.3). Responsiveness of peripheral blood lymphocytes to mitogenic stimuli has been noted as early as two weeks posttransplant in some infants whereas in others it has not occurred for three to four weeks (DuPont et al, 1974). Similarly, increases in peripheral blood lymphocytes and the appearance of delayed cutaneous reactivity have been noted between the second and third weeks in many such infants but not until four to five weeks in others. The onset of immunoglobulin production has probably been more variable than any other function, with this not appearing in some infants until around 10 weeks posttransplant. In at least two such infants this function has failed to appear altogether despite the appearance of donor cell-mediated function. Again, factors responsible for the variability of appearance of these functions are not established, but one of these appears to be the number of marrow cells administered (DuPont et al, 1974).

Table 10.3   Time course of immunologic changes[a] following successful bone marrow transplantation

1.	In vitro lymphocyte response to mitogens	2–5 weeks
2.	Increase in absolute lymphocyte count	2–3 weeks
3.	Delayed cutaneous responsiveness	2–5 weeks
4.	Immunoglobulin synthesis	3–10 weeks

[a] Variability of time course appears dependent in large part on dose of cells administered

Table 10.4   Problems observed following bone marrow transplantation in severe combined immunodeficiency

1. Graft-versus-host disease
2. Bacterial infections
3. *Pneumocystis carinii* pneumonia
4. Cytomegalovirus infection
5. Aspiration pneumonia
6. Marrow aplasia or Coombs' positive anaemia

As mentioned at the outset, there are many problems which remain with this therapeutic approach, and not all of these appear to have an immunologic basis. Some of the problems encountered are summarised in Table 10.4. Graft-versus-host disease is an almost invariable accompaniment even of histocompatible bone marrow transplants. This reaction, which is caused by immunocompetent donor cells which recognise and react against foreign tissue antigens of the recipient, usually begins within a week after the marrow cells are infused and is heralded by the appearance of a maculopapular rash beginning 5 to 12 days posttransplantation.

The reaction is characterised further by varying degrees of diarrhoea, hepatosplenomegaly, liver dysfunction, eosinophilia, protein-losing enteropathy (Cornelius, 1970), marked wasting, hypertension (Ammann et al, 1970), pneumonia, pleural nodules and effusions (Buckley et al, 1971a), bone marrow aplasia, extensive exfoliation of the skin, and marked susceptibility to infection (Solberg et al, 1971). Biopsies of skin lesions reveal small lymphocytes in the dermis.

In incompatible marrow grafting GVH disease is invariably fatal. This occurred in one dual system immunodeficiency patient after only 8×10^5/kg haploidentical nucleated marrow cells (Hong, personal communication). Hence, if there is a 'safe' number of marrow cells below which fatal GVH will not occur, it would appear to be less than this number. No immunosuppressive or other agents other than possibly some lots of antithymocyte globulin have been found effective in treating GVH from histoincompatible grafts once it begins (Storb, Gluckman and Thomas, et al, 1974). Indeed, the cell responsible for GVH is hydrocortisone-resistant (Cohen, Fischbach and Claman, 1970). Fortunately, among infants with severe combined immunodeficiency receiving compatible marrow grafts, I know of no documented examples of fatal GVH. In leukaemic patients, however, this has not been the case, since several examples of fatal GVH have been observed among such patients receiving compatible marrow (Graw et al, 1970). As with the rate of reconstitution, the severity of GVH in combined immunodeficiency seems related to the dose of nucleated marrow cells administered (DuPont et al, 1974). It is the impression of some workers in this field that one may have to tolerate a certain amount of GVH if rapid and complete reconstitution is to be achieved.

The second kind of problem, and one which has proved more difficult to contend with than GVH in matched sibling transplants, is infection in the posttransplant period. While bacterial infection due primarily to Gram-negative organisms from the infants' enteric tracts has been responsible for death in some infants, infections with *Pneumocystis carinii* or certain viruses have been the cause of death in the majority. Nearly half of the deaths among severe combined immunodeficiency patients transplanted with histocompatible marrow in Minneapolis, Boston and other centres were thought to have been due either to infection or to reactions of the infants' newly acquired immunological systems to those infections (DuPont et al, 1974).

In view of these complications, it would seem that the establishment of pathogen or germ-free states in these patients prior to and during reconstitution deserves further evaluation. The possibility that such a 'germ-free' state might lessen the severity of GVH also needs to be assessed in light of studies in experimental animals which showed that GVH could be avoided even in histo*in*compatible grafts in germ-free irradiated mice (van Bekkum et al, 1974). Similar results were also obtained in monkeys, but these animals went on to die of interstitial pneumonia, usually from cytomegalovirus. Clinical evidence to date also indicates that pathogen-free or germ-free isolation in laminar flow units provides little protection against the development of cytomegalovirus and *Pneumocystis carinii* infections seen so often in posttransplant patients (Meyers et al, 1975). It is the opinion of many workers in this field that gut decontamination with non-absorbable antibiotics should be carried out prior to transplantation in order to avoid Gram-negative infections in the posttransplant period, but again there is no uniform agreement of the efficacy of this.

Other problems that have been encountered include aspiration pneumonia (which caused the deaths of at least two of these infants who otherwise appeared to be having relatively uncomplicated posttransplant courses and had evidence of immunologic reconstitution) marrow aplasia and Coombs positive anaemia (DuPont et al, 1974). In one instance of marrow aplasia, the donor and recipient had a major mismatch for the ABO system (Gatti et al, 1968); fortunately a second transplant corrected the aplasia and donor type erythrocytes became established in the recipient (Meuwissen et al, 1969). Coombs positive anaemia was also observed in another infant who was blood type A and the donor was type O, but at least two infants have been reconstituted with ABO incompatible marrow without this problem (DuPont et al, 1974).

Since GVH disease can be caused by immunocompetent cells in blood, plasma, or platelet or granulocyte preparations (Hathaway et al, 1967), it is imperative that all such materials be irradiated prior to infusion into bone marrow recipients during the period before establishment of the graft. The exact dose of radiation required has not been established, but doses ranging from 1500 to 5000 rad have been used without evidence of GVH in the recipient after the blood products were infused (Cowan and Phillips, 1972), and these doses have been shown to have little effect on red cell, platelet, or phagocytic cell function (McCullough et al, 1969).

FETAL THYMUS TRANSPLANTATION

Fetal thymus transplantation would appear to have been used most successfully in the treatment of patients with the DiGeorge syndrome. In this condition, there is impaired development of the thymus gland and other structures derived from the third and fourth pharyngeal pouches. It is the only deficiency state in which the rationale for the use of thymus tissue for immunologic reconstitution seems well founded.

Immunologic improvement has been noted in five infants with this syndrome given either transplants of fetal thymus (August et al, 1968; Cleveland et al, 1968; Gatti et al, 1972; Steele et al, 1972; Biggar et al, 1975) or a thymus gland implanted in a millipore diffusion chamber (Steele et al, 1972). The mechanism of the improvement is unclear, however, since none of these patients had direct evidence of engraftment, and a number of DiGeorge patients have had 'spontaneous' acquisition of cellular immune function even without thymus transplantation (Kretschmer et al, 1968; Sieber et al, 1974). The latter may be related to the fact that a majority of DiGeorge patients have some thymic tissue, albeit small, and this thymic tissue appears normal histologically (Lischner and Huff, 1975).

Another puzzling aspect of the 'reconstitutions' observed following fetal thymus transplantation in these patients is the rapidity with which the immunologic improvement has been noted (within a matter of hours), implying that a humoral substance from the transplant may have been responsible for the augmented function. The improvement noted following implantation of a thymus gland in a Millipore chamber also supports this concept (Steele et al, 1972).

Fetal thymus transplants have been attempted without success many times in the past in patients with severe combined immunodeficiency (Hitzig, Kay and Cottier, 1965; Githens et al, 1973) but Ammann et al (1973) and Rachelefsky et al (1975) have reported what appears to be T-cell reconstitution by intraperitoneal infusions of minced fresh fetal thymus tissue in two infants with this disease, both of whom showed evidence of chimerism. Shearer and Hong (unpublished) also observed transient improvement in cell-mediated immune function in a third infant with that defect treated in the same manner. In each of these instances, transfer factor therapy (see below) was given prior to the thymus transplants. In contrast to previous reports that human fetal thymus tissue has little or no GVH potential (Kay, 1971), mild to very severe GVH was observed in all three of the latter infants, but none died from GVH and all are alive at the time of this writing. Cell suspensions derived from adult rodent thymuses have been showd to cause GVH in newborn or irradiated rodent recipients (Stutman et al, 1968); the age at which primate thymuses develop this potential is unknown but is probably close to 12 to 14 weeks. More recently, successful immunological reconstitution has been achieved with cultured mature thymic epithelial transplants (Hong et al, 1976).

Thymus grafting has also been attempted in patients with other types of immunodeficiency, including those with the Nezelof syndrome (Ammann et al, 1973), ataxia telangiectasia (Buckley, 1975b), and chronic mucocutaneous moniliasis (Kirkpatrick and Gallin, 1975; Aiuti, Businco and Gatti, 1975; Levy et al, 1971). Immunologic improvement was noted in one patient with the Nezelof syndrome (Ammann et al, 1975) and in one with chronic moniliasis (Aiuti et al, 1975); in several others transient improvement was observed but did not recur even after subsequent implants. Chimerism was not demonstrated in any of these patients.

The transplantation procedure is simple, with the fetal thymus gland usually being inserted intact or in fragments into a pocket created surgically between the rectus fascia and muscle. Alternatively, the thymic tissue has been minced or a cell suspension prepared from it and these preparations have been injected by various routes.

FETAL LIVER CELL TRANSPLANTATION

Reconstitution experiments in lethally irradiated mice have found fetal liver to be nearly as effective as bone marrow in restoring haematopoietic function and in permitting survival (Uphoff, 1958; Lowenberg, 1975). In addition, although GVH was noted frequently following allogeneic fetal mouse liver treatment, it always occurred later and to a much less severe degree than with allogeneic bone marrow cells (Lowenberg, 1975).

As an alternative to marrow transplantation, two infants with severe combined immunodeficiency who had no histocompatible donors were given intraperitoneal infusions of fresh liver cells from fetuses of 8 and 9 to 10 weeks (Buckley et al, 1976). Transient graft-versus-host disease began at 42 and 52 days, respectively. Both had rises in T cells and declines in B cells by three months. No functional immunologic improvement occurred in the first infant, who died of pulmonary disease 10 months later. Both clinical and functional immunologic improvement occurred in the other, who is 43 months old and 30 months posttransplantation at the time of this writing. Lymphocyte responses to phytohaemagglutinin and pokeweed mitogen were noted by three months, to concanavalin A by five months, and to allogeneic cells by eight months; delayed cutaneous responsiveness to candida developed by six months. IgM became normal by 11 months; IgA and IgG remain low. Chimerism was demonstrated by a donor marker chromosome in metaphases from recipient lymphocytes. The observation of transient graft-versus-host disease in both infants documents the GVH potential of even this very young fetal tissue.

The successful reconstitution of one of the above patients and of three additional cases of severe combined immunodeficiency by Keightley et al (1975), Ackeret, Pluss and Hitzig (1975) and Rieger, Lustig and Rothberg, (1976) stand in sharp contrast to results in some 16 other patients given fetal liver that have been reported in the literature (Hitzig et al, 1965; Githens et al, 1973; Soothill, Kay and Batchelor, 1971) or are known to the author. In none of those cases was there evidence of development of immune function, and only one is described as having findings consistent with GVH; that infant had been given both fetal thymus and fetal liver (Soothill et al, 1971). Failure of engraftment appears to have been the major reason for lack of success in most of the earlier cases. Frozen liver cells were used in a majority of those cases, undoubtedly reducing the number and function of cells administered. The successful cases all were done with very young fetal livers (4–12 weeks) given as cell suspensions by intraperitoneal infusion. Total cell numbers in the successful cases have ranged from only 3.7×10^6 to 1.23×10^9. Perhaps younger fetal livers may be more effective because of their relative enrichment for haematopoietic stem cells compared to livers of older gestational age. Another factor that must be considered as a cause for failure of both fetal thymus and fetal liver engraftment is the phenomenon of allogeneic resistance described by Cudkowicz (1975). Lowenberg's (1975) observation that higher fetal liver cell numbers were required for allogeneic reconstitution than for syngeneic would certainly support this thesis. Variations in the strength of allo-geneic resistance have been found to be genetically determined (Cudkowicz, 1975) in the mouse and, if true in man, this could account for the inconsistent human results.

The nature of the cell or cells in fetal liver responsible for immunologic reconstitution and transient GVH in patients with severe combined immunodeficiency is not known. Since fetal mouse liver is a rich source of stem cells, as defined by spleen colony forming unit (CFU-S) activity (Lowenberg, 1975) and since it has been postulated that the basic defect in patients with severe combined immunodeficiency may lie in the pluripotential stem cell, Keightley et al (1975) concluded that reconstitution must have occurred through proliferation and differentiation of fetal liver stem cells into mature T and B cells in their patient.

It is equally likely, however, that fetal liver of the gestational age used may contain cells that have already begun the differentiation pathways to become mature T and B cells and that reconstitution may take place on the basis of adoptive transfer of these cells. In sup-port of this concept is the fact that development of immunoglobulin-bearing lymphocytes was observed in organ cultures of 14 day mouse fetal liver (Owen, Cooper and Raff, 1974) and by the fact that mixed lymphocyte reactivity, a property solely of T cells, is present in human fetal liver as early as 7.5 weeks (Stites, Carr and Fudenberg, 1974). The latter reactivity could have possibly mediated the transient GVH seen in the above patients.

Whatever the mechanism by which immunlogic reconstitution occurs with fetal liver cells, the successful immunologic reconstitution of the above-mentioned infants confirms the usefulness of transplantation of this tissue as an alternative form of definitive therapy in severe combined immunodeficiency when bone marrow transplantation cannot be performed. It is obvious that fetal liver may not be as effective as bone marrow in con-ferring immune function to these patients, however, even when successful engraftment occurs. Although complete immunologic reconstitution was seen in the cases of Keightley et al (1975) and Ackeret et al (1976), evidence of only T-cell reconstitution was seen in the cases of Buckley et al (1976) and Rieger et al (1976). Moreover, the deaths of the patient described by Keightley et al (1975) at one year following transplantation, and of the patient of Ackeret et al (1976) 18 months after grafting, raise the question of how permanent the immunologic reconstitution will be. The former patient died of severe chronic renal disease (possibly secondary to GVH) and the latter of a viral pneumonia. In the first case full immune function was present at the time of death, but in the latter case immunologic function was not reassessed prior to death. With the possible exception of the case of Keightley et al (1975) GVH was mild and transient when it occurred.

Transfer factor therapy

Transfer factor is a dialysable low molecular weight ($< 10\ 000$ daltons) substance de-rived from leucocyte lysates of skin test-positive donors; it has the capacity to endow skin test-negative subjects with the ability to develop the same delayed allergic responses of the donor (Lawrence, 1969). Although its exact chemical composition is unknown, it is resistant to DNAase, RNAase and trypsin and it is thought to be a polyribonucleotide–polypeptide complex (Kirkpatrick, 1975). Its mechanism of action is also unknown, although it has been suggested that transfer factor may act on multiple cell types, including the T lymphocyte, polymorphonuclear cells and monocytes (through its chemotactic action) and on the macrophage, effecting its activation (Kirkpatrick, 1975). Certain attri-butes of this substance make it highly attractive as a potentially useful therapeutic agent for patients with cellular immunodeficiency. It contains no histocompatibility or other antigens, therefore is non-sensitising; it does not contain HbsAg; and there is no risk of GVH attendant to its use. The development of autoimmune haemolytic anaemia in a patient with the Wiskott–Aldrich syndrome (Ballow, DuPont and Good, 1973) and of polyclonal gammopathy and lymphoproliferative disease in a patient with severe combined immunodeficiency (Gelfand et al, 1973) following transfer factor therapy, however, suggest that this therapy may not be completely innocuous.

The reported clinical experiences with use of transfer factor therapy in immunodeficient patients have all been anecdotal, as no controlled studies were done, and the results have been highly variable (Kirkpatrick, 1975). Most claims of benefit from this therapy in immunodeficiency have been in patients with either chronic mucocutaneous moniliasis (Schulkind et al, 1972) or in those with the Wiskott–Aldrich syndrome (Spitler et al, 1972). The benefits have been seem primarily in conversion of delayed skin test reactivity, in increases in the number of rosette-forming cells, and in apparent clinical improvement. Impaired lymphocyte transformation has rarely been corrected; when improvement has been noted it was small and inconstant (Kirkpatrick, 1975). Little or no beneficial effect from transfer factor has been seen in patients with severe combined immunodeficiency (except in those later given fetal thymus transplants, see above) or in those with Nezelofs syndrome (Pachman et al, 1974), suggesting that a normal thymus and/or functioning T cells may be required for the action of transfer factor.

Thymosin therapy

Extracts of calf thymus and a purified substance derived from such extracts, called thymosin or thymic hormone, are capable of restoring loss of thymic function due to thymic ablation in animals and of converting cells lacking in T-cell surface markers to those bearing such characteristics (Bach et al, 1971). Because of the lack of GVH risk and the seeming innocuousness of this substance, thymosin has been considered an attractive alternative to bone marrow transplantation when no histocompatible donors are available. To date some 17 patients with immunodeficiency are known to have been treated with thymosin (Horowitz, 1976). Of these, five had severe combined immunodeficiency and no clinical or immunologic improvement was noted in any. Five had Nezelofs syndrome and all of these showed variable improvement in their clinical statuses, numbers of E rosettes, skin test reactivity or (rarely) in lymphocyte blastogenesis. Four had ataxia telangiectasia and all experienced an increase in E rosettes but only variable changes in other parameters. One with partial DiGeorge's syndrome, one with nucleoside phosphorylase deficiency, and one with the Wiskott–Aldrich syndrome all improved clinically, had increased E rosettes, and showed improved lymphocyte blastogenesis following thymosin treatment. As with transfer factor therapy, these results suggest that some pre-existing T-cell function is necessary for the action of thymosin. It is also recommended that an in vitro E rosette study of the patient's cells following incubation with thymosin be conducted prior to deciding whether to use the substance in vivo (Wara et al, 1975). In contrast to transfer factor, there appear to be certain definite risks from the use of this substance in the treatment of immunodeficiency patients, as two developed hepatitis and two cutaneous allergic reactions following its administration (Horowitz, 1976).

Glycerol-frozen erythrocytes

For those patients with the adenosine-deaminase negative form of severe combined immunodeficiency disease and no histocompatible potential donors, another alternative form of therapy has recently been described by Polmar et al (1975). The administration of glycerol-frozen packed normal erythrocytes to one such infant at monthly intervals has conferred normal reactivity to his previously unresponsive lymphocytes to a variety of mitogenic and antigenic stimuli, and the patient has been well clinically. Since the erythrocyte adenosine-deaminase activity remains fairly constant in the patient for some two to three weeks following each red cell infusion, it is thought that the transfused cells may take up and inactivate toxic products (such as adenosine) of the purine salvage pathway that inhibit lymphocyte DNA synthesis. A similar improvement in lymphocyte function was not noted following administration of glycerol-frozen erythrocytes to a child with nucleoside phosphorylase deficiency, however. The eventual usefulness of this form of therapy must await further clinical trials.

REFERENCES

Ackeret, C., Pluss, H. J. & Hitzig, W. H. (1976) Hereditary severe combined immunodeficiency and adenosine deaminase deficiency. *Pediatric Research*, **10,** 67–70.

Aiuti, F., Businco, L. & Gatti, R. A. (1975) Reconstitution of T cell disorders following thymus transplantation. In *Immunodeficiency in Man and Animals*, ed. Bergsma, D., Good, R. A., Finstad, J. & Paul, N. W., pp. 370–376. Sunderland, Mass.: Sinauer Associates, Inc.

Allen, J. C. & Kunkel, H. G. (1966) Antibodies against γ-globulin after repeated blood transfusions in man. *Journal of Clinical Investigation*, **45,** 29–39.

Ammann, A. J., Meuwissen, H. J., Good, R. A. & Hong, R. (1970) Successful bone marrow transplantation in a patient with humoral and cellular immunity. *Clinical and Experimental Immunology*, **7,** 343–353.

Ammann, A. J., Wara, D. W., Salmon, S. & Perkins, H. (1973) Thymus transplantation. Permanent reconstitution of cellular immunity in a patient with sex-linked combined immunodeficiency. *New England Journal of Medicine*, **289,** 5–9.

Ammann, A. J., Wara, D. W., Doyle, N. E. & Golbus, M. S. (1975) Thymus transplantation in patients with thymic hypoplasia and abnormal immunoglobulin synthesis. *Transplantation*, **20,** 457–466.

August, C. S., Rosen, F. S., Filler, R. M., Janeway, C. A., Markowski, B. & Kay, H. E. M. (1968) Implantation of a fetal thymus, restoring immunological competence in a patient with thymic aplasia (diGeorge's syndrome). *Lancet*, **ii,** 1210–1211.

Bach, F. H., Albertini, R. J., Joo, P., Anderson, J. L. & Bortin, M. M. (1968) Bone marrow transplantation in a patient with Wiskott–Aldrich syndrome. *Lancet*, **ii,** 1364–1366.

Bach, J. F., Dardenne, M., Goldstein, A. L., Guha, A. & White, A. (1971) Appearance of T cell markers in bone marrow rosette forming cells after incubation with thymosin, a thymic hormone. *Proceedings of the National Academy of Sciences*, **68,** 2734–2738.

Ballow, M., DuPont, B. & Good, R. A. (1973) Autoimmune hemolytic anemia in Wiskott–Aldrich syndrome during treatment with transfer factor. *Journal of Pediatrics*, **83,** 772–780.

Barandun, S., Kistler, P., Jeunet, F. & Isliker, H. (1962) Intravenous administration of human γ-globulin. *Vox Sanguinis*, **7,** 157–174.

Biggar, W. D., Park, B. H., Stutman, O., Gajl-Peczalska, K. & Good, R. A. (1975) Fetal thymus transplantation: experimental and clinical observations. In *Immunodeficiency in Man and Animals*, ed. Bergsma, D., Good, R. A., Finstad, J. & Paul, N. W., pp. 361–365. Sunderland, Mass.: Sinauer Associates, Inc.

Bruton, O. C. (1952) Agammaglobulinemia. *Pediatrics*, **9,** 722–727.

Buckley, R. H. (1971) Reconstitution: grafting of bone marrow and thymus. In *Progress in Immunology*, *I*, ed. Amos, D. B., pp. 1061–1080. New York and London: Academic Press, Inc.

Buckley, R. H., Amos, D. B., Kremer, W. B. & Stickel, D. L. (1971a) Incompatible bone marrow transplantation in lymphopenic immunologic deficiency: circumvention of fatal graft-versus-host-disease by immunologic enhancement. *New England Journal of Medicine*, **285,** 1035–1042.

Buckley, R. H., Kremer, W. P., Rowlands, D. T., Huntley, C. C., Amos, D. B. & Huang, A. (1971b) Lymphopenic immunologic deficiency in identical twins: lymphocyte allografting and graft-versus-host disease following treatment with albumin-gradient-separated bone marrow 'stem' cells. *Clinical and Experimental Immunology*, **9,** 289–304.

Buckley, R. H. (1972) Plasma therapy in immunodeficiency diseases. *American Journal of Diseases of Children*, **124**, 376–381.

Buckley, R. H. (1973) Transplantation. In *Immunologic Disorders in Infants and Children*, ed. Stiehm, E. R. & Fulginiti, V. A., pp. 591–623. Philadelphia: W. B. Saunders Co.

Buckley, R. H. (1975a) Clinical and immunological features of selective IgA deficiency. In *Immunodeficiency in Man and Animals*, ed. Bergsma, D., Good, R. A., Finstad, J. & Paul, N. W., pp. 134–142. Sunderland, Mass.: Sinauer Associates, Inc.

Buckley, R. H. (1975b) Bone marrow and thymus transplantation in ataxia telangiectasia. In *Immunodeficiency in Man and Animals*, ed. Bergsma, D., Good, R. A., Finstad, J. & Paul, N. W., pp. 421–424. Sunderland, Mass.: Sinauer Associates, Inc.

Buckley, R. H., Whisnant, J. K., Schiff, R. I., Gilbertsen, R. B., Huang, A. T. & Platt, M. S. (1976) Correction of severe combined immunodeficiency by fetal liver cells. *New England Journal of Medicine*, **294**, 1076–1081.

Christian, C. L. (1960) Studies on aggregated γ-globulin. I. Sedimentation, electrophoretic, and anticomplementary properties. *Journal of Immunology*, **84**, 112–121.

Cleveland, W. W., Fogel, B. J., Brown, W. T. & Kay, H. E. M. (1968) Fetal thymic transplant in a case of DiGeorge's syndrome. *Lancet*, **ii**, 1211–1214.

Cohen, J. J., Fischbach, M. & Claman, H. R. (1970) Hydrocortisone resistance of graft-versus-host activity in mouse thymus, spleen, and bone marrow. *Journal of Immunology*, **105**, 1146–1150.

Cohn, E. S., Gard, F. R. N., Surgenor, D. M., Barnes, B. D., Brown, R. K., Derouaux, G., Gillespie, J. M., Kahnt, F. W., Lener, W. F., Liu, C. H., Mittelman, D., Mouton, R. F., Schmid, K. & Uroma, E. (1950) A system for the separation of the components of human blood: quantitative procedures for the separation of the protein components of human plasma. *Journal of the American Chemical Society*, **72**, 465–474.

Cooper, M. D., Faulk, W. P., Fudenberg, H. H., Good, R. A., Hitzig, W., Kunkel, H. G., Rosen, F. S., Seligmann, M., Soothill, J. R. & Wedgwood, R. J. (1973) Classification of primary immunodeficiencies. *New England Journal of Medicine*, **288**, 966–967.

Cornelius, E. A. (1970) Protein-losing enteropathy in the graft-versus-host reaction. *Transplantation*, **9**, 247–252.

Cowan, D. H. & Phillips, R. A. (1972) Human bone marrow transplantation. *Medical Clinics of North America*, **56**, 433–451.

Cudkowicz, F. (1975) Genetic control of resistance to allogeneic and xenogeneic bone marrow grafts in mice. *Transplantation Proceedings*, **vii**, 155–159.

de Koning, J., Dooren, L. J., van Bekkum, D. W., van Rood, J. H., Dicke, K. A. & Radl, J. (1969) Transplantation of bone marrow cells and fetal thymus in an infant with lymphopenic immunological deficiency. *Lancet*, **i**, 1223–1227.

DuPont, B., Andersen, V., Faber, V., Good, R. A., Henriksen, K., Juhl, F., Koch, C., Berat, N. M., Park, B., Svegaard, A. & Wiik, A. (1973) Immunological reconstitution in severe combined immunodeficiency with HL-A incompatible bone marrow graft. Donor selection by mixed lymphocyte culture. *Transplantation Proceedings*, **5**, 905–908.

DuPont, B., O'Reilly, R. J., Jersild, C. & Good, R. A. (1974) Transplantation of immunocompetent cells. In *Progress in Immunology, II*, ed. Brent, L. & Holborow, J., Vol. 5, pp. 203–214. North Holland: American Elsevier.

Ellis, E. F. & Henney, C. S. (1969) Adverse reactions following administration of human gamma globulin. *Journal of Allergy*, **43**, 45–54.

Fudenberg, H. H., Good, R. A., Goodman, H. C., Hitzig, W., Kunkel, H. G., Roitt, I. M., Rosen, F. S., Rowe, D. S., Seligmann, M. & Soothill, J. R. (1971) Primary immunodeficiencies: report of a World Health Organisation committee. *Pediatrics*, **47**, 927–946.

Gatti, R. A., Meuwissen, H. J., Allen, H. D., Hong, R. & Good, R. A. (1968) Immunological reconstitution of sex-linked lymphopenic immunological deficiency. *Lancet*, **ii**, 1366–1369.

Gatti, R. A., Gershanik, J. J., Levkof, A. H., Wertelecki, W. W. & Good, R. A. (1972) DiGeorge syndrome associated with combined immunodeficiency. *Journal of Pediatrics*, **81**, 920–926.

Gelfand, E. W., Baumel, R., Huber, J., Crookston, M. C. & Shumak, K. H. (1973) Polyclonal gammapathy and lymphoproliferation after transfer factor in severe combined immunodeficiency disease. *New England Journal of Medicine*, **289**, 1385–1389.

Githens, J. H., Fulginiti, V. A., Suvatte, V., Schroter, G., Hathaway, W. E., Pearlman, D. S., Kay, H. E. M., Terasaki, P. I., Hill, G. J., Kempe, C. H. & Cox, S. T. (1973) Grafting of fetal thymus and hematopoietic tissue in infants with immunodeficiency syndromes. *Transplantation*, **15**, 427–434.

Graw, R. G., Jr, Rogentine, G. N., Jr, Leventhal, B. G., Halterman, R. H., Berard, C., Herzig, G. P., Yankee, R. A., Whang-Peng, J., Kruger, G. & Henderson, E. S. (1970) Graft-versus-host reaction complicating HL-A matched bone marrow transplantation. *Lancet*, **ii**, 1053–1055.

Hathaway, W. E., Fulginiti, V. A., Pierce, C. W., Githins, J. H., Pearlman, D. S., Muschenheim, F. & Kempe, C. H. (1967) Graft-versus-host reaction following a single blood transfusion. *Journal of the American Medical Association*, **201**, 1015–1020.

Heiner, D. C. & Evans, L. (1967) Immunoglobulins and other proteins in commercial preparations of gamma globulin. *Journal of Pediatrics*, **70**, 820–827.

Herzenberg, L. A., Herzenberg, L. A., Goodlin, R. C. & Rivera, E. C. (1967) Immunoglobulin synthesis in mice. Suppression by anti-allotype antibody. *Journal of Experimental Medicine*, **126**, 701–713.

Hitzig, W. H., Kay, H. E. M. & Cottier, H. (1965) Familial lymphopenia with agammaglobulinaemia. An attempt at treatment by implantation of foetal thymus. *Lancet*, **ii**, 151–156.

Hong, R., Santosham, M., Schulte-Wisserman, H., Horowitz, S., Hsu, S. H. & Winklestein, J. A. (1976) Reconstitution of B and T lymphocyte function in severe combined immunodeficiency disease after transplantation with thymic epithelium. *Lancet*, **ii**, 1270–1272.

Horowitz, S. D., Groshong, T., Bach, F. H. & Hong, R. (1975) Treatment of severe combined immunodeficiency with bone marrow from an unrelated, mixed leucocyte-culture-nonreactive donor. *Lancet*, **ii**, 431–433.

Horowitz, S. D. (1976) Fetal thymus and liver transplantation in immunodeficiency. In *Human Health and Disease*, Biological Handbook. Washington, DC: Federation of the American Societies for Experimental Biology and Medicine (in press).

Jager, B. V. (1967) Intravenous administration of modified gamma globulin. *Archives of Internal Medicine*, **119**, 60–64.

Janeway, C. A., Rosen, F. S., Merler, E. & Alper, C. A. (1967) *The Gamma Globulins*. Boston: Little, Brown.

Janeway, C. A., Merler, E., Rosen, F. S., Salmon, S. & Crain, J. D. (1968) Intravenous gamma globulin. Metabolism of gamma globulin fragments in normal and agammaglobulinemic persons. *New England Journal of Medicine*, **278**, 919–923.

Kay, H. E. M. (1971) Fetal thymus transplants in man. In *Ontogeny of Acquired Immunity*, a Ciba Foundation Symposium, ed. Porter, R. & Knight, J., pp. 249–268. North-Holland: Elsevier.

Keightley, R. G., Lawton, A. R., Cooper, M. D., Wu, L. Y. F. & Yunis, E. J. (1975) Successful fetal liver transplantation in a child with severe combined immunodeficiency. *Lancet*, **ii**, 850–853.

Kirkpatrick, C. H. (1975) Properties and activities of transfer factor. *Journal of Allergy and Clinical Immunology*, **55**, 411–421.

Kirkpatrick, C. H. & Gallin, J. I. (1975) Suppression of cellular immune responses following transfer factor: report of a case. *Cellular Immunology*, **15**, 470–474.

Kretschmer, R., Say, B., Brown, D. & Rosen, F. S. (1968) Congenital aplasia of the thymus gland (DiGeorge's syndrome). *New England Journal of Medicine*, **279**, 1295–1301.

Lawrence, H. S. (1969) Transfer factor. *Advances in Immunology*, **11**, 195–266.

Levy, R. L., Huang, S. W., Bach, M. L., Bach, F. H., Hong, R., Ammann, A. J., Bortin, M. M. & Kay, H. E. M. (1971) Thymic transplantation in a case of chronic mucocutaneous candidiasis. *Lancet*, **ii**, 898–900.

Lischner, H. W. & Huff, D. S. (1975) T-cell deficiency in DiGeorge syndrome. In *Immunodeficiency in Man and Animals*, ed. Bergsma, D., Good, R. A., Finstad, J. & Paul, N. W., pp. 16–21. Sunderland, Mass.: Sinauer Associates, Inc.

Lowenberg, B. (1975) *Fetal liver cell transplantation. Role and nature of the fetal haemopoietic stem cell*. Doctoral Thesis, Erasmus University (Rotterdam) Rijswijk (A.H.), pp. 1–142. The Netherlands: Publication of the Radiobiological Institute.

MacKay, M., Vallet, L. & Cambridge, B. S. (1973) The characterization and stability during storage of human immunoglobulin prepared for clinical use. *Vox Sanguinis*, **25**, 124–140.

McCullough, J., Benson, S. J., Yunis, E. J. & Quie, P. G. (1969) Effect of blood-bank storage on leucocyte function. *Lancet*, **ii**, 1333–1388.

Medical Research Council Working Party on Hypogammaglobulinaemia (1971) Hypogammaglobulinaemia in the United Kingdom. *Medical Research Council Special Report Series*, No. 310. pp. 1–319.

Meuwissen, H. J., Gatti, R. A., Terasaki, P. I., Hong, R. & Good, R. A. (1969) Treatment of lymphopenic hypogammaglobulinemia and bone marrow aplasia by transplantation of allogeneic marrow. Crucial role of histocompatibility matching. *New England Journal of Medicine*, **281**, 691–697.

Meyers, J. D., Spencer, H. C., Jr, Watts, J. C., Gregg, M. B., Stewart, J. A., Troupin, R. H. & Thomas, E. D. (1975) Cytomegalovirus pneumonia after human marrow transplantation. *Annals of Internal Medicine*, **82**, 181–188.

Miller, M. E. (1969) Uses and abuses of gammaglobulin. *Hospital Practice*, **4**, 38–43.

Nowell, P. C., Hirsch, B. E., Fox, D. H. & Wilson, D. B. (1970) Evidence for the existence of multipotential lympho-hematopoietic stem cells in the adult rat. *Journal of Cellular Physiology*, **75**, 151–158.

Owen, J. J. T., Cooper, M. D. & Raff, M. C. (1974) *In vitro* generation of B lymphocytes in mouse foetal liver, a mammalian 'bursa equivalent'. *Lancet*, **i**, 361–363.

Pachman, L. M., Kirkpatrick, C. H., Kaufman, D. B. & Rothberg, R. M. (1974) The lack of effect of transfer in thymic dysplasia with immunoglobulin synthesis. *Journal of Pediatrics*, **84**, 681–688.

Polmar, S. H., Wetzler, E. M., Stern, R. C. & Hirschorn, R. (1975) Restoration of *in vitro* lymphocyte responses with exogenous adenosine deaminase in a patient with severe combined immunodeficiency. *Lancet*, **ii**, 743–746.

Rachelefsky, G. S., Stiehm, E. R., Ammann, A. J., Cederbaum, S. D., Opelz, G. & Teraski, P. I. (1975) T-cell reconstitution by thymus transplantation and transfer factor in severe combined immunodeficiency. *Pediatrics*, **55**, 114–118.

Reynolds, H. Y. & Thompson, R. E. (1973a) Pulmonary host defenses. I. Analysis of protein and lipids in bronchial secretions and antibody responses after vaccination with *Pseudomonas aeruginosa*. *Journal of Immunology*, **111**, 358–368.

Reynolds, H. Y. & Thompson, R. E. (1973b) Pulmonary host defenses. II. Interaction of respiratory antibodies with *Pseudomonas aeruginosa* and alveolar macrophages. *Journal of Immunology*, **111**, 369–380.

Richerson, H. B. & Seebohm, P. M. (1966) Anaphylactoid reaction to human gamma globulin. *Archives of Internal Medicine*, **117**, 568–572.

Rieger, C. H. L., Lustig, J. V. & Rothberg, R. M. (1976) T-cell development after transplantation of early embryonic liver in severe combined immunodeficiency disease (SCID). *Federation Proceedings (Abstracts)*, **35**, 791.

Schmidt, A. P., Taswell, H. F. & Gleich, G. J. (1969) Anaphylactic transfusion reactions associated with anti-IgA antibody. *New England Journal of Medicine*, **280**, 188–193.

Schulkind, M. L., Adler, W. H., Altemeier, W. A. & Ayoub, E. M. (1972) Transfer factor in the treatment of chronic mucocutaneous candidiasis. *Cellular Immunology*, **3**, 606–615.

Sieber, O. F., Jr, Durie, B. G., Hattler, B., Salmon, S. E. & Fulginiti, V. A. (1974) Spontaneous evolution of immune competence in DiGeorge syndrome. *Pediatric Research*, **8**, 418.

Simons, M. J., Schumacher, M. J. & Fowler, R. (1968) Intravenous gamma globulin therapy of immunoglobulin deficiency diseases. *Australian Paediatric Journal*, **4**, 127–133.

Solberg, C. O., Meuwissen, H. J., Needham, R. N., Good, R. A. & Matsen, J. M. (1971) Infectious complications in bone marrow transplant patients. *British Medical Journal*, **i**, 18–23.

Soothill, J. F., Kay, H. E. M. & Batchelor, J. R. (1971) Graft restoration of primary immunodeficiency. In *Cell Interaction and Receptor Antibodies in Immune Responses*, ed. Makela, O., Cross, A. & Kosmen, T. E., pp. 41–52. New York: Academic Press.

Spitler, L. E., Levin, A. S., Stites, D. P., Fudenberg, H. H., Pirofsky, B., August, C. S., Stiehm, E. R., Hitzig, W. H. & Gatti, R. A. (1972) The Wiskott-Aldrich syndrome: results of transfer factor therapy. *Journal of Clinical Investigation*, **51**, 3216–3224.

Steele, R. W., Limas, C., Thurman, G. B., Schuelein, M., Bauer, H. & Bellanti, J. A. (1972) Familial thymic aplasia. Attempted reconstruction with fetal thymus in a Millipore diffusion chamber. *New England Journal of Medicine*, **287**, 787–791.

Stiehm, E. R. & Fudenberg, H. H. (1965) Antibodies to gamma globulin in infants and children exposed to isologous gamma globulin. *Pediatrics*, **35**, 229–235.

Stiehm, E. R., Vaerman, J.-P. & Fudenberg, H. H. (1966) Plasma infusions in immunologic deficiency states: metabolic and therapeutic studies. *Blood*, **28**, 918–937.

Stites, D. P., Carr, M. C. & Fudenberg, H. H. (1974) Ontogeny of cellular immunity in the human fetus. Development of responses to phytohemagglutinin and to allogeneic cells. *Cellular Immunology*, **11**, 257–271.

Storb, R., Gluckman, E. & Thomas, E. D. (1974) Treatment of established human graft-versus-host disease by antithymocyte globulin. *Blood*, **44**, 57–75.

Stutman, O., Yunis, E. J., Teague, P. O. & Good, R. A. (1968) Graft-versus-host reactions induced by transplantation of parental strain thymus in neonatally thymectomized F_1 hybrid mice. *Transplantation*, **6**, 514–523.

Thomas, E. D. & Storb, R. (1970) Technique for human marrow grafting. *Blood*, **36**, 507–515.

Thorsby, E. (1974) The human major histocompatibility system. *Transplant Reviews*, **18**, 51–129.

Uphoff, D. E. (1958) Preclusion of secondary phase of irradiation syndrome by inoculation of fetal hematopoietic tissue following lethal total body irradiation. *Journal of the National Cancer Institute*, **20**, 625–632.

van Bekkum, D. W., Roodenberg, J., Heidt, P. J. & van der Waaij, D. (1974) Mitigation of secondary disease of allogeneic mouse radiation chimeras by modification of the intestinal microflora. *Journal of the National Cancer Institute*, **52**, 401–404.

Vossen, J. M., de Koning, J., van Bekkum, D. W., Dicke, K. A., Eijsvoogel, V. P., Hijmans, W., Van Loghem, E., Radl, J., Van Rood, J. J., Van der Waaij, D. & Dooren, L. J. (1973) Successful treatment of an infant with severe combined immunodeficiency by transplantation of bone marrow cells from an uncle. *Clinical and Experimental Immunology*, **13**, 9–20.

Vyas, G. N., Perkins, H. A. & Fudenberg, H. H. (1968) Anaphylactoid transfusion reactions associated with anti-IgA. *Lancet*, **ii**, 3–12.

Vyas, G. N., Levin, A. S. & Fudenberg, H. H. (1970) Intrauterine isoimmunization caused by maternal IgA crossing the placenta. *Nature*, **225**, 275–276.

Waldmann, T. A. & Strober, W. (1969) Metabolism of immunoglobulins. *Progress in Allergy*, **13**, 1–110.

Wara, D. W., Goldstein, A., Doyle, N. E. & Ammann, A. J. (1975) Thymosin activity in patients with cellular immunodeficiency. *New England Journal of Medicine*, **292**, 70–74.

Wu, A. M., Till, J. E., Siminovitch, L. & McCulloch, E. A. (1967) A cytological study of the capacity for differentiation of normal hemopoietic colony-forming cells. *Journal of Cellular Physiology*, **69**, 177–184.

Wu, A. M., Till, J. E., Siminovitch, L. & McCulloch, E. A. (1968) Cytological evidence for a relationship between normal hemopoietic colony-forming cells and cells of the lymphoid system. *Journal of Experimental Medicine*, **127**, 455–463.

Yunis, E. J. & Amos, D. B. (1971) Three closely linked genetic systems relevant to transplantation. *Proceedings of the National Academy of Sciences*, **12**, 3031–3035.

11
IMMUNOTHERAPY OF HUMAN LEUKAEMIA

Charles B. Freeman

The treatment of human malignant disease by immunotherapy is not a new concept. The ability of neoplastic cells to provoke a response by the host immune system has received ample experimental support from studies of tumour transplantation and the induction of resistance to tumour transplantation notably by Gross (1943), Foley (1953) and Prehn and Main (1957). Until recently, methods for detecting antigens of experimentally induced tumours have depended upon transplantation resistance by preimmunised recipients of syngeneic tumour grafts (Old and Boyse, 1964; Baldwin, 1973). The antigens involved were thus defined as tumour-specific transplantation antigens (TSTA).

It has been made clear over the last few years that tumours of a spontaneous rather than induced origin are more comparable to the human situation and it is important to note that spontaneous animal tumours tend to have weak TSTA, or no detectable TSTA (Prehn, 1976). It is clearly difficult to support the dogma that human tumours have specific antigens indicative of their neoplastic nature by using transplantation methods, because of the more complex immunogenetic differences between humans, and because of the ethical objections of transplanting live or even dead tumour cells into genetically similar family members.

Evidence for human reactivity to autochthonous tumour cells in situ has partly been based upon the observation of spontaneous regression of tumours (Everson, 1964; Stephenson et al, 1971) of lymphoid cell infiltration into the tumour and neighbouring lymph nodes (Black, Opler and Speer, 1955, 1956; Black and Speer, 1958; Hamlin, 1968; di Paola et al, 1974) and the increased incidence of malignancy in primary and acquired immunological disorders (Gatti and Good, 1971; Kersey, Spector and Good, 1973). Other evidence has been derived from in vitro studies of immune responses to putative tumour antigens, although in most cases the precise specificity of the response is uncertain. These studies include work on the Burkitt lymphoma (Klein et al, 1967; Fass, Herberman and Ziegler, 1970a), on malignant melanoma (Morton et al, 1968; Lewis et al, 1969; Muna, Mattens and Smart, 1969; Jehn et al, 1970; Bluming et al, 1972; Jagarlamoody et al, 1971; Fossati et al, 1971; De Vries, Rümke and Bernheim, 1972), on neuroblastoma (Hellström et al, 1970), on sarcomata (Morton et al, 1969, 1971), on colonic and mammary neoplasms (Gold, Gold and Friedman, 1968; Baldwin et al, 1973) and on bladder tumours (Bubenik et al, 1970a, b).

In analysing the effects of immunotherapeutic manoeuvres in leukaemia, most clinical trials rely on differences in first remission length and survival, without considering differences in the residual leukaemia cell mass at the time of diagnosis of remission and differences in the proliferative properties of individual patients' blast cells. Unfortunately, the treatment is difficult to evaluate using in vitro techniques in which most of the variables between patients can be eliminated. This review will attempt to place the current clinical trials into the perspective of what is known about specific immunity in haematological neoplasia, to consider how immunotherapy can be measured in vitro, and to discuss the likely future of immunotherapy in leukaemia.

LEUKAEMIA SPECIFIC IMMUNITY

The evidence for leukaemia specific immunity, or at least leukaemia directed auto-immunity is derived from serological, cellular and delayed hypersensitivity studies. The immune reactivity by the host against his own leukaemia cells is possibly the only evidence for the existence of leukaemia-specific antigens.

Tests of Cell-mediated Responses

MIXED LEUCOCYTE REACTION (MLR)

Several authors have described the response of patients in remission to their own acute phase leukaemia blasts (Bach, Bach and Loo, 1969; Fridman and Kourilsky, 1969; Viza et al, 1969; Powles et al, 1971; Gutterman et al, 1973a; Taylor, Harris and Freeman, 1976). The response is measured by the increase in ^{3}H-thymidine incorporation by lymphocytes cultured in vitro in the presence of leukaemia blasts, compared with controls consisting either of separate lymphocytes and blast cell cultures or lymphocytes stimulated with autologous lymphocytes. The response characteristically occurs early (after 72 h in culture) (Fridman and Kourilsky, 1969; Taylor et al, 1976), and is generally weaker in magnitude than reponses to phytohaemagglutinin (PHA) or allogeneic normal leucocytes.

A positive MLR is more frequent in acute myeloid leukaemia (AML) than acute lymphoblastic leukaemia (ALL), and is correlated both with the presence of immunoglobulin on the surface of the leukaemia cells, and with the ability of the patient's serum to inhibit the reaction (Gutterman et al, 1973b). The response to ALL cells is much less frequent (Cotropia et al, 1975), and according to Schweitzer, Melief and Eijsvoogel (1973) cannot be separated from the non-specific stimulation by control cells. Lymphoblasts have a low level of releasable sialic acid in comparison with myeloblasts (Cotropia et al, 1975) and E-rosette forming lymphoblasts consistently fail to stimulate allogeneic lymphocytes (Tsukimoto, Wong and Lamplin, 1976; Leventhal, Leung and Johnson, 1976).

It is now established that human lymphoblastoid cell lines (Green and Sell, 1970; Flier et al, 1970; Knight, Moore and Clarkson, 1971; Junge, Koekstra and Deinhardt, 1971; Han, Moore and Sokal, 1971; Weksler and Birnbaum, 1972; Steel et al, 1973; Bauscher and Smith, 1973; Svedmyr et al, 1974) and PHA or conconavalin A-induced blasts (Flier et al, 1970; Weksler, 1973) can stimulate autologous peripheral blood lymphocytes to increased DNA synthesis and blast transformation similar to or even stronger than the normal allogeneic MLR and much stronger than the MLR between autochthonous leukaemia blasts and remission lymphocytes.

Rudolph, Mickelson and Thomas (1970a, b) failed to find evidence of leukaemia-associated antigens by means of the MLR when testing four sets of identical twins, when one of each pair of twins had acute leukaemia. On the other hand, such stimulation has been observed by Han and Wang (1972) in one set of twins and by Fefer et al (1974a) in 3 out of 12 sets of identical twins. Bach et al (1969) and Taylor, Harris and Jones (1975) have detected unidirectional stimulation of lymphocytes from HL-A identical siblings, although it is likely that other normal transplantation antigens may have been responsible for the response.

Thus, although there is no doubt that some autochthonous leukaemia cells are able to trigger lymphocytes, the antigen or antigens involved have not so far been characterised and assigning them the status of tumour-specific antigen may be premature.

IN VITRO CYTOTOXICITY (CMC)

Attempts have been made to measure the ability of patient and close relative lymphocytes to mediate in vitro cytotoxicity using chromium-51- (^{51}Cr) labelled leukaemic blasts as target cells (Leventhal et al, 1972). Though low-grade cytotoxicity was found there are problems in interpretation owing to the method of calculating the CMC values. Moreover the technique does not lend itself well to direct CMC assays owing to the high lymphocyte target cell ratios required, and the rapid spontaneous release of ^{51}Cr from the target cells relative to the immune cytolysis during the incubation period. A more promising technique would seem to be based upon the in vitro sensitisation of the patient's lymphocytes to the prospective targets based upon the in vitro CMC systems developed for mouse (Häyry and Defendi, 1970) and human histocompatibility studies (Solliday and Bach, 1972; Lightbody and Bach, 1972; Miggiano et al, 1972). This technique will be discussed later in relation to the in vitro assessment of the effects of immunotherapy.

SKIN TESTS

The reactions of patients to the intradermal injection of leukaemic cell extracts is currently receiving more attention. It was observed that hypotonic NaCl extracted leukaemic cells (Oren and Herberman, 1971; Char et al, 1973) were capable of eliciting delayed hypersensitivity type reactions in autologous and allogeneic leukaemic patients, whereas remission leucocytes were incapable of eliciting such responses, though this was a concentration-dependent result. There was a good correlation with the clinical state of the patient, since remission patients responded more frequently than relapsed patients. The introduction of preparative polyacrylamide gel electrophoresis to separate the skin reactive antigens of leukaemic cells (Hollinshead and Herberman, 1975) may assist further in the isolation and characterisation of tumour-associated antigens. If successful this would provide the basis for more rational immunotherapy by active immunisation, or by the administration of passively raised antisera.

Tests of Humoral Responses

Attempts have been made to identify antibodies reacting with leukaemic cells using a variety of techniques (Séligmann, Graber and Bernard, 1954; Killman, 1957; de Carvalho, 1964; Doré et al, 1967; Yoshida and Imai, 1970; Bias et al, 1972). In general autoantibodies have been found only in a minority of patients with leukaemia and in normal controls, while cross-reactivity between leukaemias of different cytomorphology and with non-leukaemic cells raises doubts as to the leukaemia-specific nature of the reacting antibodies.

PRODUCTION OF LEUKAEMIA-SPECIFIC ANTISERA

The use of leukaemic cells and membrane extracts to produce antibody in non-human species has been a fertile ground of investigation. These have usually been produced by

9

immunising rabbits (Séligmann, 1956; de Carvalho, 1960; Korngold, Van Leeuwen and Miller, 1961; Garb, Stein and Sims, 1962; Hyde, Garb and Bennett, 1967; Viza et al, 1970a, b; Yata et al, 1970; Mann et al, 1971, 1973; Harlozinska et al, 1973; Billings and Terasaki, 1974; Baker et al, 1976), but one group of workers has immunised non-human primates (Metzgar et al, 1972, 1974; Mohanakumar, Metzgar and Miller, 1974) and another group has raised antibodies in mice (Baker and Taub, 1973). These reports show considerable differences in activity and specificity between such xenoantisera, as indicated by varying degrees of cross-reactivity with normal lymphoid cells or tissue extracts, and other leukaemic cells. They suggest that several antigens may be represented on leukaemia cells only some of which may be truly leukaemia specific. These non-leukaemic antigens may include species-specific antigens, histocompatibility determinants, fetal antigens, cell cycle-specific antigens and tissue-specific or differentiation antigens. Nevertheless some of these sera offer the hope of better diagnostic tools and possibly even of passive immunotherapy.

IMMUNOTHERAPY

The long and checkered history of attempts at the immunotherapy of human malignant disease (for review see Currie, 1972) belies the difficulties both theoretical, and practical in this form of treatment. In many cases, immunotherapy is used at a late stage of disease, a time when any beneficial effects must be considered to be suboptimal. Frequently it is preceded by x-irradiation and chemotherapy which are strongly immunosuppressive, and must in many cases work against the effects of immunotherapy. Finally even where immunotherapy is contemplated, it is still not clear what form of immunotherapy should be used, and moreover, what dosage, timing and route of treatment should be employed. It is thus not surprising that so far no spectacular results have been obtained.

The various forms of immunotherapy which have been used are defined as follows:

1. *Passive immunotherapy*: transfer of immune serum from animals immunised with tumour cells, or serum taken from patients in whom the tumour has regressed.

2. *Passive cellular immunotherapy*: the transfer of lymphoid cells (a) from normal subjects, and (b) from other patients in whom the same type of tumour has either regressed or has been removed. Such lymphoid cells might have cytotoxic effects on the recipients' tumour cells. Under certain circumstances the transferred lymphoid cells could also have an adoptive role.

3. *Passive immunotherapy with immunological mediators*: the transfer of subcellular products of lymphoid cells from specifically immune animals or patients leading to the recruitment of a tumour specific immune response in the recipient, e.g., immune RNA, transfer factor.

4. *Adoptive immunotherapy*: the transfer of immunocompetent cells in the hope that the transferred cells will produce a long-lived immunity and actually replace those of the host. The most important example is bone marrow transplantation from a normal tissue-matched donor to a leukaemic patient whose own marrow and immunocompetent cells have been ablated by irradiation or cytotoxic drugs.

5. *Active immunotherapy*: the immunisation of patients with tumour material of autochthonous or allogeneic origin (specific) or with other agents, notably Bacille Calmette Guérin (BCG) (non-specific) in an attempt to stimulate a failing immune response.

Passive Immunotherapy

This probably represents the earliest form of immunotherapy of human malignant disease. The passive transfer of immune serum has long been employed in the treatment of tetanus and diphtheria, and more recently of snake bites. This concept has obvious attractions for the treatment of malignant disease since the serum can be produced easily, it can be stored for relatively long periods, and its antitumour effects are relatively easily tested in vitro. The first clinical tests of passive immunotherapy with immune serum were published in 1895 by Hericourt and Richet. There has followed a long series of studies using passive immunotherapy with immune serum in several types of human cancer including leukaemia (Lindström, 1927; Brittingham and Chaplin, 1960; de Carvalho, 1963; Fernbach, Rossen and Butler, 1960) and some investigators have treated leukaemias and lymphomas with sera containing antibodies against human lymphocytes (Laszlo, Buckley and Amos, 1968; Djerassi, 1968; Herberman et al, 1971). In contrast to the somewhat discouraging and at best anecdotal results for passive serum therapy of human leukaemia, animal studies have produced more encouraging results (Gorer and Amos, 1956; Old et al, 1967; Miller et al, 1968; Reiff and Kim, 1969; Hill et al, 1969).

The mechanism of action of passively transferred antibody is difficult to study in vivo. It has been difficult to induce the rejection of allografts using passively transferred immune serum, possibly because of dilution effects following injection, by complexing and inactivation by soluble antigen, and by rapid degradation and clearance by the liver and kidneys. Whether injected antibody is able to synergise with Fc-receptor bearing macrophages or killer (K) cells, as is known to occur in vitro in allogeneic and syngeneic tumour systems (Pollack et al, 1972; Lamon et al, 1972), is open to further investigation.

Ways of potentiating this effect have also been sought. Linking the passively transferred antibody to a drug or radioactive isotope such as ^{131}I has been proposed and animal studies have shown promise (Ghose et al, 1967, 1972). However, the results obtained in experimental systems have shown that drug and antibody injected alone produced results as good as antibody–drug complexes (Davies and O'Neill, 1973) and clinical trials in patients with malignant melanoma were disappointing. What is interesting is that cells treated with drugs may be more susceptible to killing than untreated cells and indicates that 'preconditioning' of tumour cells with systemically administered drugs, followed by brief but relatively large amounts of passive immunotherapy could point the way to future developments in this field.

Several cautionary notes however apply to passive immunotherapy. Firstly, in some experiments the immunopotentiation of tumour growth by the enhancing or blocking effects of an antiserum has been observed, and this may be a risk clinically. Secondly, there is the problem of serum sickness following repeated infusions especially of xeno-antisera although this may be less of a problem in highly immunosuppressed patients, such as those undergoing remission induction in leukaemia.

Passive Cellular Immunotherapy

Although not yet an accepted clinical form of treatment, passive cellular immunotherapy has grown out of studies in allogeneic tumour systems, which show that the transfer of lymphoid cells from an immune individual to an immunosuppressed bearer of an actively growing allogeneic tumour could abolish tumour growth (Freedman, Cerottini and Brunner, 1972). In syngeneic tumours, both in vivo (Delorme and Alexander, 1964; Hellström et al, 1969) and in vitro immunisation of lymphoid cells (Röllinghoff and Wagner, 1973; Treves, Cohen and Feldman, 1975) can have dramatic results when these cells are used to combat the tumour in vivo.

The infusion of large numbers of allogeneic and syngeneic lymphoid cells may result in a graft versus leukaemia (GVL) reaction which is incidental to the destruction of host cells by the donor cells [graft versus host reaction (GVH)]. The effectiveness was demonstrated by Mathé and his colleagues in mouse leukaemias including L1210 (Mathé and Schwarzenberg, 1968), Friend leukaemia (Mathé and Amiel, 1964) and spontaneous AKR leukaemia (Mathé, Amiel and Bernard, 1960). Schwarzenberg et al (1966) transfused lymphocytes from nonimmune allogeneic donors into acute leukaemia patients, and obtained remissions, though of relatively short duration (one week to four months).

Other studies using patient conditioning prior to the transfer of haemopoietic cells come under the heading of adoptive immunotherapy and are considered below. The distinction is simply between the short-term antileukaemic effects of the transferred cells, and the longer term effects of lymphoid cell replacement by haemopoietic cell grafting. This does not necessarily apply in the GVL protocols of Bortin (1974) who has developed sophisticated animal models for the examination of the effects of transferred immunologically competent cells. The technique is based on that described by Boranic (1968) who treated leukaemic mice with allogeneic immunocompetent cells and rescued these mice from the subsequent GVH by treatment with cyclophosphamide (CYCLO) and a syngeneic bone marrow graft.

Bortin has used this model to treat an AKR mouse leukaemia. AKR leukaemia cells were injected into syngeneic recipients, and after four days the mice were treated with sublethal doeses of CYCLO and Total Body Irradiation (TBI). Histoincompatible bone marrow and spleen cells are injected intravenously and the GVH/GVL reaction allowed to continue for 10 days, when the reaction is terminated with a small dose of CYCLO plus antiserum to the grafted cells, followed by a repopulating dose of histocompatible bone marrow. Bortin et al (1973) tested the relationship between the GVL effect and GVH effects of various strains of mice, to determine whether they were positively correlated. A clear correlation existed in three donor strains: AKR cells caused no GVH disease and had no detectable antileukaemic effect; CBA cells caused mild GVH disease amd only slight antileukaemic effect and C57BL/6 produced acute GVH disease and excellent GVL capability. However, there was a definite difference in the relationship between GVH and GVL in two other strains tested: strain A cells caused the most severe GVH disease but had only moderate antileukaemic effect and DBA/2 cells caused somewhat less GVH disease, but had the highest GVL reactivity.

The essential features of this treatment from a clinical standpoint is that histocompatible cells have little GVL effect, that selection of the donor GVL cells requires a certain degree of in vitro testing which is now possible, and that abolition of later GVH disease is not beyond the bounds of possibility. The elegant studies carried out by Bortin deserve careful clinical testing since they are based on a rational and clear appraisal of the problems involved in the immunological ablation of a weakly immunogenic leukaemia. It is possible that the utilisation of differences in the representation of histocompatability antigens in a 'controlled GVH' system such as this represents the best hope for future developments in this field.

Passive Immunotherapy with Immunological Mediators

The use of immunological mediators to combat the growth of tumours has been advocated to overcome the problems discussed above in the use of the transfer of serum or cells. Alexander et al (1967) have suggested that passively transferred lymphoid cells operate by releasing a subcellular component which has a host antitumour recruiting effect. This thesis was supported by the finding that an immune RNA extracted from the lymphoid cells of sheep immunised with rat benzpyrene induced sarcoma cells, slowed the growth of the rat tumour. The use of immune RNA extracted from syngeneic, allogeneic and xenogeneic animals has been repeatedly advocated by Pilch and deKernion (1974), for the treatment of tumours, but unfortunately the role of immune RNA as an immunotherapeutic agent has not been investigated in human leukaemia. The results are interesting enough to warrant further investigation.

A further approach is the use of transfer factor (TF), a dialysable factor of low molecular weight capable of transferring delayed hypersensitivity responses from skin-test positive donors to skin-test negative recipients. TF taken from normal lymphocytes of patients with tumours in regression, both autochthonous and allogeneic has been used to treat solid tumours (Brandes, Galton and Wiltshaw, 1971; Oettgen et al, 1974). Neidhart and LoBuglio (1974) treated five patients with ALL using TF from family donors who had positive in vitro MIF assays to leukaemia cells. There was no effect on the clinical course of the disease.

Adoptive Immunotherapy

Adoptively acquired immunity can be distinguished from passively acquired immunity be it serum or cells, by the fact that the immunity is long lived, and replaces that of the host. In practice the distinction is less easy to make especially in the patient, since both types of immunity could theoretically have immediate antitumour effects, and long-term replacement effects, in immunosuppressed patients. Nevertheless it is pertinent to consider adoptive immunotherapy as a form of antitumour therapy since the conditioning of the patient to receive the graft is usually accompanied by immunosuppressive drugs and irradiation which have strong antitumour effects. Moreover, the grafted cells may have a variable GVL effect, though the object is to match the donor and recipient HLA antigens to eliminate fatal GVH disease. Excellent reviews of bone marrow transplantation can be found by van Bekkum (1972), Mathé and Schwarzenberg (1974), Good and Bach (1974) and Thomas et al (1975). The essential criteria of bone marrow transplantation in immune deficiency disorders, aplastic anaemia and leukaemia are described by Thomas et al (1975) and can be divided into selection of the donor, by HL-A and MLR matching with the recipient by irradiation and/or chemotherapy and in some cases postgrafting immunotherapy of donor white cells.

SYNGENEIC TRANSPLANTS

Although it is rare for a leukaemic patient to have an identical twin, such a patient is a logical candidate for attempts to eradicate the leukaemia by TBI with or without additional chemotherapy and immunotherapy followed by twin marrow transplantation. In early clinical studies by Thomas et al (1961) normal haematopoiesis was restored in three ALL patients following TBI and syngeneic transplants, but all three relapsed within 7 to 12 weeks. In later studies (Fefer, Mickelson and Thomas, 1974b) 'immunotherapy' was added to the basic regimen of TBI and twin marrow transplantation with the hope of delaying leukaemic recurrence, 'immunotherapy' consisted of infusions of normal twin buffy-coat lymphocytes three times per week for three weeks and weekly subcutaneous injections of irradiated (10 000 rad) autologous leukaemic cells in the hope of providing an antigenic stimulus to the infused donor lymphocytes. A 15-year-old patient with ALL relapsed within a month, a 26-year-old patient with AML went into remission but died of interstitial pneumonitis at seven weeks and a 33-year-old patient with AML relapsed at 10 months. Subsequently, high-dose chemotherapy with CYCLO 60 mg/kg on two days was added to the protocol in an attempt to provide more effective initial tumour cell reduction. Twenty patients received CYCLO, TBI and twin marrow transplants and 13 of these additional 'immunotherapy'. Seventeen patients entered complete remission and eight (three ALL, four AML and one lymphosarcoma/leukaemia) remain in complete remission at 3 to 49 months without any maintenance chemotherapy.

The main problem with syngeneic transplants would appear to be the persistence of residual leukaemic cells in the patient and this would seem to call for more intensive combination chemotherapy prior to CYCLO and TBI.

ALLOGENEIC TRANSPLANTS

The majority of marrow grafts for acute leukaemia have been performed between ABO compatible, HL-A identical siblings and siblings not reactive in MLR. Of various conditioning schedules so far tried high-level chimerism and sustained remissions have been obtained only with CYCLO in doses of at least 45 mg/kg day for four days (Graw et al, 1972) high dose chemotherapy with BACT [bischloroethylnitrosurea (BCNU), cytosine arabinoside (Ara-C), CYCLO and thioguanine (6TG)] (Graw et al, 1974) and TBI alone or in combination with CYCLO (Thomas et al, 1975).

Thomas and his colleagues (1975) have reported on five years' experience of marrow grafts given to a total of 70 patients, 36 with AML and 34 with ALL. All these patients received their transplants at a time when more conventional chemotherapy was considered as failing. Sixty-six patients obtained functional grafts and 46 of these (73 per cent) developed varying degrees of GVH disease. The percentage of patients surviving beyond 50 days has increased from less than 50 per cent in those receiving transplants between 1969 and 1971 to 100 per cent in those with transplants in the first six months of 1974. The improved results are attributed to improvement in the supportive care of patients and more effective conditioning regimes. Nineteen of the original 70 patients remain in complete remission beyond three months, nine for one to four years after transplantation.

The rather limited, if encouraging results of marrow transplantation and the need for highly sophisticated facilities for supportive care are major factors in inhibiting the spread of such treatment facilities.

Active Immunotherapy

Most of the current clinical trials in leukaemia utilise some form of active immunotherapy, such as BCG, or *Corynebacterium parvum*, either alone or with tumour cells, or cell lines. It would be premature to say that this form of immunotherapy offers the best hope for the future, but by far the most effort in the immunotherapy of leukaemia has been directed to this form of treatment. It is time to review the progress in this area with a view to determining the direction of future studies.

BCG IMMUNOPROPHYLAXIS IN MAN

Reports that BCG may inhibit the development of experimental neoplasms have prompted certain groups to consider the possibility that BCG vaccination might protect children not only from tuberculosis but also lead to a lowering of the incidence of malignant disease including leukaemia. Davignon et al (1970, 1971) reported a 50 per cent reduction in risk of leukaemia death among Canadian children vaccinated neonatally and a report from Chicago indicated an 85 per cent reduction in the risk of death from leukaemia among black children vaccinated neonatally (Rosenthal et al, 1973).

Objections have been raised, however, to the epidemiological methods used in both these studies. Comstock, Livesay and Webster (1971) were unable to find a decreased incidence of leukaemia, Hodgkin's disease or lymphosarcoma in BCG vaccinated individuals. A study from Great Britain (MRC, 1972) and one from Puerto Rico (Comstock, Martinez and Livesay, 1975) showed no statistically significant deficit of leukaemia deaths or cases respectively. It should be noted, however, in view of the early onset at least of acute lymphoblastic leukaemia, that none of these studies involved neonatal vaccination.

There is no evidence from overall population statistics that leukaemia mortality is lower in Quebec, Canada, or Glasgow, Scotland, where BCG is given to a large proportion of the newborn, than in areas without this policy (Kinlen and Pike, 1971) and in Scandinavia where the Swedes vaccinate the newborn, the Danes school entrants (age seven) and the Norwegians school-leavers (13–14) there is no difference in the age specific mortality rates for leukaemia between each country (Waaler, 1971).

It is thus doubtful whether BCG vaccination even in the neonatal period confers any significant protection against leukaemia.

THERAPY

In animal studies, BCG, with or without tumour cells, have been admin..iered successfully prior to the inoculation of tumour grafts although established tumour grafts are generally refractory to systemic BCG immunisation. However, Mathé and his colleagues (Mathé, 1968; Mathé, Pauillart and Lapayraque, 1969a) taking the grafted syngeneic murine leukaemia L1210 have shown that treatment of animals with BCG or irradiated leukaemia cells applied even after the grafting of 10^4 leukaemia cells delays and reduces mortality. Irradiated leukaemia cells appear more effective than BCG but the combination was superior to either used alone. However, this type of immunotherapy was ineffective if the number of leukaemia cells grafted was over 10^5.

Therapy of Acute Lymphoblastic Leukaemia (ALL)

Prompted by his studies using the L1210 leukaemia, Mathé and his colleagues (1969b) embarked on a clinical trial of active immunotherapy in ALL patients. These patients received induction chemotherapy consisting either of prednisolone (Pred.) alone or with vincristine (VCR) and rubidomycin (DNR), followed by up to 18 months' consolidation chemotherapy using several agents in sequence in order to produce minimal residual disease. The 30 patients between 3 and 50 years who were in complete remission after this chemotherapy were randomised into four groups receiving either no treatment (10 patients)

BCG alone (eight patients), pooled irradiated allogeneic ALL cells alone (five patients), or BCG plus cells (seven patients). All the 'no treatment' patients had relapsed after 130 days, whereas only 9/20 patients receiving the various forms of immunotherapy had relapsed. No difference was found between the three types of immunotherapy and in any case all immunotherapy patients received both cells and BCG after a few months.

Mathé and his colleagues have tested eight other treatment protocols in which leukaemia cells + BCG have been given with or without other adjuvants such as *Corynebacterium parvum*, Poly I Poly C, (synthetic polynucleotides) or *C. granulosum* (Mathé et al, 1972, 1973). Concurrent changes in the chemotherapy and treatment of central nervous system (CNS) disease and the lack of controls in these studies makes the assessment of the relative merits of the immunotherapy schedules very difficult. Poly I Poly C was poorly tolerated and is no longer used by these workers, while the addition of adamantadine and VCR to one of their immunotherapy protocols produced shorter remission lengths (Mathé et al, 1971). Patients with relatively well-differentiated cytological types of ALL are said to respond more favourably to immunotherapy, but the morphological classification proposed by Mathé's group has not met with universal approval.

In 1971, the United Kingdom Medical Research Council published the results of a multicentre randomised clinical trial in ALL (Concord trial). Of 191 cases entered, 177 (93 per cent) achieved remission on Pred. and VCR, and after a further five months of intensive chemotherapy, the patients were randomised to receive either BCG, twice weekly methotrexate (MTX) or no further treatment. The BCG used was the Glaxo freeze-dried preparation, administered by percutaneous inoculation using a 20 needle Heaf gun set at 2 mm (1 mm in children under two years) fired twice. Maintenance MTX was given twice a week either orally or intramuscularly in the maximum tolerated dose up to 30 mg/m^2. There was no evidence from this trial that BCG had any significant effect on first remission duration. Similar conclusions were reached by the United States Children's Cancer Study Group A (Heyn et al, 1975) which also showed that BCG alone was relatively ineffective whereas maintenance chemotherapy with MTX twice weekly, and reinduction courses of VCR and Pred. significantly prolonged the median duration of remission.

This failure to confirm Mathé's observations in the Concord and US Children's Cancer Study Group A trials may be related to the type of BCG used and the method of administration. Mathé used the liquid Pasteur strain, while the Concord trial used Glaxo BCG and the US group a Chicago strain originally derived from the Pasteur Institute in Paris. Moreover, Mathé's group used scarification as the method of BCG application whilst the UK and US trials used multiple puncture techniques. In the US trial fewer viable BCG organisms were used in comparison with the other two trials. Comparison of the results with Mathé's is therefore difficult and this illustrates the danger of setting up trials to repeat work which claims the effectiveness of a certain protocol, unless that protocol is adhered to exactly, including the use of precisely the same reagents.

Leventhal et al (1973) compared ALL patients who had relapsed on conventional treatments, and following reinduction with L-asparaginase (L-Asp) with or without actinomycin D. Nine patients who received weekly irradiated allogeneic ALL cells with Pasteur BCG administered by scarification had remission lengths not significantly different to seven patients receiving allogeneic cells plus methotrexate in five-day pulses. If methotrexate contributed to remission maintenance in these cases BCG was no less effective.

The same group (Poplack et al, 1975) compared the effects of chemotherapy alone (four months of intermittent Pred. + VCR, weekly MTX and daily 6-mercaptopurine (6-MP) alternating with two months of MTX alone) and chemoimmunotherapy (four months Pred., VCR, MTX and 6-MP alternating with two months' immunotherapy). The immunotherapy was fresh Pasteur BCG given by multiple puncture plus intradermal irradiated allogeneic cells from a single donor given in four weekly doses for the first month of the two months. Unlike their previous study only previously untreated ALL patients were entered into this study. Initial remission induction was with Pred., VCR, MTX and 6-MP (POMP) followed by cranial irradiation plus intrathecal MTX. There was additional consolidation in half the patients with two five-day courses of Ara-C and 6TG prior to randomisation. There was no significant difference in relapse rate between patients on maintenance chemotherapy and chemotherapy + immunotherapy.

IMMUNISATION WITH RAJI CELLS

The detection of a human leukaemia-associated antigen shared with RAJI cells (Mann et al, 1971, 1973; Billings and Terasaki, 1974) led to a randomised clinical trial of RAJI immunisation in patients with ALL (Sacks et al, 1975). All patients who had relapsed at least once were reinduced with L-Asp, VCR, DNR and Pred. Patients in remission were then randomised to receive either chemotherapy alone [CYCLO, VCR, Ara-C and Pred. (COAP)] or COAP + RAJI cell immunisation. There was no evidence of any clinical benefit from the immunotherapy.

The EORTC Haemopathies Working Party (1976) have presented preliminary results of a trial of active immunotherapy in ALL. Patients in a chemotherapy-induced-remission after one year received either maintenance chemotherapy (MTX interspersed with Pred. + VCR) or immunotherapy consisting of Pasteur BCG with non-irradiated allogeneic ALL cells. There was no significant difference between the chemotherapy and immunotherapy maintenance groups although three deaths occurred out of the 24 patients in the chemotherapy maintenance arm of the trial. It is unfortunate that this group has compared immunotherapy with chemotherapy, since it is impossible to decide whether immunotherapy is as beneficial as chemotherapy in maintaining remission, or whether neither treatment is necessary after such intensive preliminary chemotherapy.

Median survivals of children with ALL is now three to five years using the latest chemotherapy protocols and prophylactic CNS irradiation. Whether active immunotherapy adds anything to the present more conventional treatment is still subject to speculation and it may be time to consider other immunotherapeutic approaches in this disease.

Therapy of Acute Myeloid Leukaemia (AML)

Powles and his colleagues (1973) have adapted the Mathé protocol for the active immunotherapy of adult acute myeloid leukaemia in which patients from St Bartholomew's Hospital, London, given induction chemotherapy consisting of DNR and Ara-C then received either monthly chemotherapy (19 patients) or chemotherapy and weekly immunotherapy with 10^9 allogeneic irradiated AML blasts and Glaxo BCG by Heaf gun (23 patients). The chemotherapy group had a median remission length of 188 days, and the chemoimmunotherapy group 375 days. The median survival figures after attaining remission were respectively 303 and 545 days.

Powles (1973) reported on a group of nine patients at the Royal Marsden Hospital who were maintained with weekly irradiated allogeneic AML blasts + BCG alone following remission induction with DNR and Ara-C and consolidation chemotherapy with 6TG

+ CYCLO for six weeks. As with the previous trial the BCG was administered into one limb using a 20 needle Heaf gun fired twice and the irradiated allogeneic cells were injected partly subcutaneously, partly intradermally into the other three limbs. These patients did at least as well as the patients receiving immunotherapy + chemotherapy at

Table 11.1   Manchester Immunotherapy Trial 1: duration and frequency of remissions and survival

Patient	1st rem	2nd rem	3rd rem	4th rem	5th rem	6th rem	Survival
A1	23	11	15	15	14	7[c]	141
A6	28	—	—	—	—	—	44
A14	18	(2)	7	—	—	—	71
A19	86	112[a]					205[b]
A21	14	169[a]					203[b]
A26	18	39	(4)	12	(3)		155
A29	183[a]						188[b]

Figures in brackets indicate doubtful remissions. All figures in weeks
[a] In remission
[b] Alive
[c] Died in remission from cardiac failure

Table 11.2   Summary of results of Manchester Immunotherapy Trials 1 and 2

	1 IMM	2 IMM	IMM + CHEM
Patients	7	20	9
First remission duration (weeks) median (range)	23(14–183)	12(3–39)	18(8–68)
Second remission	5/6	14/20	4/8
Third remission	2/3	7/14	1/2
Alive	3	6	4
Survival (weeks) mean (range)	143(44–205)	78(23–161)	81(35–155)
Median	155	74	58

IMM—immunotherapy alone
IMM + CHEM—immunotherapy plus chemotherapy

St Bartholomew's Hospital both in terms of first remission duration and survival. The results of such a small group are clearly difficult to evaluate and do not give us a clear answer as to whether immunotherapy alone is as good as chemoimmunotherapy, or whether both forms of maintenance are unnecessary.

Following these trials Freeman et al (1973) published the results of a pilot study using an identical protocol to that of Powles (1973). Seven of eight patients in remission following initial induction and consolidation chemotherapy were given weekly irradiated leukaemia cells + BCG. The median duration of first remission was 23 weeks which was similar to that of St Bartholomew's Hospital patients receiving chemotherapy alone, and patients in the MRC fourth and fifth AML trials (MRC, 1974). In other words there was no increase in first remission length as compared with patients on maintenance chemotherapy alone. Nevertheless, there was a remarkably high rate of remission reinduction following relapse (5/6 second remissions and one with six remissions) prolonged survival (median three years) and excellent quality of life in patients treated in this way (Tables 11.1 and 11.2).

The United Kingdom Medical Research Council is presently assessing the relative merits of immunotherapy, immunotherapy + chemotherapy and chemotherapy alone as maintenance for patients entering remission with DNR and Ara-C (MRC sixth AML trial). Most centres in this trial have been comparing combined therapy with chemotherapy alone in an attempt to confirm the original results from St Bartholomew's Hospital and to date there is no evidence of any difference in either duration of first remission or survival in these two groups.

Table 11.3   Manchester Immunotherapy Trial 2: duration and frequency of remissions and survival —immunotherapy alone

Patient	1st rem	2nd rem	3rd rem	4th rem	5th rem	Survival
B3	20	11	6	—	—	80
B7	11	10	8			161[b]
B18	3	4	—	—	—	37
B23	18	20	—	—	—	77
B30	4	9	49	45[a]		140[b]
B33	12	(4)	—	—	—	57
B34	7	—	—	—	—	29
B37	24	11	—	—	—	65
B40	35	31[c]	—	—	—	95
B45	5	6	—	—	—	70
B48	5	16	62[a]			122[b]
B52	6	—	—	—	—	23
B56	10	—	—	—	—	57
B60	12	11	—	—	—	77
B65	11	17	13	10	16	107[b]
B66	39	12	22[a]			107[b]
B75	13	—	—	—	—	47
B77	11	—	—	—	—	63
B79	17	(4)	(5)	10	—	68
B87	16	22	10			81[b]

N.B. All figures in weeks; rem = remission
[a] In remission
[b] Alive
[c] Died in remission from disseminated carcinoma of bronchus

In Manchester, we have been comparing immunotherapy alone with the combined therapy. One feature of this new trial which differs from that of our original pilot study in Manchester is the exclusion of a consolidation phase of chemotherapy, apart from one extra ('*n* + 1') course of DNR + Ara-C. This could explain the relatively short remission duration of 12 weeks in patients receiving chemotherapy alone as compared with 23 weeks in our pilot trial (Table 11.2). Whether the inclusion of consolidation reduces the leukaemic cell population to a level more amenable to immunotherapy effects is still open to speculation. In spite of a short duration of remission the survival figures for patients on immunotherapy alone in the MRC trial are equivalent to those in the other groups, mainly because of again a high reinduction rate following relapse. To date 14 out of 20 patients randomised to immunotherapy alone have achieved second remissions. Seven have achieved a third remission, two a fourth and one patient had five remissions (Table 11.3). As may be seen in Tables 11.1, 11.3 and 11.4 a number of patients had second or subsequent remissions of longer duration than their original remission. We are not yet however in a position to attribute this to a particular response to immunotherapy.

The confirmation of the high rate of reinduction in patients receiving immunotherapy alone in the MRC sixth AML trial is of considerable interest. This may result from a beneficial effect of immunotherapy, the avoidance of drug resistance or drug-induced immunosuppression, the earlier diagnosis of relapse or a combination of these factors. There is some suggestion both from our trials and those of St Bartholomew's Hospital, that patients receiving immunotherapy + chemotherapy have a higher second remission rate than those receiving chemotherapy alone. A reanalysis of the St Bartholomew's Hospital data suggests that there is no statistical difference between immunotherapy + chemotherapy and

Table 11.4   Manchester Immunotherapy Trial 2: duration and frequency of remissions and survival—immunotherapy and chemotherapy

Patient	1st rem	2nd rem	3rd rem	4th rem	Survival
B9	21	(3)	—	—	54
B14	28	(9)	68[a]		155[b]
B15	18	—	—	—	45
B32	8	106[a]			139[b]
B44	9	—	—	—	35
B47	37	64[a]	—	—	124[b]
B51	9	5	—	—	58
B71	10	—	—	—	40
B91	68[a]	—	—	—	76[b]

N.B. All figures in weeks. After 52 weeks' continuous remission patients receive weekly immunotherapy alone until relapse
[a] In remission
[b] Alive

chemotherapy alone in terms of first remission duration but they still have a significant difference in survival (Hamilton-Fairley, 1975). The longer survival may be related to a higher second remission rate or greater bone marrow reserve in patients receiving immunotherapy in addition to drugs. If confirmed the higher reinduction rate of patients on combined therapy compared with chemotherapy alone could only be explained if immunotherapy itself plays a positive role.

A third Manchester trial has now been started and is designed to build upon the experience previously gained in the first two trials. Thus consolidation has been reintroduced, and the patients have been randomised to immunotherapy alone or no treatment. This protocol is basically a direct comparison of the effects of immunotherapy and no immunotherapy, but without maintenance chemotherapy, and recalls Mathé's (1969) original ALL trial. Paradoxically none of the trials of active immunotherapy had until now repeated Mathé's original design by incorporating a no treatment arm. Although this may be considered unethical in ALL, because of the proven effectiveness of maintenance chemotherapy, this is not the case in AML where maintenance therapy, at least of the type used at St Bartholomew's Hospital and in the MRC sixth AML trial, is of uncertain value.

Clearly, it is crucial to determine whether immunotherapy has any positive effect in prolonging first remission length and whether it affects ease of reinduction. Both groups randomised in our third trial are subjected to monthly bone marrow examination and weekly blood counts and clinical assessment. So hopefully the two groups will be truly comparable.

The optimistic picture presented by the original St Bartholomew's Hospital results has been tempered by the largely negative results with respect to duration of first remission emerging from current trials of immunotherapy in AML in the United Kingdom. There have been two reports from the US suggesting that BCG may be of some value in the maintenance of patients with AML. Vogler and Chan (1974) found that Tice-strain BCG alone given weekly for four weeks before maintenance chemotherapy with twice weekly MTX, was associated with a significant prolongation of remission as compared with a group given MTX alone and Gutterman et al (1974), reported that patients receiving intermittent chemoimmunotherapy with Ara-C, VCR and Pred. (OAP) + liquid Pasteur BCG, administered by scarification, did significantly better than an historical control of patients receiving only OAP. However, the use of historical controls, has been criticised as most centres achieve better results in time using the same protocol (EORTC, 1974).

THE USE OF AN EXTRACT OF BCG

MER is a methanol extraction residue of BCG that has been found to be capable of immune modulation and to be of therapeutic value in certain animal tumour systems (Hopper, Pimm and Baldwin, 1975; Weiss, 1976). MER has the advantages over BCG of being non-living material and thus unable to produce progressive infectious disease, and of being stable at refrigerator temperatures for many years. It does have the disadvantage, however, of being painful to administer and tending to produce severe local ulceration.

MER is being used in several clinical trials in man and two pilot studies have been reported in AML. Weiss and his colleagues (1975) have provided preliminary evidence that monthly intradermal injections of MER together with maintenance chemotherapy results in a prolongation of remission and survival as compared with patients receiving chemotherapy alone. In a study reported by Cuttner et al (1975) six AML patients treated with chemotherapy alone relapsed in from 63 to 162 days while five later patients treated with identical drugs plus MER had remissions ranging from 92+ to 193+ days. Although promising, controlled clinical trials with this material are indicated as for example in the US Acute Leukaemia Group B No. 7521 Protocol.

USE OF MODIFIED LEUKAEMIC CELLS

Most trials of 'specific' active immunotherapy in acute leukaemia have used irradiated cells to reduce the risk of the tumour graft establishing itself and disseminating. It has been suggested that irradiation by modifying the cell surface antigens could reduce the efficacy of the vaccine and some workers have used non-irradiated cells including the EORTC group mentioned above. Mathé's group (unpublished) have presented evidence of occasional local spread of the immunotherapy cells in ALL, but the precise risk of dissemination is uncertain and other centres have used non-irradiated cells without obvious harm. Modification of the cell surface may under certain circumstances increase the immunogenicity of tumour cells and such appears to be the case with neuraminidase treated cells. Bekesi et al (1976) have reported on the results of a trial in AML where patients received as maintenance either neuraminidase treated allogeneic myeloblasts or treated blasts + MER, together with cyclical chemotherapy every month, or just monthly chemotherapy. Median remission duration for the control group was 20 weeks whilst neither forms of chemoimmunotherapy have reached a median remission duration at 78 weeks. Chemoimmunotherapy also influenced survival: 17 of 25 patients in the chemotherapy group died by 90 weeks compared with 5 of 32 patients in the other two groups.

Several other centres are assessing the role of various forms of active immunotherapy In AML, it is still uncertain whether BCG with or without leukaemia cells is of value in prolonging remission in this disease. The success of this form of treatment will depend on several factors including type of BCG used, dosage, mode and frequency of administration of the cells and BCG, immunogenicity of cells, and timing in relation to chemotherapy and the extent of residual disease. Optimal conditions for this type of immunotherapy will only be achieved by patient and gradual modification of current protocols hopefully aided by some breakthrough in our methods of assessing responses in vitro.

Therapy of Chronic Myeloid Leukaemia (CML)

Sokal, Aungst and Grace (1973) have treated CML patients with mixtures of BCG and cultured cells of lines from leukaemic patients in blast crisis (probably lymphoblastoid cell lines). There were 15 patients considered to have well-controlled and uncomplicated Philadelphia chromosome-positive CML. Survival was prolonged in this group as compared with an historical control of unimmunised Philadelphia-positive patients treated between 1960 and 1969. Not only must great caution be taken in accepting the results of such a trial using historical controls, but it must also be made clear that the cell lines used are almost certainly not derived directly from leukaemia cells. There is thus no evidence that these workers are dealing with specific immunisation.

IN VITRO STUDIES ON THE EFFECTS OF IMMUNOTHERAPY

CELLULAR RESPONSES

Many of the problems surrounding the evaluation of immunotherapy would be solved if there were adequate methods for the evaluation of its effect in vitro. Attempts have been made to do this by Powles et al (1971) and Gutterman et al (1973a). Both groups studied the intensity of the response by patients to autochthonous blasts before and after auto-immunisation with these cells. Although the results indicated that there was an increase in the intensity of the response, Gutterman et al (1973a) also observed an increased PHA response, which suggested that the effect was due to a postchemotherapy rebound by T cells rather than a specific effect of immunotherapy. Unfortunately no untreated controls were used so it is difficult to evaluate these results in terms of their use in monitoring immunotherapy.

This rebound in T cells following the cessation of chemotherapy has been observed in ALL patients by Borella, Green and Webster (1972) using E rosetting as the assay of T cells. A similar rebound in MLR response to autochthonous blast cells has been observed at 10 to 20 days after five-day courses of high-dose chemotherapy by Leventhal et al (1972). It is more likely that the response to immunotherapy could be better measured using studies of the kinetics of the response to autochthonous and allogeneic immuno-therapy blasts. We have been studying these responses in our new trial and our initial observations show a shift in the peak response to autochthonous blasts in both untreated and immunotherapy patients.

ANTIBODY RESPONSES

Immunotherapy may lead to the formation of antibody to HL-A antigens (Klouda et al, 1975) and although Sacks et al (1975) were unable to show any clinical benefit from RAJI cell immunisation in patients with ALL, they did demonstrate the development of complement-dependent cytotoxic antibody to RAJI and both allogeneic and autologous acute leukaemia cells in five of eight immunised patients, but in none of eight controls receiving chemotherapy only. Hersey et al (1973) have shown that immunotherapy sera can be used to sensitise immunotherapy blasts, which are then killed by K cells. There is no evidence yet that tumour-specific antibodies are involved, but it is possible that the techniques used to detect antibodies are still not sensitive enough. A renewed examination of this problem, perhaps using isotopic antiglobulin technique, might yield valuable results.

DIRECT CYTOTOXICITY

We have recently published data showing that the stimulation of normal and patients' lymphocytes in vitro with immunotherapy blasts leads to the development of direct cell-mediated cytotoxicity by patients' lymphocytes to the immunotherapy blasts (Taylor et al, 1976). This response had a degree of specificity, since both normal and patient lymphocytes responded similarly to RAJI and lymphoblastoid cell lines. Using this technique we are presently studying the cross-reactivity of autochthonous and allogeneic blasts, and the effects of immunotherapy, on the patients in the third Manchester trial in comparison with the patients receiving no immunotherapy.

In spite of the investment of clinical time and resources in the performance of immunotherapy trials, and studies in tumour immunology in general, there have been relatively few attempts to develop methods for the in vitro monitoring of specific responses. This is in part due to technical difficulties which could undoubtedly be overcome, and in part due to the limited number of centres involved in these trials. Nevertheless, there are conspicuous advantages in studying the responses of acute leukaemia patients, since tumour cells can easily be collected and stored until required for in vitro testing and skin testing. Moreover, trials are now being designed in which the positive effects of immunotherapy can be compared with untreated controls. This is an important precedent for cancer in general; clearly the organisation of clinical immunotherapy trials should be accompanied by realistic in vitro studies of the specific or allogeneic antitumour responses.

CONCLUSIONS

The plethora of antigens detected on the surface of leukaemic cells as detected by in vitro assays and skin testing raises doubts as to the existence of truly specific human tumour antigens, and in such a situation the efficacy of immunotherapy must also be in doubt.

The organisation of clinical trials in leukaemia have obviously depended heavily upon the extent of immunological knowledge and theory at the time of the initiation. Since the leukaemias are relatively rare neoplasms, and remission rates, at least in AML, dependent upon good supportive care facilities, the number of patients entered into these trials may be relatively small, and consequently it may take time to achieve a result. The developments in theoretical immunology and in the clinical treatment may render the original concept of the trial outdated by the time it is finalised and may lead to a general lessening of interest in this form of treatment. It is crucial to bear these facts in mind when considering the results of current trials in human leukaemia.

It cannot be argued that active immunotherapy using BCG or allogeneic blasts has resulted in any cures of leukaemia. With the increased effectiveness of current chemotherapy in ALL, one may question whether current immunotherapeutic techniques are likely to add significantly to remission length or survival in these patients. AML is still an intractable disease, in which chemotherapy has made limited inroads; there is clearly a need for continuation of present immunotherapy trials and possible new approaches.

This may be the time to reappraise the effectiveness of passive immunotherapy using either xenogeneic adsorbed antisera or possibly sera from patients who have received active immunotherapy in which there is HLA antibody. Passive cellular immunotherapy either using normal lymphocytes, lymphocytes from patients in remission following active immunotherapy, or in vitro sensitised lymphocytes obtained in bulk from cell separators is another approach which may offer possibilities at least as good as in the present trials. The evaluation of graft versus leukaemia protocols would depend upon there being good clinical facilities for this difficult procedure. Adoptive immunotherapy using bone marrow transplants is also subject to the availability of sophisticated clinical facilities, specifically for the critical transplantation stages, and for selection of appropriate donors. Developments in the transplantation field suggest that the latter may not be very difficult in the near future.

There are many problems to be overcome in the treatment of leukaemia, and immunotherapy though not a new concept has clear advantages for the future. There is still much to be learned in applied immunology which may be of help to the immunotherapist in ways not yet fully understood, and it is essential that clinical trials of these new concepts should continue.

REFERENCES

Alexander, P., Delorme, E. J., Hamilton, L. D. G. & Hall, J. G. (1967) Effect of nucleic acids from immune lymphocytes on rat sarcomas. *Nature*, **213**, 569–572.

Bach, M. L., Bach, F. H. & Joo, P. (1969) Leukaemia associated antigens in the mixed leucocyte culture test. *Science*, **166**, 1520–1522.

Baker, M. A. & Taub, R. N. (1973) Production of antiserum in mice to human leukaemia-associated antigens. *Nature New Biology*, **241**, 93–94.

Baker, M. A., Falk, R. E., Falk, J. & Greaves, M. F. (1976) Detection of monocyte specific antigen on human leukaemia cells. *British Journal of Haematology*, **32**, 13–19.

Baldwin, R. W. (1973) Immunological aspects of chemical carcinogenesis. *Advances in Cancer Research*, **18**, 1–75.

Baldwin, R. W., Embleton, M. J., Jones, J. S. P. & Langman, M. J. S. (1973) Cell mediated and humoral immune reactions to human tumours. *International Journal of Cancer*, **12**, 73–83.

Bauscher, J. C. & Smith, R. T. (1973) Studies of the Epstein–Barr virus–host relationship: autochthonous and allogeneic lymphocyte stimulation by lymphoblast cell lines in mixed cell culture. *Clinical Immunology and Immunopathology*, **1**, 270–281.

Bekesi, J. G., Holland, J. F., Cultner, J., Silver, R., Coleman, M., Jarowski, C. & Vinceguerra, V. (1976) Immunotherapy in acute myelocytic leukemia with neuraminidase treated allogeneic myeloblasts with or without MER. *Proceedings of the American Association for Cancer Research*, **17**, 184 (Abstract).

Bekkum, D. W. van (1972) Use and abuse of hemopoietic cell grafts in immune deficiency diseases. *Transplantation Reviews*, **9**, 3–53.

Bias, W. B., Santos, G. W., Burke, P. J., Mullins, G. M. & Humphrey, R. L. (1972) Cytotoxic antibody in normal human serums reactive with tumor cells from acute lymphocytic leukaemia. *Science*, **178**, 304–306.

Billings, R. & Terasaki, P. T. (1974) Human leukemia antigen. I. Production and characterization of antisera. *Journal of the National Cancer Institute*, **53**, 1635–1638.

Black, M. M., Opler, S. R. & Speer, F. D. (1955) Survival in breast cancer cases in relation to the structure of the primary tumor and regional lymph nodes. *Surgery, Gynecology and Obstetrics*, **100**, 543–551.

Black, M. M., Opler, S. R. & Speer, F. D. (1956) Structural representation of tumor–host relationships in gastric carcinoma. *Surgery, Gynecology and Obstetrics*, **102**, 599–603.

Black, M. M. & Speer, F. D. (1958) Sinus histiocytosis of lymph nodes in cancer. *Surgery, Gynecology and Obstetrics*, **106**, 163–175.

Bluming, A. Z., Vogel, C. L., Ziegler, J. L. & Kiryabwive, J. W. M. (1972) Delayed cutaneous sensitivity reactions to extracts of autologous malignant melanoma: a second look. *Journal of the National Cancer Institute*, **48**, 17–24.

Boranic, M. (1968) Transient graft-versus-host reaction in the treatment of leukaemia in mice. *Journal of the National Cancer Institute*, **41**, 421–437.

Borella, L., Green, A. A. & Webster, R. E. (1972) Immunologic rebound after cessation of long-term chemotherapy in acute leukaemia. *Blood*, **40**, 42–51.

Bortin, M. M., Rimm, A. A., Saltzstein, E. C. & Rodey, G. E. (1973) Graft versus leukaemia. III. Apparent independent antihost and antileukemic activity of transplanted immunocompetent cells. *Transplantation*, **16**, 182–188.

Bortin, M. M. (1974) Graft versus leukaemia. In *Clinical Immunobiology*, ed. Bach, F. H. & Good, R. A., Vol. 2, pp. 287–306. New York: Academic Press.

Brandes, L. J., Galton, D. A. G. & Wiltshaw, E. (1971) New approach to immunotherapy of melanoma. *Lancet*, **ii**, 293–295.

Brittingham, T. F. & Chaplin, H. (1960) Production of a human 'anti-leukemic leukocyte' serum and its therapeutic trial. *Cancer*, **13**, 412–418.

Bubenik, J., Perlmann, P., Helmstein, K. & Moberger, G. (1970a) Immune response to urinary bladder tumors in man. *International Journal of Cancer*, **5**, 39–46.

Bubenik, J., Perlmann, P., Helmstein, K. & Moberger, G. (1970b) Cellular and humoral immune responses to human urinary bladder carcinomas. *International Journal of Cancer*, **5**, 310–319.

Carvalho, S. de (1960) Segregation of antigens from human leukaemic and tumoral cells by fluorocarbon extraction. *Journal of Laboratory and Clinical Medicine*, **56**, 333–341.

Carvalho, S. de (1963) Preliminary experimentation with specific immunotherapy of neoplastic disease in man. I. Immediate effects of hyperimmune equine gamma globulins. *Cancer*, **16**, 306–330.

Carvalho, S. de (1964) Identity of reaction of an autologous antibody in leukaemic children in remission with a heterologous antibody produced with leukemic antigens. *Proceedings of American Association of Cancer Research*, **5**, 14.

Char, D. H., Lepourhiet, A., Leventhal, B. G. & Herberman, R. B. (1973) Cutaneous delayed hypersensitivity responses to tumor-associated and other antigens in acute leukaemia. *International Journal of Cancer*, **12**, 409–419.

Comstock, G. W., Livesay, V. T. & Webster, R. G. (1971) Leukaemia and BCG. *Lancet*, **ii**, 1062–1063.

Comstock, G. W., Martinez, I. & Livesay, V. T. (1975) Efficacy of BCG vaccination in prevention of cancer. *Journal of the National Cancer Institute*, **54**, 835–839.

Cotropia, J. P., Gutterman, J. U., Hersh, E. M., Granatek, C. H. & Mavligit, G. M. (1975) Antigen expression and cell surface properties of human leukemic blasts. *International Conference on Immunobiology of Cancer* (Abstract). New York: New York Academy of Sciences.

Currie, G. A. (1972) Eighty years of immunotherapy: a review of immunological methods used for the treatment of human cancer. *British Journal of Cancer*, **26**, 141–153.

Cuttner, J., Holland, J. F., Bekesi, J. G., Ramachandar, K. & Donovan, O. (1975) Chemoimmunotherapy of acute myelocytic leukemia. *Proceedings of the American Association for Cancer Research and American Society of Clinical Oncology*, **16**, 264.

Davies, D. A. L. & O'Neill, G. J. (1973) *In vivo* and *in vitro* effects of tumor specific antibodies with chlorambucil. *British Journal of Cancer*, **28** (Suppl. I), 285–298.

Davignon, L., Lemonde, P., Robillard, P. & Frappier, A. (1970) BCG vaccination and leukaemia mortality. *Lancet*, **ii**, 638.

Davignon, L., Lemonde, P., St Pierre, J. & Frappier, A. (1971) BCG vaccination and leukaemia mortality. *Lancet*, **i**, 80–81.

Delorme, E. J. & Alexander, P. (1964) Treatment of primary fibrosarcoma in the rat with immune lymphocytes. *Lancet*, **ii**, 117–120.

Djerassi, I. (1968) Transfusion of lymphocyte antibodies and lymphocytes from multitransfused donors. *Clinical Pediatrics*, **7**, 272–273.

Doré, J. F., Marholes, L., Colas de la Noue, H., de Vassal, F., Motta, R., Hrsak, I., Seman, G. & Mathé, G. (1967) New antigens in human leukaemic cells and antibody in the serum of leukaemic patients. *Lancet*, **ii**, 1396–1398.

EORTC Leukaemia and Haematosarcoma Cooperative Group (Malpas, J., Mathé, G., Hayat, M. et al) (1974) A second comparative trial of remission induction (by cytosine arabinoside given every 12 hours, or CAR and thioguanine or CAR and daunorubicin) and maintenance therapy (by CAR or methylgag) in acute myeloid leukaemia. *European Journal of Cancer*, **10**, 413–418.

264 RECENT ADVANCES IN CLINICAL IMMUNOLOGY

EORTC Haemopathies Working Party (presented by Stryckmans, P. A. & Otten, J.) (1976) Immunotherapy in acute lymphoblastic leukemia. *Proceedings of the American Association for Cancer Research and American Society of Clinical Oncology*, **17**, 217 (Abstract).

Everson, T. C. (1964) Spontaneous regression of cancer. *Annals of the New York Academy of Science*, **114**, 721–735.

Fass, L., Herberman, R. B. & Ziegler, J. (1970) Delayed cutaneous hypersensitivity reactions to autologous extracts of Burkitt-lymphoma cells. *New England Journal Medicine*, **282**, 776–780.

Fefer, A., Einstein, A. B., Thomas, E. D., Buckner, C. D., Clift, R. A., Glucksberg, H., Neiman, P. E. & Storb, R. (1974a) Bone-marrow transplantation for hematological neoplasia in 16 patients with identical twins. *New England Journal of Medicine*, **290**, 1389–1393.

Fefer, A., Mickelson, E. & Thomas, E. D. (1974b) Leukaemia antigens: mixed leucocyte culture tests on twelve patients with identical twins. *Clinical and Experimental Immunology*, **18**, 237–242.

Fernbach, D. J., Rossen, R. D. & Butler, W. T. (1970) Studies of antilymphocyte globulin (ALG) treatment of children with acute leukemia. *Proceedings of the American Association for Cancer Research*, **11**, 25.

Flier, J. S., Glade, P. R., Broder, S. W. & Hirschhorn, K. (1970) Lymphocyte stimulation by allogeneic and autochthonous cultured cell lines. *Cellular Immunology*, **1**, 596–602.

Foley, E. J. (1953) Attempts to induce immunity against mammary adenocarcinoma in inbred mice. *Cancer Research*, **13**, 578–580.

Fossati, A., Colnaghi, M. I., Porta, G. D., Cascinelli, N. & Veronesi, U. (1971) Cellular and humoral immunity against human malignant melanoma. *International Journal of Cancer*, **8**, 344–350.

Freedman, L. R., Cerottini, J.-C. & Brunner, K. T. (1972) *In vivo* studies of the role of cytotoxic T cells in tumor allograft immunity. *Journal of Immunology*, **109**, 1371–1378.

Freeman, C. B., Harris, R., Geary, C. G., Leyland, M. J., MacIver, J. E. & Delamore, I. W. (1973) Active immunotherapy used alone for maintenance of patients with acute myeloid leukaemia. *British Medical Journal*, **iv**, 571–573.

Fridman, W. H. & Kourilsky, F. M. (1969) Stimulation of lymphocytes by autologous leukaemia cells in acute leukaemia. *Nature*, **224**, 277–279.

Garb, S., Stein, A. A. & Sims, G. (1962) The production of anti-human leukaemic serum in rabbits. *Journal of Immunology*, **88**, 142–152.

Gatti, R. A. & Good, R. A. (1971) Occurrence of malignancy in immunodeficiency diseases. *Cancer (Philadelphia)*, **28**, 89–98.

Ghose, T., Cerini, M., Carter, M. & Nairn, R. C. (1967) Immunoradioactive agent against cancer. *British Medical Journal*, **i**, 90–93.

Ghose, T., Norrell, S. T., Guilu, A., Cameron, D., Bodurlha, A., & MacDonald, A. S. (1972) Immunotherapy of cancer with chlorambucil-carrying antibody. *British Medical Journal*, **iii**, 495–499.

Gold, P., Gold, J. M. & Freedman, J. O. (1968) Cellular location of carcinoembryonic antigens of the human digestive system. *Cancer Research*, **28**, 1331–1334.

Good, R. A. & Bach, F. H. (1974) Bone marrow and thymus transplants: cellular engineering to correct primary immunodeficiency. In *Clinical Immunobiology*, ed. Bach, F. H. & Good, R. A., Vol. 2, pp. 63–114. New York: Academic Press.

Gorer, P. A. & Amos, D. B. (1956) Passive immunity in mice against C57BL leukosis E.L.4 by means of iso-immune serum. *Cancer Research*, **16**, 338–343.

Graw, R. G., Jr, Yankee, R. A., Rogentine, G. N., Leventhal, B. G., Herzig, G. P., Halterman, R. H., Merritt, C. B., McGinniss, M. H., Krueger, G. R. D., Whang-Peng, J., Carolla, R. L., Gullion, D. S., Lippman, M. E., Gralnick, H. R., Berard, C. W., Terasaki, P. I. & Henderson, E. S. (1972) Bone marrow transplantation from HL-A matched donors to patients with acute leukemia: toxicity and antileukemic effect. *Transplantation*, **14**, 79–90.

Graw, R. G., Jr, Lohrmann, H. P., Bull, M. I., Decter, J., Herzig, G. P., Bull, J. M., Leventhal, B. G., Yankee, R. A., Herzig, R. H., Krueger, G. R. F., Bleyer, W. A., Buja, M. L., McGinniss, M. H., Alter, H. J., Whang-Peng, J., Gralnick, H. R., Kirkpatrick, C. H. & Henderson, E. S. (1974) Bone marrow transplantation following combination chemotherapy-immunosuppression (B.A.C.T.) in patients with acute leukemia. *Transplantation Proceedings*, **VI**, 349–354.

Green, S. S. & Sell, K. W. (1970) Mixed leukocyte stimulation of normal peripheral leukocytes by autologous lymphoblastoid cells. *Science*, **170**, 989–990.

Gross, L. (1943) Intradermal immunization of C3H mice against a sarcoma that originated in an animal of the same line. *Cancer Research*, **3**, 326–333.

Gutterman, J. U., Mavligit, A., McCredie, K. B., Freireich, E. J. & Hersh, E. M. (1973a) Autoimmunization with acute leukemia cells: demonstration of increased lymphocyte responsiveness. *International Journal of Cancer*, **11**, 521–526.

Gutterman, J. U., Rossen, R. D., Butler, W. T., McCredie, K. B., Bodey, G. P., Freireich, E. J. & Hersh, E. M. (1973b) Immunoglobulins on tumour cells and tumour-induced lymphocyte blastogenesis in human leukaemia. *New England Journal of Medicine*, **288**, 169–173.

Gutterman, J. U., Hersh, E. M., Rodriguez, V., McCredie, K. B., Mavligit, G., Reed, R., Burgess, M. A., Smith, T., Gehan, E., Bodey, G. P. & Freireich, E. J. (1974) Chemoimmunotherapy of adult acute leukaemia. *Lancet*, **ii**, 1405–1409.

Hamilton Fairley, G. (1975) Verbal communication.

Hamlin, I. M. E. (1968) Possible host resistance in carcinoma of the breast: a histological study. *British Journal of Cancer*, **22**, 383–401.

Han, T., Moore, G. E. & Sokal, J. E. (1971) *In vitro* lymphocyte response to autologous cultured lymphoid cells (35409). *Proceedings of the Society for Experimental Biology (New York)*, **136**, 976–979.

Han, T. & Wang, J. (1972) 'Antigenic' disparity between leukaemia lymphoblasts and normal lymphocytes in identical twins. *Clinical and Experimental Immunology*, **12**, 171–175.

Harlozinska, A., Kotlarek-Haus, S., Richter, R. & Brodzka, W. (1973) Preliminary studies on antigenicity of chronic lymphatic leukemia cells in humans. *Archivum Immunologiae et Therapiae Experimentalis*, **21**, 403–415.

Häyry, P. & Defendi, V. (1970) Mixed lymphocyte cultures produce effector cells: model *in vitro* for allograft rejection. *Science*, **168**, 133–135.

Hellström, I., Hellström, K. E., Pierce, G. E. & Fefer, A. (1969) Studies on immunity to autochthonous mouse tumors. *Proceedings of the Transplantation Society*, **i**, 90–94.

Hellström, I., Hellström, K. E., Bill, A. H., Pierce, G. E. & Yang, J. P. S. (1970) Studies on cellular immunity to human neuroblastoma cells. *International Journal of Cancer*, **6**, 172–188.

Herberman, R. B., Oren, M. E., Rogentine, G. N. & Fahey, J. L. (1971) Cytolytic effects of alloantiserum in patients with lymphoproliferative disorders. *Cancer*, **28**, 365–371.

Hericourt, J. & Richet, C. (1895) 'Physiologie–Pathologique'—de la serotherapie dans la le traitement du cancer. *Comptes rendus hebdomadaire des séances de l'Académie des sciences*, **121**, 567–569.

Hersey, P., MacLennan, I. C. M., Campbell, A. C., Hanis, R. & Freeman, C. B. (1973) Cytoxicity against human leukaemic cells. *Clinical and Experimental Immunology*, **14**, 159–166.

Heyn, R. M., Joo, P., Karon, M., Nesbit, M., Shore, N., Breslow, N., Weiner, J., Reed, A. & Hammond, D. (1975) BCG in the treatment of acute lymphocytic leukemia. *Blood*, **46**, 431–442.

Hill, G. J., Atkins, R. C., Parks, S., Littlejohn, K. & Eiseman, B. (1969) Immunotherapeutic effect of sensitized leukocytes and antiserum on mouse leukemia. *Surgical Forum*, **20**, 122–124.

Hollinshead, A. C. & Herberman, R. B. (1975) Identification and characterization: cell membrane antigens associated with the blast phase of human adult leukemia. In *Comparative Leukemia Research 1973 Leukemogensis*, ed. Ito, Y. & Dutcher, R. M., pp. 339–348. Tokyo: University of Tokyo Press; Basel: Karger.

Hopper, D. G., Pimm, M. V. & Baldwin, R. W. (1975) Methanol extraction residue of BCG in the treatment of transplanted rat tumour. *British Journal of Cancer*, **31**, 176–181.

Hyde, R. M., Garb, S. & Bennett, A. J. (1967) Demonstration by immunoelectrophoresis of antigen in human myelogenous leukaemia. *Journal of National Cancer Institute*, **38**, 909–919.

Jagarlamoody, S. M., Aust, J. C., Tew, R. H. & McKhann, C. F. (1971) *In vitro* detection of cytotoxic cellular immunity against tumour-specific antigens by a radioisotope technique. *Proceedings of the National Academy of Sciences, U.S.A.*, **68**, 1346–1350.

Jehn, U. W., Nathanson, L., Schwartz, R. S. & Skinner, M. (1970) *In vitro* lymphocyte stimulation by soluble antigen from malignant melanoma. *New England Journal of Medicine*, **283**, 329–333.

Junge, U., Koekstra, J. & Deinhardt, F. (1971) Stimulation of peripheral lymphocytes by allogeneic and autochthonous mononucleosis lymphocyte cell lines. *Journal of Immunology*, **106**, 1306–1315.

Kersey, J. H., Spector, B. D. & Good, R. A. (1973) Immunodeficiency and cancer. *Advances in Cancer Research*, **18**, 211–230.

Killmann, S. A. (1957) Leukocyte-auto-agglutinin in a case of acute monocytic leukaemia. *Acta haematologica*, **17**, 360–374.

Kinlen, L. J. & Pike, M. C. (1971) BCG vaccination and leukaemia. *Lancet*, **i**, 398–402.

Klein, G., Clifford, P., Klein, E., Smith, R. T., Minowada, J., Kourilsky, F. M. & Burchenal, J. (1967) Membrane immunofluorescence reactions of Burkitt lymphoma cells from biopsy specimens and tissue cultures. *Journal of the National Cancer Institute*, **39**, 1027–1044.

Klouda, P. T., Lawler, S. D., Powles, R. L., Oliver, R. T. D. & Grant, C. K. (1975) HL-A antibody response in patients with acute myelogenous leukaemia treated by immunotherapy. *Transplantation*, **19**, 245–249.

Knight, S. C., Moore, G. E. & Clarkson, B. D. (1971) Stimulation of autochthonous lymphocytes by cells from normal and leukaemic lines. *Nature New Biology*, **229**, 185–187.

Korngold, L., Van Leeuwen, G. & Miller, D. G. (1961) The antigens of human leukocytes. II. The specificity of leukocyte antigens. *Journal of the National Cancer Institute*, **26**, 557–567.

Lamon, E. W., Skurzak, H. M., Klein, E. & Wigzell, M. (1972) *In vitro* cytotoxicity by a nonthymus processed lymphocyte population with specificity for a virally determined tumour cell surface antigen. *Journal of Experimental Medicine*, **136**, 1072–1079.

Laszlo, J., Buckley, C. E. & Amos, B. D. (1968) Infusion of isologous immune plasma in chronic lymphocytic leukemia. *Blood*, **31**, 104–110.

Leventhal, B. G., Herberman, R. B., Rosenberg, E. B. & Halterman, R. (1972) Immune reactivity of leukaemia patients to autologous blast cells. *Cancer Research*, **32**, 1820–1825.

Leventhal, B. G., Lepourhiet, A., Halterman, R. H., Henderson, E. S. & Herberman, R. B. (1973) Immunotherapy in previous treated acute lymphatic leukemia. *National Cancer Institute Monograph*, **39**, 177–187.

Leventhal, B. G., Leung, E. & Johnson, G. E. (1976) E rosette forming lymphoblasts fail to stimulate allogeneic donors in mixed leukocyte culture (MLC). *Proceedings of the American Association for Cancer Research and the American Society of Clinical Oncology*, **17**, 271 (Abstract C-137).

Lewis, M. G., Idonopisov, R. L., Nairn, R. C., Phillips, T. M., Fairley, H. G., Bodenham, D. C. & Alexander, P. (1969) Tumour-specific antibodies in human malignant melanoma and their relationship to the extent of the disease. *British Medical Journal*, **iii**, 547–562.

Lightbody, J. J. & Bach, F. H. (1972) Specificity of destruction by lymphocytes activated in mixed leukocyte culture. *Transplantation Proceedings*, **4**, 307–310.

Lindström, G. A. (1927) An experimental study of myelotoxic sera. Therapeutic attempts in myeloid leukaemia. *Acta medica scandinavica*, Suppl. 22, 1–169.

Mann, D. L., Rogentine, G. N., Halterman, R. & Leventhal, B. (1971) Detection of an antigen associated with acute leukaemia. *Science*, **174**, 1136–1137.

Mann, D. L., Halterman, R. & Leventhal, B. G. (1973) Cross reactive antigens on human cells infected with Rauscher leukaemia virus and on human acute leukaemia cells. *National Academy of Science, Proceedings*, **70**, 495–497.

Mathé, G., Amiel, J. L. & Bernard, J. (1960) Traitement de souris AKR à l'age de six mois par irradiation totale suivie de transfusion de cellules hématopoietiques allogéniques incidences respectives de la leucémie et du syndrome secondaire. *Bulletin du Cancer*, **47**, 331–340.

Mathé, G. & Amiel, J. L. (1964) Immunologie. Réduction de la concentration plasmatique leucémigène de Charlotte Friend par immunothérapie adoptive. *Comptes rendus hebdomadaires des séances de l'Acadamie des sciences*, **164**, 4408–4413.

Mathé, G. & Schwarzenberg, L. (1968) Immunothérapie adoptive locale de la leucémie L1210 ascitique. Analyse des facteurs de son efficacité. *European Journal of Cancer*, **4**, 211–218.

Mathé, G. (1968) Immunothérapie active de la leucémie L1210 appliquée après la greffe tumorale. *Revue française d'etudes cliniques et biologiques*, **13**, 881–883.

Mathé, G., Pouillart, P. & Lapeyraque, F. (1969a) Active immunotherapy of L1210 leukaemia applied after the graft of tumour cells. *British Journal of Cancer*, **23**, 814–824.

Mathé, G., Amiel, J. L., Schwarzenberg, L., Schneider, M., Cattan, A., Schlumberger, J. R., Hagert, M. & de Vassal, F. (1969b) Active immunotherapy for acute lymphoblastic leukaemia. *Lancet*, **i**, 697–699.

Mathé, G., Amiel, J. L., Schwarzenberg, L., Schneider, M., Hayat, M., de Vassal, F., Jasmin, C., Rosenfeld, C. & Pouillart, P. (1971) Preliminary results of a new protocol for the active immunotherapy of acute lymphoblastic leukaemia: inhibition of the immunotherapeutic effect by vincristine or adamantadine. *European Journal of Clinical and Biological Research*, **16**, 216–224.

Mathé, G., Pouillart, P., Schwarzenberg, L., Amiel, J. L., Schneider, M., Hayat, M., de Vassal, F., Jasmin, C., Rosenfeld, C., Weiner, R. & Rappaport, H. (1972) Attempts at immunotherapy of 100 patients with acute lymphoid leukaemia: some factors influencing results. *National Cancer Institute Monograph*, **35**, 361–374.

Mathé, G., Weiner, R., Pouillart, P., Schwarzenberg, L., Jasmin, C., Schneider, M., Hayat, M., Amiel, J. L., de Vassal, F. & Rosenfeld, C. (1973) BCG in cancer immunotherapy: experimental and clinical trials of its use in treatment of leukemia minimal and/or residual disease. *National Cancer Institute Monograph*, **39**, 164–175.

Mathé, G. & Schwarzenberg, L. (1974) Bone marrow transplantation in France, 1958–1973. *Transplantation Proceedings*, **VI**, 335–343.

Medical Research Council, Preliminary Report by the Leukaemia Committee and the Working Party on Leukaemia in Childhood (1971) Treatment of acute lymphoblastic leukaemia—comparison of immunotherapy (BCG) intermittent methotrexate, and no therapy after a 5 month intensive cytotoxic regimen (Concord Trial). *British Medical Journal*, **iv**, 189–194.

Medical Research Council (1972) BCG and vole bacillus vaccines in the prevention of tuberculosis in adolescence and early adult life. *Bulletin of the World Health Organisation*, **46**, 371–385.

Medical Research Council's Working Party on Leukaemia in Adults (1974). Treatment of acute myeloid leukaemia with daunorubicin, cytosine arabinoside, mercaptopurine, L-asparaginase, prednisone and thioguanine: results of treatment with five multiple-drug schedules. *British Journal of Haematology*, **27**, 373–389.

Metzgar, R. S., Mohanakumar, T. & Miller, D. S. (1972) Antigens special for human lymphocytic and myeloid leukaemia cells: detection by nonhuman primate antiserums. *Science*, **178**, 986–988.

Metzgar, R. S., Mohanakumar, T., Green, R. W., Miller, D. S. & Bolognesi, D. P. (1974) Human leukemia antigens: partial isolation and characterization. *Journal of the National Cancer Institute*, **52**, 1445–1452.

Miggiano, V. C., Bernoco, D., Lightbody, J., Trinchieri, G. & Ceppellini, R. (1972) Cell mediated lympholysis (CML) *in vitro* with normal lymphocytes as target. Specificity and cross reactivity of the test. *Transplantation Proceedings*, **4**, 231–237.

Miller, D. G., Moldovanu, G., Kaplan, A. & Tocci, S. (1968) Antilymphocytic leukaemic serum and chemotherapy in the treatment of murine leukaemia. *Cancer*, **22**, 1192–1198.

Mohanakumar, T., Metzgar, R. S. & Miller, D. S. (1974) Human leukemia cell antigens: serologic characterization with xenoantisera. *Journal of the National Cancer Institute*, **52**, 1435–1444.

Morton, D. L., Malmgren, R. A., Holmes, E. C. & Ketcham, A. S. (1968) Demonstration of antibodies against human malignant melanoma by immunofluorescence. *Surgery*, **64**, 232–240.

Morton, D. L., Malmgren, R. A., Hall, W. T. & Schidlovsky, G. (1969) Immunlogic and virus studies with human sarcomas. *Surgery*, **66**, 152–161.

Morton, D. L., Holmes, E. C., Eilber, F. R. & Wood, W. C. (1971) Immunological aspects of neoplasia: a rational basis for immunotherapy. *Annals of Internal Medicine*, **74**, 587–604.

Muna, N. M., Marrcus, S. & Smart, C. (1969) Detection by immunofluorescence of antibodies specific for human malignant melanoma cells. *Cancer*, **23**, 88–93.

Neidhart, J. A. & LoBuglio, A. F. (1974) Transfer-factor therapy of malignancy. *Seminars in Oncology*, **1**, 379–385.

Oettgen, H. F., Old, L. J., Farrow, J. H., Valentine, F., Lawrence, H. S. & Thomas, L. (1974) Effects of dialyzable transfer factor in patients with breast cancer. *Proceedings of the National Academy of Sciences (U.S.A.)*, **71**, 2319–2323.

Old, L. J. & Boyse, F. A. (1964) Immunology of experimental tumors. *Annual Review of Medicine*, **15**, 167–186.

Old, L. J., Stockert, E., Boyse, F. A. & Geering, G. (1967) A study of passive immunization against a transplanted G+ leukemia with specific antiserum (31667). *Proceedings of the Society for Experimental Biology and Medicine*, **124**, 63–68.

Oren, M. E. & Herberman, R. B. (1971) Delayed cutaneous hypersensitivity reactions to membrane extracts of human tumour cells. *Clinical and Experimental Immunology*, **9**, 45–56.

Paola, M. di, Angelini, L., Bertolotti, A. & Calizza, S. (1974) Host resistance in relation to survival in breast cancer. *British Medical Journal*, **iv**, 268–270.

Pilch, Y. H. & deKernion, J. B. (1974) Immunotherapy of cancer with 'immune' RNA: current status. *Seminars in Oncology*, **1**, 387–395.

Pollack, S., Heppner, G., Brown, R. J. & Nelson, K. (1972) Specific killing of tumour cells *in vitro* in the presence of normal lymphoid cells and sera from hosts immune to the tumour antigens. *International Journal of Cancer*, **9**, 316–323.

Poplack, D. G., Graw, R. G., Pomeroy, T. C., Henderson, E. S. & Leventhal, B. G. (1975) Chemotherapy and immunotherapy in childhood acute lymphatic leukemia. *Proceedings of the American Society of Clinical Oncology*, **16**, (Abstract 1038).

Powles, R. L., Balchin, L. A., Hamilton Fairley, G. & Alexander, P. (1971) Recognition of leukaemia cells as foreign before and after autoimmunisation. *British Medical Journal*, **i**, 486–489.

Powles, R. (1973) Immunotherapy for acute myelogenous leukaemia. *British Journal of Cancer*, **28** (Suppl. 1) 262–265.

Powles, R. L., Crowther, D., Bateman, C. J. T., Beard, M. E. J., McElwain, T. J., Russell, J., Lister, T. A., Whitehouse, J. M. A., Wrigley, P. F. M., Pike, M., Alexander, P. & Hamilton Fairley, G. (1973) Immunotherapy for acute myelogenous leukaemia. *British Journal of Cancer*, **28**, 365–376.

Prehn, R. T. & Main, J. M. (1957) Immunity to methylcholanthrene-induced sarcomas. *Journal of the National Cancer Institute*, **18**, 769–778.

Prehn, R. T. (1976) Do tumors grow because of the immune response of the host? *Transplantation Reviews*, **28**, 34–42.

Reiff, A. E. & Kim, C.-A. H. (1969) Therapy of transplantable mouse leukaemias with antileukaemia sera. *Nature*, **223**, 1377–1379.

Röllinghoff, M. & Wagner, H. (1973) *In vivo* protection against murine plasma cell tumor growth by *in vitro* activated syngeneic lymphocytes. *Journal of the National Cancer Institute*, **51**, 1317–1318.

Rosenthal, S. R., Crispen, R. G., Thorne, M. G., Piekavski, M., Raisys, N. & Rettig, P. (1973) BCG vaccination and leukemia mortality. *National Cancer Institute Monograph*, **39**, 189–194.

Rudolph, R. H., Mickelson, E. & Thomas, E. D. (1970a) A study by mixed leukocyte culture of leukemic twins. In *Proceedings of Vth Leucocyte Culture Conference*, ed. Harris, J. F., pp. 319–327. New York and London: Academic Press.

Rudolph, R. H., Mickelson, E. & Thomas, E. D. (1970b) Mixed leukocyte reactivity and leukaemia: study of identical siblings. *Journal of Clinical Investigation*, **49**, 2271–2275.

Sacks, K. L., Olweny, C., Mann, D. L., Simon, R., Johnson, G. E., Poplack, D. G. & Leventhal, B. G. (1975) A clinical trial of chemotherapy and RAJI immunotherapy in advanced acute lymphatic leukemia. *Cancer Research*, **35**, 3715–3720.

Schwarzenberg, L., Mathé, G., Schneider, M., Amiel, J. L. & Schumberger, J. R. (1966) Attempted adoptive immunotherapy of acute leukaemia by leucocyte transfusions. *Lancet*, **ii**, 365–368.

Schweitzer, M., Melief, C. J. M. & Eijsvoogel, V. P. (1973) Failure to demonstrate immunity to leukaemia associated antigens by lymphocyte transformation *in vitro*. *International Journal of Cancer*, **11**, 11–18.

Séligmann, M., Grabar, P. & Bernard, J. (1954) Présence d'anticorps précipitants anti-leucocytaire (leuco-précipitines dans le sérum de sujets atteints de leucose aiguë. *Presse médicale*, **62**, 1700–1702.

Séligmann, M. (1956) Mise en évidence d'antigènes leucocytaires dans le sérum humain normal et dans certains sérums de leucémiques. *Comptes rendus hebdomodaires des séances de l'Académie des sciences*, **243**, 531–534.

Sokal, J. E., Aungst, C. W. & Grace, J. T. (1973) Immunotherapy of chronic myelocytic leukemia. *National Cancer Institute Monograph*, **39**, 195–198.

Solliday, S. & Bach, F. H. (1972) Lymphocyte reactivity *in vitro*. VI. Specificity of target cell destruction following *in vitro* sensitization in mixed leukocyte cultures. *European Journal of Immunology*, **2**, 68–72.

Steel, C. M., Hardy, D. A., Ling, N. R., Dick, H. M., Mackintosh, P. & Crichton, W. B. (1973) The interaction of normal lymphocytes and cells from lymphoid cell lines. III. Studies on activation in an autochthonous system. *Immunology*, **24**, 177–189.

Stephenson, H. E., Delmez, J. A., Renden, D. I., Kimpton, R. S., Todd, P. C., Charron, T. L. & Lindberg, D. A. B. (1971) Host immunity and spontaneous regression of cancer evaluated by computerized data reduction study. *Surgery, Gynecology and Obstetrics*, **133**, 649–655.

Svedmyr, E. A., Deinhardt, F., Gatti, R. A., Golub, S., Gunvén, P., Hoekstra, J., Klein, G., Leibold, W., Menezes, J. & Wigzell, H. (1974) Sensitization of human lymphocytes with autologous lymphoblastoid cell line. In *Lymphocyte Recognition and Effector Mechanisms*. Proceedings of the 8th Leucocyte Culture Conference 1973, ed. Lindahl-Kessling, K. & Osaba, D., pp. 217–222. New York and London: Academic Press.

Taylor, G. M., Harris, R. & Jones, S. V. (1975) Unpublished data.

Taylor, G. M., Harris, R. & Freeman, C. B. (1976) Cell-mediated cytotoxicity as a result of immunotherapy in patient with acute myeloid leukaemia. *British Journal of Cancer*, **33**, 137–143.

Thomas, E. D., Herman, E. C., Jr, Greenough, W. B., III, Hager, E. B., Cannon, J. H., Sahler, O. D. & Ferrebee, J. W. (1961) *Archives of Internal Medicine*, **107**, 829–845.

Thomas, E. D., Storb, R., Clift, R. A., Fefer, A., Johnson, L., Neiman, P. E., Lerner, K. G., Glucksberg, H. & Buckner, C. D. (1975) Bone marrow transplantation (Parts 1 and 2). *New England Journal of Medicine*, **292**, 832–843, 895–902.

Treves, A. J., Cohen, I. R. & Feldman, M. (1975) Immunotherapy of lethal metastases by lymphocytes sensitized against tumor cell *in vitro*. *Journal of the National Cancer Institute*, **54**, 777–780.

Tsukimoto, I., Wong, K. Y. & Lamplin, B. C. (1976) Surface markers and prognostic factors in acute lymphoblastic leukaemia. *New England Journal of Medicine*, **294**, 245–248.

Viza, D. C., Bernard-Degani, O., Bernard, C. & Harris, R. (1969) Leukaemia antigens. *Lancet*, **ii**, 493–494.

Viza, D., Davies, D. A. L. & Harris, R. (1970a) Solubilization and partial purification of human leukaemic specific antigens. *Nature*, **227**, 1249–1251.

Viza, D., Davies, D. A. L., Todd, R., Bernard-Degani, O., Bernard, C. L. & Harris, R. (1970b) Mise en évidence isolement et purification partielle d'antigènes leucémiques chez l'homme. *Presse médicale*, **78**, 2259–2264.

Vogler, W. R. & Chan, Y.-K. (1974) Prolonging remission in myeloblastic leukaemia by tice-strain bacillus Calmette–Guérin. *Lancet*, **ii**, 128–131.

Vries, J. E. de, Rümke, P. & Bernheim, J. C. (1972) Cytotoxic lymphocytes in melanoma patients. *International Journal of Cancer*, **9**, 567–576.

Waaler, H. T. (1971) BCG and leukaemia mortality. *Lancet*, **ii**, 1314.

Weiss, D. W., Stupp, Y., Manny, N. & Izak, G. (1975) Treatment of acute myelocytic leukemia patients with the MER tubercle bacillus fraction: A preliminary report. *Transplantation Proceedings*, **VII** (1) (Suppl. 1), 545–552.

Weiss, D. W. (1976) MER and other mycobacterial fractions in the immunotherapy of cancer. *Medical Clinics: Symposium on Immunotherapy in Malignant Disease*, ed. Terry, W. D. Philadelphia, London, Toronto: W. B. Saunders Co.

Weksler, M. E. & Birnbaum, G. (1972) Lymphocyte transformation induced by autologous cells: stimulation by cultured lymphoblast lines. *Journal of Clinical Investigation*, **51**, 3124–3132.

Weksler, M. E. (1973) Lymphocyte transformation induced by autologous cells. *Journal of Experimental Medicine*, **137**, 799–806.

Yata, J., Klein, G., Kobayashi, N., Furukawa, T. & Yanagisawa, M. (1970) Human thymus-lymphoid tissue antigen and its presence in leukaemia and lymphoma. *Clinical and Experimental Immunology*, **7**, 781–792.

Yoshida, T. O. & Imai, K. (1970) Auto-antibody to human leukaemic cell membrane as detected by immune adherence. *European Journal of Clinical and Biological Science*, **XV**, 61–65.

12

THE TREATMENT OF ALLERGIC DISEASE

J. Morrison Smith

In discussing the current treatment of allergic disease most attention will be paid to asthma and conditions which are associated with it such as allergic rhinitis. The ideal treatment for allergic disease is avoidance of the identified allergen or allergens, before any destructive element in the immunological process has developed. Thus in farmer's lung, exposure to mouldy hay should cease as soon as the condition is recognised, preferably before pulmonary fibrosis and irreversible impairment of lung function has occurred. In most cases of drug allergy a suitable alternative drug can be substituted. Only occasionally will suppressive treatment with corticosteroids or antihistamines be an acceptable alternative in such conditions. Allergen avoidance is, however, impractical in many cases of asthma and our knowledge of the aetiology of atopic eczema is so poor that specific treatment is virtually impossible. The only practical approach is to treat the condition symptomatically.

Most of the recent advances in the treatment of allergic disease have been pharmacological rather than immunological and although these advances are of great importance to those who suffer from the conditions they are essentially suppressive rather than curative. New concepts and improved understanding of immunological mechanisms do hold some promise that the antigen–antibody reaction may be controlled, and even that the prevalence of allergic disease is subject to environmental influences which may not be beyond our power to change (Morrison Smith, 1972–73). The main developments so far have come from drugs such as sodium cromoglycate which influence the consequences of the antigen–antibody reaction with release of mediators, or from corticosteroids which reduce inflammatory tissue reactions resulting from the action of these mediators and from other mechanisms. The great hopes of specifically reducing allergic disease by desensitisation have, after more than 60 years, gone largely unrealised. Much research and a widespread use of injections of allergen extracts throughout the world has continued.

Between 1960 and 1966 there was an alarming rise in deaths from asthma in England, and in certain other countries, proportionally affecting young people between 5 and 25 years to a greater extent than older people and leaving unaffected children under five (Morrison Smith, 1966; Speizer, Doll and Heaf, 1968). The rise in deaths coincided with a rise in the use of aerosols of isoprenaline and the fall occurred shortly after these aerosols became no longer available in England without a doctor's prescription. The stimulation of interest resulting from these events probably contributed to an improvement in the treatment of acute asthma and to a more general awareness that avoidable deaths were not uncommon.

THE TREATMENT OF ACUTE ASTHMA

The development of units for intensive care and mechanical ventilation has made it possible to save the lives of patients who would otherwise die (Ambiavagar and Sherwood

Jones, 1967). Many deaths from asthma occur, however, at home due to a failure on the part both of the patient and of his medical attendant to appreciate the risk to life (Speizer, et al, 1968). Deterioration often occurs at night and at weekends when help is least readily available so that there is a tendency to put off seeking advice, particularly in patients who have long continued airways obstruction and have had a number of acute attacks in the past which have resolved.

Patients most at risk are those whose airways are never completely normal, who have had previous severe episodes, who find their normal bronchodilator has become markedly less effective, have noted difficulty in carrying on a conversation, show signs of tiredness through prolonged distress and difficulty in sleeping, have persistent tachycardia and overinflation of the chest so that the tidal volume is being maintained at the top of the inspiratory cycle giving rise in some cases to pulsus paradoxus. Routine use of simple tests of ventilatory capacity when patients attend for repeat prescriptions are useful and indicate those at risk. Clinical assessment, and even auscultation, can be misleading. A less easily audible wheeze may not indicate clinical improvement if less air is gaining entry to the lungs. Young people often remain ambulant, denying distress, when a very marked reduction in ventilatory capacity has occurred.

In hospital it may be assumed that assessment and treatment will be fully adequate but this is not always so, as reported by Cochrane and Clark (1975) in a survey of asthma mortality in patients aged 35 to 64 in the Greater London hospitals in 1971. They found assessment of severity incomplete and lacking in accuracy. Estimations of electrolytes, and particularly serum potassium, were frequently omitted and when abnormal, were left uncorrected. Measurements of blood–gas tensions which should have been routine in patients with severe asthma were also frequently omitted or inaccurately recorded, in particular no record was made of whether oxygen therapy was being given when blood was taken. Although chest radiographs were usual, electrocardiography was often omitted.

They found that 68 per cent of the deaths occurred between midnight and 8.0 a.m. Of 19 patients whose records they were able to study after death only one was admitted to the intensive care unit and that was for a period of two days only, after which this patient was transferred to a general medical ward and died there six days later. They found treatment given in the 24 h prior to death suggested a gross underuse of corticosteroids both before and after admission with, in some cases, the use of inappropriate preparations such as corticotrophin. Moreover, no less than 15 out of 19 had received sedation. In the hospitals concerned there were about 2000 admissions for asthma in 1971 in patients between 35 and 64 years of age and of these 47 were recorded as dying of asthma (2.4 per cent), although Cochrane and Clark concluded from a study of the death certificates that only 19 (1 per cent) died of acute asthma while in hospital. It is likely that only a small proportion of all asthmatics are at serious risk and they are often admitted repeatedly.

Admission to a specialised unit of patients considered to be at risk as reported from Edinburgh by Crompton and Grant (1975) would probably improve the general level of care. Mechanical ventilation should be used depending on the level of consciousness, the amount of distress, the duration of the attack and evidence of tiredness. Absolute indications for assisted ventilation are difficult to define so that they cover all patients. Loss of consciousness, exhaustion and obvious cyanosis would virtually always require mechanical ventilation. Carbon dioxide tension of over 8 kPa or an oxygen tension under 5 kPa without rapid improvement would again call for mechanical ventilation. Blood–gas tensions and ventilatory function tests may have to be repeated after using adequate bronchodilator and steroid treatment. Response monitored by restoration of arterial oxygen and carbon dioxide to safe levels is very varied, the younger atopic patients respond more rapidly and usually require less steroid both in total dosage and in duration than older patients.

Care must be taken to avoid overdosage of toxic drugs such as aminophylline which may be given before admission more than once and repeated on admission. Adequate corticosteroid by intravenous or intramuscular injection should be given while awaiting transport to hospital. Initially intravenous hydrocortisone is recommended in a dose of 3 mg/kg of body weight repeated every 3 h until intramuscular or oral preparations can be safely used.

Intubation and intermittent positive pressure ventilation with a volume-cycled ventilator is now established practice. Patients usually require restoration of blood volume and correction of electrolyte imbalance. Opinion is somewhat divided on the question of the value of bronchial lavage, but tracheotomy is rarely required as mechanical ventilation seldom need be continued over six days when adequate steroid and supportive treatment is given. The continued use of intravenous bronchodilators is of doubtful value. A response will be obtained in less than 6 h if it is possible, and where none occurs it is best to wait until responsiveness may be restored and try again. Sedatives can be given safely only when mechanical ventilation has been established.

CORTICOSTEROIDS—SYSTEMIC AND INHALED

Systemic

'When acute severe asthma does not respond to bronchodilators, corticosteroids are essential and should be given in adequate dose without delay' (*Lancet*, 1975b). With this there is now little disagreement but the long-term use of corticosteroids does arouse some doubt and disagreement. The mode of action of corticosteroids is not precisely known. They do resolve infiltrative and inflammatory processes but have little effect on IgE-mediated allergic reactions, failing to block significantly skin, nasal or bronchial immediate reactions to allergens while effectively blocking delayed, type III, reactions. They may stabilise cell membranes and protect smooth muscle, vascular endothelium and leucocytes from injury. They restore responsiveness to catecholamines, a rise in intracellular $3':5'$-cyclic AMP occurs which may reduce mediator release from mast cells and suppress inflammatory responses (Szentivanyi, 1968).

Corticosteroids are given more readily to adults than to children, although children usually respond to small doses and often require only temporary treatment. There has also been some reluctance to treat seasonal hay fever and pollen asthma with steroids, although again, in spite of the obvious presence of a type I sensitivity, response to treatment is generally good and only a short period of treatment, carrying little risk, is required.

Maunsell, Bruce Pearson and Livingstone (1968) studied 170 patients with severe asthma and found no tendency for the effectiveness of corticosteroid treatment to diminish, even after 10 years. Side effects occurred in 20 per cent and were related to dosage rather than duration of treatment. Rees and Williams (1962) reported striking improvement in 56 per cent of their 317 patients with asthma and complete failure in only 5 per cent. An undue pessimism regarding the use of corticosteroids in asthma resulted from a Medical Research Council trial in 1956 which concluded that the value of steroids in chronic asthma was uncertain. In spite of many reports to the contrary there was for many years a widespread reluctance to use corticosteroids in asthma and an undue fear of side-effects.

In status asthmaticus corticosteroid treatment is essential and must be absorbed as quickly as possible since action will be delayed by several hours at least. Intravenous hydrocortisone hemisuccinate, initially 3 mg/kg of body weight repeated every 3 h until some improvement is noted, is recommended (*British Medical Journal*, 1975). In less severe cases intramuscular hydrocortisone 100 mg six-hourly, or oral prednisolone, may be adequate. When very high doses are used, particularly by intravenous drip, potassium supplements should be added. Potassium depletion and muscular weakness may result in hypoxia due to hypoventilation when the patient is taken off a ventilator, even when the airways obstruction has been relieved. For oral use it is unlikely that other preparations have any real advantage over prednisolone. Dosage must be tailored to the needs of each patient and may vary from time to time. The aim is to use the smallest dose over the shortest period consistent with safety and the relief of serious distress. A short course of oral steroid treatment may be necessary as a prelude to establishing effective maintenance on inhaled treatment with sodium cromoglycate or with a steroid aerosol.

Corticotrophin has the disadvantage of having to be given by injection and may occasionally result in sensitisation (Hill and Swinburn, 1954). This risk is much reduced with tetracosactrin but not entirely eliminated. In patients who may have adrenal suppression the action of corticotrophin is uncertain. Friedman and Strang (1966) showed that in children corticotrophin was less likely to give rise to growth suppression than corticosteroids given orally. Although this report gave rise to considerable interest corticotrophin has not gained great popularity. Even depot preparations of corticotrophin and tetracosactrin may be unsatisfactory in controlling severe asthma and they do give rise to marked fluid retention.

Long-term use of corticosteroids in children has given much anxiety, not all of it justified. Growth suppression is fairly common but in asthmatic children other complications are rare, which is in contrast to children with juvenile rheumatism who are more constitutionally ill and require larger doses than asthmatic children. Morrison Smith and Pizarro (1973) followed 145 children who required long-term steroid treatment and found none died of complications of the treatment although four died of asthma in circumstances where there had been a failure to increase the dose of steroid in time of need. Growth was retarded by the disease in 25 per cent before steroid treatment was given; further retardation due to treatment occurred in 20 per cent but in 18 per cent some degree of improvement occurred while 62 per cent showed no change in growth status.

In considering the need for steroid treatment it is necessary to consider not only the risk to life but the quality of life for the patient and his family. In children there is a marked tendency towards improvement in most cases so that steroid treatment may only be required for a limited period. Intermittent treatment may reduce the incidence of side-effects but is not suitable for all cases (Walsh and Grant, 1966). Children who cannot attend school properly and adults who cannot support or attend to their families may suffer deprivation and distress which far outweighs the risks of steroid treatment.

Inhaled corticosteroids in asthma

There is nothing new about the idea of using inhaled corticosteroid preparations to obtain a direct effect on the lung or the nose without the disadvantages of systemic absorption. Early trials by Brockbank and Pengelly (1958), Helm and Heyworth (1958), Morrison Smith (1958), Langlands and McNeil (1960) failed to show any effect from inhalation of hydrocortisone in solution or cortisone acetate as a powder, although

Herxheimer, McAllen and Williams (1958) did report a favourable response. Favourable results in hay fever were reported by Morris-Owen and Truelove (1958) and by Herxsheimer and McAllen (1956). This form of treatment did not however really give very good results in subsequent years. A dramatic change in the effectiveness of local steroid treatment came with the use of beclomethasone dipropionate and betamethasone 17-valerate which had been previously used as local applications in ointments for skin conditions. It is simpler to discuss in detail beclomethasone dipropionate since most work has been published on this and the pharmacological properties are very similar to those of betamethasone 17-valerate. The metered aerosol of beclomethasone dipropionate (Becotide) delivers a dose of 50 μg.

When applied to the skin beclomethasone dipropionate has a high degree of anti-inflammatory activity with little systemic effect (Caldwell et al, 1968; Raffle and Frain-Bell, 1967). Since about 90 per cent of an aerosol dose is swallowed it was important to establish the dose of beclomethasone dipropionate which would cause measurable adrenal suppression when given by mouth. Harris et al (1973) found that although it is well-absorbed only doses over 1 mg gave measurable suppression and that it was about 500 times more active topically than dexamethasone.

Morrow-Brown, Storey and George (1972) reported 60 cases of asthma treated with the aerosol with good results. The standard dose was two inhalations four times a day, a total of 400 μg. The only important side-effects were due to steroid withdrawal. Similar results were reported by many authors. Gaddie et al (1973) studied 15 patients with chronic asthma and found no further benefit resulting from increasing the dose above 400 μg per day. In children clinical trials were particularly successful (Morrison Smith, 1973b Dickson et al, 1973; Jones, 1973; Godfrey and König, 1973). Similar results were reported with betamethasone 17-valerate in adults (McAllen, Kochanowski and Shaw, 1974) and in children (Frears, Wilson and Friedman, 1973).

Candidiasis of the pharynx and occasionally of the larynx was found. McAllen et al (1974) reported pharyngeal candidiasis in 13 per cent and the larynx was affected in 5 per cent. It was absent at doses of 200 μg/day or less. This complication is probably more likely in patients who have been receiving oral as well as inhaled steroid but is practically unknown in children (Gwynn and Morrison Smith, 1974). Treatment can usually be continued while the candidiasis is treated concurrently, or the steroid aerosol can be temporarily withdrawn. A very rapid increase in growth velocity in children is noted when aerosol is substituted for oral treatment (Gwynn and Morrison Smith, 1974). The warning given by Morrow-Brown et al (1972) regarding the need for rapid resumption of systemic treatment in the event of a serious, if temporary, relapse has been amply borne out and fatal consequences of failure to do this have occurred (Gwynn and Morrison Smith, 1974).

Very frequent candidiasis was reported in a trial by the Brompton Hospital and Medical Research Council (1974). This trial carried out in 101 patients, and preliminarily reported at 28 weeks, was in patients whose mean age was 48 years and who were all on oral steroids. The main aim was to compare the effect of 800 μg daily with 400 μg, and a placebo. Both levels of dosage gave significantly better results than the placebo in allowing reduction in oral steroid to be made, but only in those having 16 mg of predisolone or more daily was 800 μg better than 400 μg. The preliminary report was made because of a cumulative increase in oropharyngeal candidiasis, significantly greater in those on 800 μg (77 per cent) than in those on 400 μg (45 per cent) and much greater than in those on placebo (9 per cent).

The fact that 9 per cent of patients on the placebo did develop candidiasis suggests that in this relatively elderly group, all having prednisolone, there was a marked predisposition to the development of candidiasis compared with younger patients and those who had not already received oral steroids over long periods. No patient had to stop the aerosol steroid because of candidiasis, the complication being controlled by giving amphotericin tablets. Precipitins to Candida were found in 25 per cent of patients before entering the trial and a further 16 per cent developed precipitins during the trial. No evidence of systemic candidiasis occurred, but those with precipitins before the trial seemed particularly liable to develop clinical evidence of candidiasis.

The risks of candidiasis are considered to be greatly outweighed by the benefits of a reduction in oral steroid dosage. Milne and Crompton (1974) noted that positive throat swab cultures for candidiasis were frequent in patients with respiratory disease, occurring in 27.2 per cent of patients receiving no corticosteroid treatment at all and in 41 per cent of those on beclomethasone dipropionate. Only 5.5 per cent of their patients on inhaled steroid and 0.7 per cent on oral steroid had clinical evidence of candidiasis.

There is some anxiety that long continued inhaled steroids might eventually lead to mucosal atrophy in the respiratory tract similar to the atrophic changes which can occur in the skin with long continued use but there has been no evidence that this is a risk (Andersson and Smidt, 1974). The doses involved are relatively minute compared with those involved in treatment of widespread skin conditions.

Aerosol corticosteroids in allergic rhinitis

Beclomethasone dipropionate has also been used successfully in allergic rhinitis and hay fever (Morrow-Brown and Storey, 1974; Morrison Smith et al, 1975; Löfkvist and Svensson, 1975). No side-effects were reported but with long continued use in chronic perennial rhinitis candidiasis might occur although this seems very unlikely in hay fever.

BRONCHODILATORS

A bronchodilator may relax smooth muscle but the immunopathological process continues. Bronchodilators can be divided into those which stimulate beta two adrenergic receptors, the methyl zanthine derivatives which are phosphodiesterase inhibitors and lead to an increase in intracellular cyclic $3':5'$-adenosine monophosphate, anticholinergic drugs which block vagal efferent tone, and α-adrenergic blocking drugs (Fig. 12.1). In some circumstances α-blocking drugs such as thymoxamine, phentolamine and phenoxybenzamine may potentiate the effect of β-stimulating drugs such as isoprenaline (Patel and Kerr, 1975a, b). Methyl zanthine drugs such as theophylline and aminophylline given by mouth are not very effective, although given intravenously in status asthmaticus, or even per rectum in less severe attacks, may have dramatic results. Preparations containing theophylline and ephedrine remain popular probably because these drugs have a synergistic action.

Patel and Kerr (1975a) showed that in status asthmaticus adenyl-cyclase activity in leucocytes (now identified with β-receptor function) is reduced and there is a diminished response of the enzyme system to isoprenaline which can be raised towards normal by α-receptor blocking drugs such as thymoxamine. They studied these effects clinically in 10 patients and found that their results supported their biochemical work suggesting that α-receptor blocking drugs in combination with β-receptor stimulants may have a place in the management of asthma. Thymoxamine is the most specific α-blocking agent available for clinical use but its short duration of action when given intravenously and irritant effect if inhaled may limit its usefulness.

Of the more specific β_2-stimulating drugs orciprenaline, salbutamol, terbutaline and rimiterol are in common use. All are used as pressurised aerosols with metered doses giving comparable effect. Orciprenaline, salbutamol and terbutaline are available for oral use but

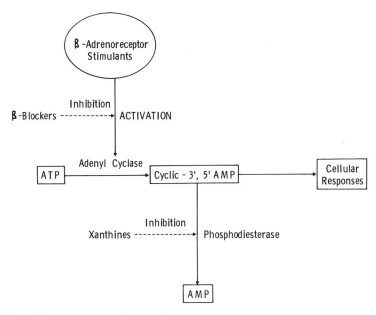

Figure 12.1 β-adrenoreceptor stimulants and cyclic-3′,5′-adenosine monophosphate(cyclic-3′5′-AMP). ATP, adenosine triphosphate; AMP, adenosine monophosphate. (Reproduced from D. Jack (1971) *Postgraduate Medical Journal*, Suppl., **47,** 8)

are less effective by this route so that the larger dose required may give side-effects such as tremor. Although this is disturbing it is unlikely to be dangerous and is probably produced by a local effect on skeletal muscle rather than an effect on the sympathetic nervous system. A rise in pulse rate may occur but this is less than occurs with isoprenaline. Both salbutamol and terbutaline are available for intravenous administration and may be valuable in some patients who may respond better to intravenous salbutamol than to intravenous aminophylline with fewer side effects (Williams, Parrish and Seaton, 1975). Salbutamol or terbutaline may be used in conjunction with assisted respiration using a Bird ventilator with a face mask in patients not sufficiently severely ill to require intubation.

Routine frequent measurements of ventilatory capacity using a dry spirometer to measure forced expiratory volume and forced vital capacity or the Wright peak flow meter to measure peak expiratory flow may give warning of deterioration and failure to respond to bronchodilators. The inappropriate use of aerosol bronchodilators was thought to have contributed to the rise in deaths from asthma in England between 1960 and 1966 (*Lancet*, 1968). Patients with severe asthma are in a dangerous physiological state (Read, 1968), and the degree of dyspnoea is a poor guide to the level of arterial oxygen tension (Rees, Millar and Donald, 1968). Pulse rate is a much better index of the physiological state, although this does not imply that cardiac failure is the primary cause of death in fatal cases.

Bronchodilator sympathomimetic drugs are known to cause pulmonary vasodilatation and this in turn can cause a fall in arterial oxygen tension by perfusion of poorly ventilated lung. This fall in arterial oxygen tension associated with ventilation–perfusion imbalance is not of clinical importance in patients with normal, or near normal, oxygen tension but may be of serious consequence in those with reduced oxygen tension who are on the point where the oxygen dissociation curve falls steeply with a small further reduction in oxygen tension.

During the 'epidemic' rise in deaths isoprenaline was the drug used in bronchodilator aerosols. The rise in deaths affected England, Scotland, Ireland, New Zealand and Australia but the United States, Canada and the Netherlands were not affected and some other European countries and Japan only slightly affected (Fraser and Doll, 1971; *British Medical Journal*, 1972). It has been suggested by Stolley (1972) that the strong isoprenaline aerosols delivering a dose of 0.4 mg could account for this uneven geographical distribution. However, as pointed out by Herxheimer, (1972) the question cannot be answered so simply and there are too many exceptions to this theory to make it acceptable. There is a lack of convincing evidence that isoprenaline is cardiotoxic in clinical circumstances and many other factors may have played a part in the excess deaths in the 1960s.

The use of aerosol bronchodilators has not been greatly reduced in England since 1966 but the use of salbutamol has increased steeply whereas that of isoprenaline has declined. The possibility of fatal consequences arising from repeated inhalation of fluorocarbon propellants in bronchodilator aerosols has been reviewed by the *Lancet* (1975a).

Animal experiments have shown that aerosol propellants may cause ventricular arrhythmias and that these occur at lower concentrations in animals given intravenous adrenaline or exercised on a treadmill. Some animals were more sensitive than the majority so that it is possible that some human beings are also more at risk than others. It was concluded that, although gross overuse of aerosol bronchodilators could give concentrations of fluorocarbons in the human myocardium of the same order as those in the experimental dogs who got ventricular arrhythmias, aerosols used in the recommended manner were not likely to be dangerous. The fact that the use of aerosols is almost as high as it was when the peak of deaths occurred in England without a return to the same high numbers of deaths tends to support this.

DISODIUM CROMOGLYCATE
(Cromolyn Sodium; Sodium Cromoglycate BP)

Experimental background

The synthesis of this drug in 1965 was the result of a study of khellin, the active principal of the plant *Ammi visnaga*. The research programme leading to the development of the drug was extensive and required both perseverance and courage (Cox, 1970).

It was originally thought that its effect was specifically antiallergic in the sense that it inhibited only the IgE antigen–antibody reaction but recent evidence indicates that it can inhibit a variety of agents which trigger the release of mediator substances from mast cells. It does not affect either the specific fixation of antibodies to mast cells or the interaction of antigen with cell-fixed antibody. It is however capable of preventing release of pharmacological mediators during desensitisation of tissues by antigen.

Antigen challenge studies by Pepys and his colleagues (1968, 1973) have demonstrated that the drug inhibits type-I reactions and can also inhibit type-III reactions, possibly by inhibiting the introductory type-I reaction without which the late type-III reaction cannot proceed. Orr and his colleagues (1970) have demonstrated that it acts at a stage following antigen–antibody reaction prior to the release of pharmacological mediators from the mast cell. Since it is capable of inhibiting histamine release from mast cells induced by a variety of non-antigenic trigger agents, this may have a bearing on some of its clinical applications such as its use in preventing exercise-induced asthma in man.

Disodium cromoglycate may also have an α-adrenergic blocking effect. Kerr, Govindara and Patel, (1970) have shown that it can block the effect of slow intravenous histamine infusion which results in a fall in forced expiratory volume and vital capacity in asthmatic patients in a manner apparently similar to prior intravenous administration of the α-adrenergic blocking drugs phentolamine and phenoxybenzamine.

Much of the courage and perseverance which went into the discovery of disodium cromoglycate was contributed by Dr R. E. C. Altounyan. Being an asthmatic, he devised a suitable antigen challenge test for use on himself and over a period of some six years carried out a large series of tests on blocking activity of chemical derivatives of khellin. An appliance ('Spinhaler') was developed by Altounyan which enabled a patient with a relatively small inspiratory effort to inhale a 20 mg dose from a capsule. If the inspiratory effort is too small, as in a patient with severe asthma or in a small child, the device is ineffective and even in a patient capable of using the device effectively an inadequate rate of inspiration may deposit the whole dose in the mouth. The maximum amount of the dose which does reach the main bronchi and beyond has been calculated as 10 per cent of the total, even in fit volunteers. Thus careful instruction and supervision of the patient on this treatment is essential to its success. About 50 per cent of the amount absorbed into the circulation from the lungs is excreted by the kidney and most of it appears in the urine within 2 h of inhalation. Most of the remainder is excreted in the bile. There is virtually no tissue-storing of this drug. Although it is highly water soluble it is hardly absorbed at all from the gastrointestinal tract.

The possibility of the occurrence of rare immunological reactions to sodium cromoglycate is raised by a report of Sheffer, Rocklyn and Goetzl (1975) describing six patients who experienced reactions with an apparently immunological background while on the drug. Patients with intolerance who experience irritation of the upper airways, and in some cases, exacerbation of asthma on disodium cromoglycate are encountered not uncommonly but the cases described by Sheffer et al were more serious. The three who had acute reactions had all been on corticosteroid treatment which had been withdrawn because of an initial favourable response to disodium cromoglycate. Further observation on such rare reactions will be of interest and control studies to eliminate the effect of rapid reduction or withdrawal of corticosteroids are desirable before reaching too firm a conclusion on this evidence.

Use of disodium chromoglycate in asthma

The first clinical trial of the drug in asthma by Howell and Altounyan (1967) was carried out in 10 patients severely disabled with allergic bronchial asthma on a double blind cross-over basis in which they received 20 mg of disodium cromoglycate plus 20 mg of lactose powder four times a day for two weeks and 40 mg of lactose powder for two weeks.   In both the active and placebo capsules 0.1 mg of isoprenaline was included to counteract the possible effect of inhalation of a drug powder in causing bronchospasm. Most later trials used capsules which also contained 5 mg of sodium sulphate in the placebo so that the slightly bitter taste of the disodium cromoglycate would be reproduced and the patients as far as possible kept in ignorance of any difference in the capsules other than that noted by their therapeutic effect.

Howell and Altounyan assessed their results by means of the physician's opinion of each patient's progress and terminated their trial as indicated by a sequential analysis graph. The results were confirmed on analysis of symptom score cards but only 4 of 10 patients showed greater than 20 per cent change in FEV_1. In other trials it has always been easier

Table 12.1   Long-term disodium chromoglycate

Definite improvement	Doubtful	Not improved	Total
157 (65°$_0$)	51 (21°$_0$)	34 (14°$_0$)	242

Steroid Cases	
Steroid stopped	57
Steroid decreased	20
Steroid increased	5
Steroid unchanged	14
Total	96
Steroid started during treatment	7

to show clinical benefit than to demonstrate physiological improvement. Kidner et al (1968) in a trial involving 28 patients and using capsules which did not contain isoprenaline were able to demonstrate a statistically significant improvement in FEV_1 during treatment.

In 44 children Morrison Smith and Devey (1968) carried out a double blind cross-over trial during two four-week periods assessing the results in the second two weeks of each period to avoid a carry-over effect of the drug, which has since become generally recognised. Analysis of the patients' symptom records showed a significant advantage for the period on disodium cromoglycate. Use of aerosol bronchodilators (23 patients) was significantly reduced and steroids were also less used. Ventilatory function tests showed significant improvement while on treatment, particularly in those whose FEV_1 or FVC were under 80 per cent of the predicted value during the period on placebo.

Subsequent follow-up on open treatment for one year showed no evidence of loss of effect in the 44 children, indeed in most respects further improvement was seen (Morrison Smith, 1970b). Long-term results are generally excellent (Table 12.1) and many children who previously required continuous steroid treatment to enable them to lead reasonably normal lives in safety were able to stop or decrease the dosage with benefit in regard to their general health and growth (Morrison Smith and Pizarro, 1972b).

The steroid-sparing effect of disodium cromoglycate has been confirmed by others (Engström and Kraepelien, 1971) but care must be taken to reintroduce or increase the dosage of steroid treatment in patients with severe asthma who were previously steroid-dependent in the event of an acute severe attack occurring, as it may do in such cases, in spite of generally satisfactory control. Although only a small number of patients may be at risk, failure to give adequate steroids in time has resulted in fatalities.

Another risk which is difficult to quantify is that after a period of improvement on regular use of disodium cromoglycate some patients fail to continue inhaling the drug regularly and relapse may occur suddenly days or weeks later owing to the variability of the carry-over effect. By examination of random urine samples and further urine collection an hour after taking a capsule under supervision Morrison Smith and Pizarro found that about 25 per cent of patients thought to be taking the treatment regularly were not in fact doing so. This problem is present in most types of long-continued therapy and was first investigated extensively in relation to antituberculosis treatment. The more troublesome or unpleasant the medication the more likely it may be that patients will 'forget' to take it regularly.

Although little doubt was present regarding the efficacy of disodium cromoglycate in children and adolescents some workers expressed doubts about its clinical value in general (Grant, Channell and Drever, 1967; Grant, 1969; Gebbie et al, 1972). Herxheimer and Bewersdorff (1969) even doubted its effect experimentally. Many hundreds of clinical trials have, however, now established its value beyond doubt. A long-term double blind controlled trial carried out by the Brompton Hospital and Medical Research Council (1972) in a group of severe adult asthmatics, both with and without evidence of extrinsic allergic sensitivity, over a period of a year showed significant benefit both from disodium cromoglycate with isoprenaline and disodium cromoglycate alone compared with a placebo. It was often possible to reduce the dose after eight weeks from four capsules to two capsules daily without relapse. The capsules were well tolerated and toxicity to the drug was not observed.

This absence of evidence of toxicity is general in reported trials apart from cases of irritation of the throat and occasional bronchial irritation with exacerbation of asthma which can preclude treatment. Patients previously maintained only on corticosteroid treatment may suffer withdrawal effects as the steroid dose is reduced under cover of disodium cromoglycate and may have reappearance of rhinitis or eczema which were previously suppressed as well as pulmonary eosinophilia. These effects may be wrongly attributed to disodium cromoglycate itself (Hargreve, McCarthy and Pepys, 1969). So far as is known there is no risk to the fetus in pregnancy. In long-term use Morrison Smith and Pizarro (1972b) found no evidence of adverse effect on examination of chest radiographs, liver function, urine, blood or growth. No evidence of immediate-type sensitivity to the drug was found either. There have, however, been patients who have developed an urticarial rash round the mouth on inhalation of the powder but this has not been established to be a truly allergic phenomenon.

The duration of action of the drug is limited to about 6 h and falls off quite rapidly after 3 h. It has not been shown convincingly that increase in the number of capsules per day beyond the usual four at six-hourly intervals will lead to success in otherwise unresponsive patients (Morrison Smith, 1973a). Altounyan (1967) demonstrated experimentally that the degree of protection given by disodium cromoglycate depends on the level of antigen challenge and this may be obvious clinically in that pollen-sensitive patients may experience protection during most of the pollen season but relapse for a few days when the pollen count is very high.

However, in clinical circumstances other factors besides allergen exposure may affect the patient and give rise to fluctuation in the level of symptoms. Knowledge of such factors is at present insufficient to quantify or even to adequately identify them. In the selection of patients suitable for treatment the most satisfactory method is to give the drug a month's trial. The most severe and persistent cases are less likely to show a satisfactory clinical response but even in such cases measurable benefit may be obtained (Brompton Hospital/Medical Research Council, 1972). Children tend to respond well and most have extrinsic asthma but Engström and Kraepelien (1971) were unable to correlate response to the drug with IgE levels in the serum.

Disodium cromoglycate reduced the fall in FEV_1 in patients with exercise-induced asthma (Davies, 1968; Godfrey, 1975). An interesting extension of the work by Godfrey is the study of the inhibition of exercise-induced asthma by particles of the drug of different size. Particles 2 μm in diameter gave much better protection than those of 11.7 μm diameter. It is suggested that only the smaller particles reach the terminal airways and thus the site of occurrence of airways obstruction in exercise-induced asthma is in the terminal airways and that the commercially available preparation given by the 'Spinhaler' effectively reaches the terminal airways.

Use of disodium chromoglycate in allergic rhinitis

Experimental work on the reduction of nasal blockage on allergen challenge has shown that disodium cromoglycate is capable of reducing the response to such challenge (Pelikan et al, 1970; Taylor and Shivalkar, 1971; Jenssen, 1973). The drug has been used clinically both as a powder ('Rynacrom') and as a 2 per cent solution ('Lomusol'). Taylor and Shivalkar (1971) found that the powder reduced symptoms in subjects with hay fever; Morrison Smith (1971) also found reduction in symptoms of hay fever but during the peak of the pollen season there was not a significant difference compared with a placebo. Holopainen, Bachman and Salo (1971) carried out a double-blind trial in 27 patients with seasonal allergic rhinitis and found significant symptomatic benefit as did Capel and McKelvie (1971). Blair and Herbert (1973) in a double-blind trial of the 2 per cent solution in hay fever found it of significant benefit.

In perennial rhinitis Holopainen and colleagues (1975) carried out a double-blind trial of four weeks on 2 per cent disodium cromoglycate administered six times a day and four weeks of a placebo on a cross-over basis, with significant improvement in symptoms when on treatment. Their cases were divided into extrinsic and intrinsic rhinitis on the basis of skin tests and provocation tests. There was no difference in the response of the two groups symptomatically. It was also noted that the number of eosinophils in the nasal secretions was not significantly different while the patients were on disodium cromoglycate or placebo. Fagerberg and Zetterström (1975) also found clinical improvement in perennial rhinitis with disodium cromoglycate compared with placebo, but they could not correlate this with the results of investigations of allergic aetiology or IgE measurements. They concluded that the best clinical approach is a therapeutic trial.

Use in other conditions

Mani et al (1976) reported a successful trial of disodium cromoglycate in proctocolitis. Frost (1973) used it successfully in a toothpaste in treating aphthous ulceration of the mouth. Kingsley (1974) reported its use in a case of gastrointestinal allergy associated with urticaria in a woman of 33 while Freier and Berger (1973) have successfully treated infants with intolerance to cow's milk. One per cent eye drops have been used with benefit in vernal keratoconjunctivitis (Easty, Rice and Jones, 1972).

SPECIFIC TREATMENT

Allergen Avoidance

Clinicians rarely have the satisfying experience of providing advice on the avoidance of a single allergen which will be successful in relieving symptoms—in fact, more rarely than most patients expect. Allergens associated with asthma and rhinitis are usually so much part of the enrivonment as to be very difficult to avoid. Air filtration has not provided a practical escape even from the discomfort of hay fever, despite the clarity of the aetiological diagnosis. Reduction of exposure to house dust allergens is even more difficult.

A cross-over controlled trial by Bar, St Leger and Neale (1976) in a group of 32 adult asthmatics with positive skin reactions to *Dermatophagoides pteronyssinus* was undertaken. The mite control measures consisted of vacuum-cleaning the mattress, pillows and base of the bed and laundering of the blankets, sheets and pillowcases at the same time. The mattress was then enclosed completely in a plastic cover for six weeks. The control procedure which also lasted six weeks was to vacuum-clean all upholstered chairs and carpets in the living-room while leaving the bedroom, the main source of mite-containing dust, unchanged. No significant difference was observed during the treatment period when mite control measures were applied to the bedroom compared with the placebo period when measures were confined to the living-room (and assumed to be ineffective). Assessment was made by observation of daily peak flow readings and by the level of medication used to relieve the asthma. Sarsfield et al (1974) did claim improvement in asthmatic children with mite control measures and it may be that such measures are more worthwhile in children although success is certainly difficult to measure convincingly.

Radical changes in environment can certainly give results (Morrison Smith, 1970a), and differences in aerobiology have been shown to exist between such places as London and an Alpine valley (Davies, 1969), which could account for changes in symptoms in individual patients. The study of mites in house dust from different environments has also given results consistent with clinical experience. Mite-sensitive patients with asthma and rhinitis often improve greatly in hospital where mite counts are very low compared with the domestic environment (Blythe, Williams and Morrison Smith, 1974; Blythe et al, 1975). Many children with atopic eczema also show improvement in an institutional environment or at high altitude for reasons which are obscure.

Measures to limit exposure to mite allergens rely mainly on good housekeeping with vacuum-cleaning of mattresses, good dust control and low humidity. Chemical means of reducing the population of pyroglyphid mites in the domestic environment do exist but the clinical value remains to be established (Penaud et al, 1975). While many workers have estimated the mite content of dust from various sources there is as yet no satisfactory method of estimating the amount of mite allergen in dust. A rapid immunological method would be of great value in epidemiological studies which might clarify the role of the mites in the causation of allergic disease and help to monitor methods of reducing exposure.

Immunotherapy

The term immunotherapy has become popular to describe hyposensitisation or desensitisation and has a highly scientific sound which is probably not fully justified. The introduction of this form of treatment by Leonard Noon (1911) was based on a mistaken scientific idea. Noon considered that hay fever was due to an idiosyncratic reaction to a toxin in grass pollen which could be controlled by inoculations inducing an antitoxin, in the same way as diphtheria prophylaxis. In the early years of this century when the foundations of modern medical science were being laid, it is not surprising that over-simplification and unjustified optimism in relation to allergic disease was common or that it resulted in later years in a period when all specific treatment of allergic disease, and indeed the whole concept of allergy, came under ill-informed scepticism.

Noon died early but his collaborator, John Freeman, lived to a great age. They showed that injections of pollen extract could give clinical relief of summer hay fever and such relief might be accompanied by a reduction in the sensitivity of the conjunctiva to pollen. Injections might be accompanied by reactions containing one or all of the following elements; a local wheal and flare, a rapid anaphylactic reaction, a rapid asthmatic or urticarial reaction or a delayed increase in symptoms.

The standardisation of allergen extracts has always been difficult since they are a complex mixture of proteins and polysaccharides of widely different allergic potency. In spite of this weight/volume standardisation has been generally used. One Noon unit is the extract from 1 μg of grass pollen. Roughly equivalent is the protein nitrogen unit introduced by Cooke which is equivalent to 0.00001 mg of nitrogen. Titration of batches of extract by skin testing on known human sensitive subjects still provides the most practical guide to the potency of extracts but subjects vary greatly and each may be inconstant in response from time to time. The most accurately standardised extract is antigen-E derived from ragweed (King and Norman, 1962). This substance has a potency of about 200 times the whole extract on skin testing and about 20 times that of the total protein in the extract.

The original allergen extracts were aqueous and were sterilised by filtration. The aims of recent developments have been to reduce unpleasant and dangerous reactions and to improve effectiveness. The methods used have been to give prolonged, and presumably beneficial antigenic stimulus, with a small dose by delaying absorption. Oil and silicone emulsions were popular for a time but gave unacceptable local and occasional general reactions. More recently attempts to 'detoxify' extracts have owed much to diphtheria prophylaxis. Alum precipitation and pyridine extraction have resulted in extracts which are much easier to use and are widely reported to give good clinical results. More recently tyrosine adsorption has been used. Tyrosine is a natural amino acid and thus fully metabolised, has a low solubility but powerfully adsorbs macromolecules. It thus has the advantage of being unlikely to cause antigenic reactions or foreign body reactions itself while providing slow release of allergen.

Results of immunotherapy

The antitoxin effect postulated by Noon and Freeman is clearly invalid but almost nothing else is clear. Cooke et al (1935) demonstrated the production of a relatively heat-stable serum factor capable of blocking the passive transfer reaction, popularly termed a 'blocking antibody'. Maunsell (1946) showed that dilutions of the patient's own serum with constant amounts of allergen gave varying degrees of inhibition of the whealing reaction on the same patient's skin. This simple experiment has been confirmed by many others and the blocking effect has been shown to occur after alum precipitated extracts as well as aqueous extracts (Munro-Ashman, McEwen and Feinberg, 1971). There is however considerable doubt if the production of 'blocking antibody' can be correlated with clinical results.

D'Sousa et al (1973) in a double-blind trial of hyposensitisation with an extract of *Dermatophagoides pteronyssinus* found a rise in specific IgE in 58 per cent of treated patients compared with 20 per cent of controls. Specific IgG antibody was present in 30 per cent of patients prior to treatment and more treated patients showed a rise in IgG than controls. Clinical improvement appeared to be associated with the presence of IgG but little or no rise in IgE. There was a diminution in histamine release from leucocytes on antigen challenge in more of the treated patients (6 out of 10) than of the controls (3 out of 11). There was no difference in lymphocyte transformation or in the liberation of leucocyte inhibiting agents.

It may be that long courses of treatment give an initial rise in specific IgE followed by a fall, accompanied by clinical improvement. Stanworth (1975) also noted that in some patients given grass pollen hyposensitisation with a pollen-tyrosine adsorbate there was a rise in specific IgG antipollen antibody which was restricted to the IgG4 subclass—likely to be the IgG anaphylactic antibody of Parish (1974). Berg and Johannson (1971) found successful immunotherapy prevented the usual seasonal rise in specific IgE in pollen sensitive subjects. Blair, Ezeoke and Hobbs (1975) using alum-precipitated pyridine extract of grass pollen found good clinical results associated with an increase in serum-blocking activity and prevention of the seasonal rise in IgE. Lichtenstein, Norman and Winkenwerder (1971) using ragweed antigen E correlated clinical improvement with decreased histamine release from patients' leucocytes but not with 'blocking antibody'.

Although there can be no reasonable doubt that some patients obtain benefit from immunotherapy it is difficult to predict which patients will benefit, which extracts are worth using, and which regimens are best. Both grass pollen and ragweed sensitive patients are likely to obtain some relief of symptoms of hay fever or seasonal asthma but this is unlikely to extend beyond one season without repetition of the treatment. House dust-sensitive subjects do less well either with crude extracts or with mite extracts. This type of treatment is unsuitable for patients with sensitivity to animals, foods or moulds.

Good clinical trials are few and the difficultues formidable. Even pollen counts give a poor index of the individual patient's antigen challenge; clinical assessment is large subjective, extracts are not uniform except perhaps in the case of antigen E and patients vary widely both clinically and immunologically. Frankland and Augustin (1954) found almost 80 per cent of treated patients improved but up to 40 per cent of controls also reported relief of symptoms. Reduced bronchial sensitivity has been demonstrated following hyposensitisation (Citron, Frankland and Sinclair, 1958; Aas, 1971). The British Tuberculosis Association (1968) in a large controlled trial failed to show significant benefit from courses of house-dust extract compared with carbol saline and Morrison Smith and Pizarro (1972a) compared a similar house dust extract with a dilute extract of *Dermatophagoides pteronyssinus* in dust mite-sensitive children and could find no significant difference.

REACTIONS TO TREATMENT

The question of immunological ill effects, other than immediate local or general reactions, has received less attention. With long courses of house dust and even pollen extract, a delayed local reaction resulting in a swelling at the site of injection lasting up to a week may become evident and in some cases a deterioration in symptoms instead of an improvement occurs. More unusual is the case of a 62-year-old woman reported by Woodroffe (1972) who developed multiple myelomatosis, possibly precipitated by many years of hyposensitisation. So far as is known this is not a risk that need influence a decision whether or not to use immunotherapy, but such treatment should not be continued for long periods if it is not beneficial and allergen extracts used should be limited to a few and be as pure as is technically possible.

Local hyposensitisation

Reduction in bronchial reactivity after repeated exposure to aerosols of allergen extract was reported by Herxheimer and Prior (1952) and by McAllen (1961). Taylor and Shivalkar (1972) reported reduction in nasal sensitivity and clinical improvement in hay fever from repeated nasal spraying with pollen extract. Mehta and Morrison Smith (1975) carried out a controlled trial of local nasal hyposensitisation in 42 patients and concluded that the method was simple, safe and gave results comparable with those of preseasonal injections.

Desensitisation in certain types of drug allergy

The paradox of the high degree of success which is associated with desensitisation to certain types of antituberculosis drugs and the poor results of such treatment in naturally occurring allergic conditions has not been adequately resolved. Streptomycin, para-aminosalicylic acid and isoniazid give rise to rashes and febrile reactions which have some of the characteristics of allergic responses in that they occur after a fairly well-defined period of sensitisation and can be reproduced by a single dose. Successful desensitisation can usually be accomplished and is apparently permanent (Morrison Smith and Zirk, 1961). The reason for this high degree of success may lie in the size of the sensitising dose or in some difference in the mechanism of the reaction. Desensitisation is seldom attempted in other forms of drug allergy since alternative drugs exist in most cases and reactions of anaphylactic type may be very dangerous.

Hyposensitisation to insect stings

In the 10 years 1962–1971 there were 47 deaths in England and Wales as a result of insect stings (*British Medical Journal*, 1974). The most effective treatment for severe reactions to insect stings is injected adrenaline but the prevention of subsequent reactions with the possibility of death may warrant the use of immunotherapy. Extracts from whole insects may be less effective than those from pure venom. Long courses with permanent maintenance may be necessary (Frankland, 1963) but a high degree of success is claimed by Barr (1974) in 245 patients sensitive to various insects with 191 patients achieving a top dose of 0.25 ml of a 1 in 10 dilution. The risks and the need for immunotherapy are greater in the United States than in England except perhaps among dedicated bee-keepers. Before undertaking this treatment careful consideration should be given to the risks it may involve and the fact that maintenance injections may be required as long as exposure to further stings remains likely.

Enzyme-potentiated hyposensitisation

McEwen has described a method of hyposensitisation used for pollen allergy (McEwen et al, 1975) and for food allergy (McEwen, 1975) based on the intradermal application of the allergen together with β-glucuronidase with cyclohexane diol, protamine, hyaluronidase, chondroitin sulphate and buffer. Considerable success is claimed for this non-invasive method but adequate clinical trials are still awaited.

Possible Future Developments

It has been shown that Praunitz–Küstner (PK) reactions in humans and passive cutaneous anaphylaxis (PCA) reactions in monkeys can be blocked by myeloma IgE and by proteolytic clearage fragments of myeloma IgE (Stanworth et al, 1967, 1968). The crucial stages in the course of immediate hypersensitivity reactions are the identification and sensitisation of the target cells (i.e. mast cells or basophils), the reaction with specific allergen and the resultant effect on the target cell leading to mediator release. Evidence has been produced to indicate that the sites on the mast cell are subject to attachment of IgE molecules by the Fc part of the molecule and that triggering of the enzyme system resulting in mediator release requires the attachment of the specific allergen molecule between two IgE molecules at their Fab end as shown in Stanworth's diagram (1973) (Fig. 12.2).

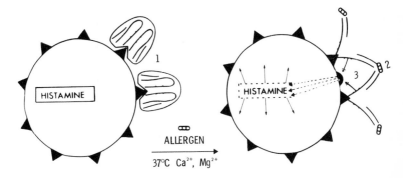

Figure 12.2 Schematic representation of three crucial steps in immediate-hypersensitivity reactions: 1, target cell sensitisation; 2, interaction with specific antigen (allergen); 3, triggering of histamine release. (Reproduced with permission from Stanworth (1973) Immediate hypersensitivity. *Frontiers of Biology*, Vol. 28. Amsterdam: North-Holland)

It would seem possible to interfere with the mechanism at various stages and in particular to block some of the binding sites by incomplete antigen molecules. Attempts are also being made to predict the antibody effector sites on the molecule by comparing the capacity of various polypeptides to cause histamine release (Jasani et al, 1973).

It might therefore be possible to inhibit or disrupt sensitisation of mast cells by a polypeptide fragment smaller than the Fc fragment. Hamburger (1975) has however reported that a pentapeptide comprising an amino acid sequence contained within another area, the CH2 domain, of the human IgE molecule is capable of inhibiting passive cutaneous sensation sites of human skin. Another approach (Stanworth, 1975) is to produce structures antagonistic to the effector groups supposedly mobilised within the Fc regions of the mast cell-bound anaphylactic antibody molecule on interaction with specific allergen, thus preventing the activation of the enzyme system within the mast cell which leads to the release of histamine, SRS-A, and other mediators.

REFERENCES

Aas, K. (1971) Hyposensitisation in house dust allergy asthma. A double blind controlled study with the evaluation of the effect on bronchial sensitivity to house dust. *Acta paediatrica scandinavica*, **60**, 264–268.

Altounyan, R. E. C. (1967) Inhibition of experimental asthma by a new compound—disodium cromoglycate-'Intal'. *Acta Allergologica*, **22**, 487.

Ambiavagar, M. & Jones, E. S. (1967) Resuscitation of the moribund asthmatic: use of intermittent positive pressure ventilation, bronchial lavage and intravenous infusions. *Anaesthesia*, **22**, 375–391.

Anderson, J. B., Halberg, P. & Mygend, N. (1975) Beclomethasone dipropionate aerosol treatment of hay fever. A dose response investigation. *Acta allergologica*, **30**, 316–325.

Andersson, E. & Smidt, C. M. (1974) An investigation of the bronchial mucous membrane after long-term treatment with beclomethasone diproprionate (Becotide). *Acta allergologica*, **29**, 354–364.

Barr, Solomon E. (1974) Allergy to hymenoptera stings. *Journal of the American Medical Association*, **228**, 718–720.

Berg, T. & Johannson, S. G. (1971) In vitro diagnosis of atopic allergy. Iv. Seasonal variations of IgE antibodies in children allergic to pollens. *International Archives of Allergy and Applied Immunology*, **41**, 452–462.

Blair, H., Ezeoke, A. & Hobbs, J. R. (1975) IgE, IgG and patient-self tests during slow hyposensitisation to grass pollen. *Clinical Allergy*, **5**, 263–270.

Blair, H. & Herbert, R. L. (1973) Treatment of seasonal allergic rhinitis with 2 per cent sodium cromoglycate (BP) solution. *Clinical Allergy*, **3**, 283–288.

Blythe, M. E. (1976) Some aspects of the ecological study of the house dust mites. *British Journal of Diseases of the Chest*, **70**, 1–29.

Blythe, M. E., Williams, J. D. & Morrison Smith, J. (1974) Distribution of pyroglyphid mites in Birmingham with particular reference to *Euroglyphus maynei*. *Clinical Allergy*, **4**, 25–33.

Blythe, M. E., Ubaydi, F. Al., Williams, J. D. & Morrison Smith, J. (1975) Study of dust mites in three Birmingham hospitals. *British Medical Journal*, **i**, 62–64.

British Medical Journal (1972) Asthma deaths: a question answered. *British Medical Journal*, **iv**, 443–444.

British Medical Journal (1974) Fatal insect stings. *British Medical Journal*, **ii**, 345.

British Medical Journal (1975) Management of acute asthma. *British Medical Journal*, **iv**, 65–66.

British Tuberculosis Association Research Committee (1968) Treatment of house dust allergy. *British Medical Journal*, **iii**, 774–777.

Brockbank, W. & Pengelly, C. D. (1958) Chronic asthma treated with powder inhalations of hydrocortisone and prednisolone. *Lancet*, **i**, 187–188.

Brompton Hospital/Medical Research Council Collaborative Trial (1972) Long-term study of disodium cromoglycate in treatment of severe extrinsic or intrinsic bronchial asthma in adults. *British Medical Journal*, **iv**, 383–388.

Brompton Hospital/Medical Research Council Collaborative Trial (1974) Double-blind trial comparing two dosage schedules of beclomethasone diproprionate aerosol in the treatment of chronic bronchial asthma. *Lancet*, **ii**, 303–307.

Caldwell, I. W., Hall-Smith, S. P., Main, R. A., Ashurst, P. J., Kirton, V., Simpson, W. T. & Williams, G. W. (1968) Clinical evaluation of a new topical corticosteroid, beclomethasone diproprionate. *British Journal of Dermatology*, **80**, 111–117.

Capel, L. H. & McKelvie, P. (1971) Disodium cromoglycate in hay fever. *Lancet*, **i**, 575–576.

Citron, K. M., Frankland, A. W. & Sinclair, J. D. (1958) Inhalation tests of bronchial hypersensitivity in pollen asthma. *Thorax*, **13**, 229–232.

Cochrane, G. M. & Clark, T. J. H. (1975) A survey of asthma mortality in patients between ages 35 and 64 in the Greater London hospitals in 1971. *Thorax*, **30**, 300–305.

Cooke, R. A., Barnard, J. H., Hebald, S. & Stull, A. (1935) Serological evidence of immunity with co-existing sensitisation in type of human allergy (hay fever). *Journal of Experimental Medicine*, **62**, 733–750.

Cox, J. S., Orr, T. S., Pollard, M. C. & Gwilliam, J. (1970) Mode of action of disodium cromoglycate studies on immediate type hypersensitivity reactions using 'double sensitisation' with two antigenically distinct rat reagins. *Clinical and Experimental Immunology*, **7**, 745–757.

Cox, J. S. G. (1970) Review of chemistry, pharmacology, toxicity, metabolism, specific side-effects, anti-allergic properties in vitro and in vivo of disodium cromoglycate. In *Disodium Cromoglycate in Allergic Airways Disease*, ed. Pepys, J. & Frankland, A. W., pp. 13–25. London: Butterworths.

Cox, J. S. G. (1975) Personal communication.

Cox, J. S. G., Beach, J. E., Blake, A. M. J. N., Clarke, A. J., King, J., Lee, T. B., Loveday, D. E. E., Moss, G. F., Orr, T. S. C., Riches, J. T. & Sheard, P. (1972) Disodium cromoglycate (Intal). *Advances in Drug Research*, **5**, 115–196.

Crompton, G. K. & Grant, I. W. B. (1975) Edinburgh emergency asthma admission service. *British Medical Journal*, **iv**, 680–682.

Davies, R. R. (1969) Aerobiology and the relief of asthma in an alpine valley. *Acta allergologica*, **24**, 377–395.

Davies, S. E. (1968) Effect of disodium cromoglycate on exercise induced asthma. *British Medical Journal*, **iii**, 593–594.

Dickson, W., Hall, C. E., Ellis, M. & Horrocks, R. H. (1973) Beclomethasone diproprionate aerosol in childhood asthma. *Archives of Disease in Childhood*, **48**, 671–675.

D'Sousa, M. F., Pepys, J., Wells, I. D., Tai, E., Palmer, F., Overell, B. G., McGrath, I. T. & Megson, M. (1973) Hyposensitisation with *Dermatophagoides pteronyssinus* in house dust allergy: a controlled study of clinical and immunological effects. *Clinical Allergy*, **3**, 177–193.

Easty, D. L., Rice, N. S. C. & Jones, B. R. (1972) Clinical trial of topical disodium cromoglycate in vernal keratoconjunctivitis. *Clinical Allergy*, **2**, 99–107.

Engström, I. & Kraepelien, S. (1971) The corticosteroid sparing effect of disodium cromoglycate in children and adolescents with bronchial asthma. *Acta allergologica*, **26**, 90–100.

Fagerberg, E. & Zetterström, O. (1975) A trial of disodium cromoglycate in perennial rhinitis. *Acta allergologica*, **30**, 63–72.

Frankland, A. W. (1963) Treatment of bee sting reactions. *Bee World*, **44**, 9–12.

Frankland, A. W. & Augustin, R. (1954) Prophylaxis of summer hay fever and asthma; controlled trial comparing crude grass-pollen extracts with isolated main protein component. *Lancet*, **i**, 1055–1057.

Fraser, P. & Doll, R. (1971) Geographical variations in the epidemic of asthma deaths. *British Journal of Preventive and Social Medicine*, **25**, 34–36.

Frears, J. F., Wilson, L. C. & Friedman, M. (1973) Beclomethasone 17-valerate by aerosol in childhood asthma. *Archives of Disease in Childhood*, **48**, 856–863.

Freier, S. (1973) Paediatric gastrointestinal allergy. *Clinical Allergy*, **3**, (Suppl.), 597–618.

Freier, S. & Berger, H. (1973) Disodium cromoglycate in gastrointestinal protein intolerance. *Lancet*, **i**, 913–915.

Friedman, M. & Strang, L. B. (1966) Effect of long-term corticosteroids and corticotrophin on the growth of children. *Lancet*, **ii**, 568–572.

Frost, M. (1973) Cromoglycate in aphthous stomatitis. *Lancet*, **ii**, 389.

Gaddie, J., Reed, I. W., Skinner, C., Petrie, G. R., Sinclair, D. J. M. & Palmer, K. N. V. (1973) Aerosol beclomethasone diproprionate: a dose response study in chronic bronchial asthma. *Lancet*, **ii**, 280–282.

Gebbie, T., Harris, E. A., O'Donnell, T. V. & Spears, G. F. S. (1972) Multicentre, short term therapeutic trial of disodium cromoglycate with and without prednisolone in adults with asthma. *British Medical Journal*, **iv**, 576–580.

Godfrey, S. (1975) The suppression of exercise-induced asthma by disodium cromoglycate. *Acta allergologica*, Suppl. 12, Bronchial asthma and its treatment with disodium cromoglycate, ed. Engström, I. & Uvnäs, B., pp. 51–61.

Godfrey, S. & König, P. (1973) Beclomethasone aerosol in childhood asthma. *Archives of Disease in Childhood*, **48**, 665–670.

Grant, I. W. B. (1969) Disodium cromoglycate in bronchial asthma. *British Medical Journal*, **i**, 842.

Grant, I. W. B., Channell, S. & Drever, J. C. (1967) Disodium cromoglycate in asthma. *Lancet*, **ii**, 673.

Gwynn, C. M. & Morrison Smith, J. (1974) A 1 year follow-up of children and adolescents receiving regular beclomethasone diproprionate. *Clinical Allergy*, **4**, 325–330.

Hamburger, R. N. (1975) Peptide inhibition of the Prausnitz–Küstner reaction. *Science*, **189**, 389–390.

Hargreave, F. E., McCarthy, D. S. & Pepys, J. (1969) Steroid 'pseudorheumatism' in asthma. *British Medical Journal*, **i**, 443–444.

Harris, D. M., Martin, L. E., Harrison, C. & Jack, D. (1973) The effect of oral and inhaled beclomethazone dipropionate on adrenal function. *Clinical Allergy*, **3**, 243–248.

Helm, W. H. & Heyworth, F. (1958) Bronchial asthma and chronic bronchitis treated with hydrocortisone acetate inhalations. *British Medical Journal*, **ii**, 765–769.

Herxheimer, H. (1972) Asthma deaths. *British Medical Journal*, **iv**, 795.

Herxheimer, H. & Bewersdorff, H. (1969) Disodium cromoglycate in the prevention of induced asthma. *British Medical Journal*, **ii**, 220–222.

Herxheimer, H. & McAllen, M. (1956) Treatment of hay fever with hydrocortisone snuff. *Lancet*, **i**, 537–539.

Herxheimer, H., McAllen, M. K. & Williams, D. A. (1958) Local treatment of bronchial asthma with hydrocortisone powder. *British Medical Journal*, **ii**, 762–765.

Herxheimer, H. & Prior, F. N. (1952) Further observations on induced asthma and bronchial hyposensitisation. *International Archives of Allergy and Applied Immunology*, **3**, 189–207.

Hill, B. H. R. & Swinburn, P. D. (1954) Death from corticotrophin. *Lancet*, **i**, 1954–1959.

Holopainen, E., Backman, A. & Salo, O. P. (1971) Effect of disodium cromoglycate on seasonal allergic rhinitis. *Lancet*, **i**, 55–57.

Holopainen, E., Viner, T., Backman, A., Salo, O., Hannuksela, M. & Malmberg, H. (1975) Clinical trial of a two per cent solution of D.S.C.G. in perennial rhinitis. *Acta allergologica*, **30**, 216–226.

Howell, J. B. L. & Altounyan, R. E. C. (1967) A double blind trial of disodium cromoglycate in the treatment of allergic bronchial asthma. *Lancet*, **ii**, 539–542.

Jasani, B., Stanworth, D. R., Mackler, B. & Kreil, G. (1973) Studies on the mast cell triggering action of certain artificial histamine liberators. *International Archives of Allergy and Applied Immunology*, **45**, 74–81.

Jenssen, A. O. (1973) Measurement of resistance to air flow in the nose in a trial with sodium cromoglycate (BP) solution in allergen-induced nasal stenosis. *Clinical Allergy*, **3**, 277–282.

Jones, R. S. (1973) Beclomethasone in childhood asthma. *Archives of Disease in Childhood*, **48**, 663–664.

Kerr, J. W., Govindara, M. & Patel, K. R. (1970) Effect of alpha-receptor-blocking drugs and disodium cromoglycate on histamine hypersensitivity in bronchial asthma. *British Medical Journal*, **ii**, 139–141.

Kidner, P. H., Price, M. B., Meisner, P. & Bruce Pearson, R. S. (1968) Disodium comoglycate in the treatment of bronchial asthma. *Lancet*, **ii**, 655–657.

King, T. P. & Norman, P. S. (1962) Isolation studies of allergens from ragweed pollen. *Biochemistry*, **1**, 709–720.

Kingsley, P. J. (1974) Oral sodium cromoglycate in gastrointestinal allergy. *Lancet*, **ii**, 1011.

Lancet (1968) Death from asthma. *Lancet*, **i**, 1412–1413.

Lancet (1975a) Fluorocarbon aerosol propellants. *Lancet*, **i**, 1073–1074.

Lancet (1975b) Corticosteroids in acute severe asthma. *Lancet*, **ii**, 166–167.

Langlands, J. H. M. & McNeill, R. S. (1960) Hydrocortisone by inhalation effects on lung function in bronchial asthma. *Lancet*, **ii**, 404–406.

Lichtenstein, L. M., Norman, P. S. & Winkenwerder, W. L. (1971) A single year of immunotherapy for ragweed hay fever. *Annals of Internal Medicine*, **75**, 663–671.

Löfkvist, T. & Svensson, G. (1975) An open assessment of Becotide (beclomethasone diproprionate) nasal spray in seasonal allergic rhinitis. *Acta allergologica*, **30**, 227–238.

McAllen, M. K. (1961) Bronchial sensitivity testing in asthma: an assessment of the effect of hyposensitisation in house-dust and pollen-sensitive subjects. *Thorax*, **16**, 30–35.

McAllen, M. K., Kochanowski, S. J. & Shaw, K. M. (1974) Steroid aerosols in asthma: an assessment of betamethasone 17-valerate and a 12-month study of patients on maintenance treatment. *British Medical Journal*, **i**, 171–175.

McEwen, L. M. (1975) Enzyme potentiated hyposensitisation: V. Five case reports of patients with acute food allergy. *Annals of Allergy*, **35**, 98–103.

McEwen, L. M., Nicholson, M., Kitchen, I., O'Gorman, J. & White, S. (1975) Enzyme potentiated hyposensitisation: IV. Effect of protamine on the immunological behavior of beta glucuronidase in mice and patients with hay fever. *Annals of Allergy*, **34**, 290–295.

Mani, V., Lloyd, G., Green, F., Fox, H. & Turnberg, L. A. (1976) Treatment of ulcerative colitis with disodium cromoglycate: a long-term double blind clinical trial. British Society of Gastroenterology. *Gut*, **16**, 832.

Maunsell, K. (1946) Direct test for blocking antibody in treated hay fever. *Lancet*, **ii**, 199–201.

Medical Research Council—Subcommittee on Clinical Trials in Asthma. (1956) Controlled trial of effects of cortisone acetate in chronic asthma. *Lancet*, **ii**, 798–803.

Mehta, S. B. & Morrison Smith, J. (1975) Nasal hyposensitisation and hay fever. *Clinical Allergy*, **5**, 279–284.

Milne, L. J. R. & Crompton, G. K. (1974) Beclomethasone diproprionate and oropharyngeal candidiasis. *British Medical Journal*, **iii**, 797–798.

Morris-Owen, R. M. & Trulove, S. C. (1958) Treatment of hay fever with local hydrocortisone hemisuccinate sodium. *British Medical Journal*, **i**, 969–972.

Morrison Smith, J. (1958) Hydrocortisone by inhalation in children with asthma. *Lancet*, **ii**, 1248–1250.

Morrison Smith, J. (1966) Death from asthma. *Lancet*, **i**, 1042.

Morrison Smith, J. (1970a) Treatment of asthmatic children away from home. *Public Health*, **84**, 286–290.

Morrison Smith, J. (1970b) Long-term results with disodium cromoglycate in the treatment of children with asthma. In *Disodium Cromoglycate in Allergic Airways Disease*, ed. Pepys, J. & Frankland, A. W., pp. 97–103. London: Butterworths.

Morrison Smith, J. (1971) Disodium cromoglycate in hay fever. *Lancet*, **i**, 295–296.

Morrison Smith, J. (1972–73) Is atopic disease preventable ? *Prevent*, 1, 25–28.

Morrison Smith, J. (1973a) Increased dosage of disodium cromoglycate. *British Medical Journal*, ii, 303–304.

Morrison Smith, J. (1973b) A clinical trial of beclomethasone diproprionate aerosol in children and adolescents with asthma. *Clinical Allergy*, 3, 249–253.

Morrison Smith, J., Clegg, R. T., Cook, N. & Butler, A. G. (1975) Intranasal beclomethasone diproprionate in allergic rhinitis. *British Medical Journal*, ii, 255.

Morrison Smith, J. & Devey, G. F. (1968) Clinical trial of disodium cromoglycate in treatment of asthma in children. *British Medical Journal*, ii, 340–344.

Morrison Smith, J. & Pizarro, Y. A. (1972a) Hyposensitisation with extracts of *Dermatophagoides pteronyssinus* and house dust. *Clinical Allergy*, 2, 281–283.

Morrison Smith, J. & Pizarro, Y. A. (1972b) Observations on the safety of disodium cromoglycate in long-term use in children. *Clinical Allergy*, 2, 143–151.

Morrison Smith, J. & Pizarro, Y. A. (1973) Evaluation of systemic steroid treatment in children with asthma. *Practitioner*, 311, 664–668.

Morrison Smith, J. & Zirk, M. H. (1961) Toxic and allergic drug reactions during the treatment of tuberculosis. *Tubercule*, 42, 287–296.

Morrow-Brown, H., Storey, G. & George, W. H. S. (1972) Beclomethasone diproprionate: a new steroid aerosol for the treatment of allergic asthma. *British Medical Journal*, i, 585–590.

Morrow-Brown, H. & Storey, G. (1974) Beclomethasone diproprionate aerosol in the treatment of seasonal asthma and hay fever. *Clinical Allergy*, 4, 331–341.

Munro-Ashman, D., McEwen, H. & Feinberg, J. G. (1971) The patient self (P-S) test. Demonstration of a rise in blocking antibodies after treatment with Allpyral. *International Archives of Allergy and Applied Immunology*, 40, 448–453.

Noon, L. (1911) Prophylactic inoculation for hay fever. *Lancet*, i, 1572.

Palmer, K. N. V. (1974) Drugs in the treatment of asthma. In *Evaluation of Bronchodilator Drugs.* An Asthma Research Council Symposium, ed. Burley, D. M., Clarke, S. W., Cuthbert, M. F., Paterson, J. W. & Shelley, J. H., pp. 263–271. London: The Trust for Education and Research in Therapeutics.

Parish, W. E. (1974) Human anaphylactic IgG (IgG S-TS). *Proceedings of the Ninth European Congress of Allergology and Clinical Immunology*, ed. Ganderton, M. A. & Frankland, A. W., pp. 164–169. Tunbridge Wells: Pitman Medical.

Patel, K. R. & Kerr, J. W. (1975a) Effect of alpha-receptor-blocking drug thymoxamine on allergen-induced broncho-construction in bronchial asthma. *Clinical Allergy*, 5, 311–316.

Patel, K. R. & Kerr, J. W. (1975b) Alpha-receptor-blocking drugs in bronchial asthma. *Lancet*, i, 348–349.

Pelikan, Z., Snock, W. J., Booij-Noord, H., Orie, N. G. M. & de Vries, K. (1970) Protective effect of disodium cromoglycate on the allergen provocation of the nasal mucosa. *Annals of Allergy*, 28, 548–553.

Penaud, A., Nourrit, J., Autran, P., Timon-David, P., Jacquet-Francillon, M. & Charpin, J. (1975) Methods of destroying house dust pyroglyphid mites. *Clinical Allergy*, 5, 109–114.

Pepys, J., Hargreave, F. E., Chan, M. & McCarthy, D. S. (1968) Inhibitory effects of disodium cromoglycate on allergen inhalation tests. *Lancet*, ii, 134–137.

Pepys, J. (1973) Effects of disodium cromoglycate and beclomethasone diproprionate on asthmatic reactions to bronchial provocation tests. *Acta allergologica*, Suppl. 12, 33–50.

Raffle, E. J. & Frain-Bell, W. (1967) The effect of topically applied beclomethasone diproprionate on adrenal function. *British Journal of Dermatology*, 79, 487–490.

Read, J. (1968) The reported increase in mortality from asthma: a clinico-functional analysis. *Medical Journal of Australia*, 1, 879–884.

Rees, H. A., Millar, J. S. & Donald, K. W. (1968) A study of the clinical course and arterial blood gas tensions of patients in status asthmaticus. *Quarterly Journal of Medicine*, 37, 541–561.

Rees, H. A. & Williams, D. A. (1962) Long-term steroid therapy in chronic intractable asthma. *British Medical Journal*, i, 1575–1579.

Sarsfield, J. K., Gowland, G., Toy, R. & Norman, A. L. E. (1974) Mite-sensitive asthma of childhood: trials of avoidance measures. *Archives of Disease in Childhood*, 49, 716–721.

Speizer, F. E., Doll, R. & Heaf, P. (1968) Investigation into the use of drugs preceding death from asthma. *British Medical Journal*, i, 339–343.

Stanworth, D. R. (1975) IgE and allergy. *Folia allergologica et immunologica clinica*, 22, 270–283.

Stanworth, D. R., Humphrey, J. H., Bennich, H. & Johansson, S. G. O. (1967) Specific inhibition of Prausnitz–Küstner reaction by an atypical human myeloma protein. *Lancet*, ii, 330–332.

Stanworth, D. R., Humphrey, J. H., Bennich, H. & Johansson, S. G. O. (1968) Inhibition of Prausnitz–Küstner reaction by proteolytic-cleavage fragments of a human myeloma protein of immunoglobulin class E. *Lancet*, ii, 17–18.

Stolley, P. D. (1972) Asthma mortality. Why the United States was spared an epidemic of deaths due to asthma. *American Review of Respiratory Disease*, **105**, 883–890.

Szentivanyi, A. (1968) The beta adrenergic theory of the atopic abnormality in bronchial asthma. *Journal of Allergy*, **42**, 203–232.

Taylor, G. & Shivalkar, P. R. (1971) Disodium cromoglycate: Laboratory studies and clinical use in allergic rhinitis. *Clinical Allergy*, **1**, 189–198.

Taylor, G. & Shivalkar, P. R. (1972) Local nasal desensitisation in allergic rhinitis. *Clinical Allergy*, **2**, 125–136.

Walsh, S. D. & Grant, I. W. B. (1966) Corticosteroids in treatment of chronic asthma. *British Medical Journal*, **ii**, 796–802.

Williams, S. J., Parrish, R. W. & Seaton, A. (1975) Comparison of intravenous aminophylline and salbutamol in severe asthma. *British Medical Journal*, **iv**, 685.

Woodroffe, A. J. (1972) Multiple myeloma associated with long history of hyposensitisation with allergen vaccines. *Lancet*, **i**, 99.

INDEX